Depression in Primary Care

Depression in Primary Care

Screening and Detection

Edited by C. Clifford Attkisson
and Jane M. Zich

ROUTLEDGE: NEW YORK & LONDON

Published in 1990 by

Routledge, an imprint of
Routledge, Chapman and Hall, Inc.
29 West 35th Street
New York, NY 10001

Published in Great Britain by

Routledge
11 New Fetter Lane
London EC4P 4EE

Note:
Several chapters in this volume were developed with special services contracts between the authors and the National Institute of Mental Health. The opinions expressed in these selected chapters (Chapters 2, 4, 5, 6, 8, 13 and 17) are the views of the authors and do not necessarily reflect the official position of the National Institute of Mental Health or any other part of the US Department of Health and Human Services. All material in these chapters is in the public domain and may be used or reproduced without permission from the Institute or the author.

Library of Congress Cataloging in Publication Data

Depression in primary care : screening and detection / edited by C.
    Clifford Attkisson, Jane M. Zich.
        p.   cm.
    Based on the majority of papers presented at the Tiburon
conference held in June 1987; jointly sponsored by the National
Institute of Mental Health and the University of California, San
Francisco.
    ISBN 0-415-90125-1
    1. Depression, Mental—Diagnosis—Congresses. 2. Family medicine—
Congresses. 3. Depressive Disorder—diagnosis—congresses.
I. Attkisson, C. Clifford. II. Zich, Jane M. III. National
Institute of Mental Health (U.S.) IV. University of California, San
Francisco.
    [DNLM: 1. Depression—diagnosis—congresses. 2. Primary Health
Care—congresses.   WM 171 D4233 1987]
RC537.D4384   1990
616.85′27075—dc20   90-8508
                                                            CIP

British Library cataloguing in publication data also available

Contents

Foreword

The majority of papers included in this volume were presented at the Tiburon Conference jointly sponsored by the National Institute of Mental Health and the University of California, San Francisco. Other papers were subsequently requested to supplement those presented in Tiburon. The editors and authors wish to acknowledge the support and encouragement provided by key individuals at NIMH, including especially Barbara J. Burns, Kenneth G. Lutterman, Thomas L. Lalley, and Jack D. Burke. Douglas B. Kamerow, as an NIMH representative and contributor to the volume, played a key role in the creation of the Tiburon Conference. Four other persons made invaluable contributions to the production of the volume and we are very grateful to them for their outstanding professional and technical assistance: Albert J. Fernandez, María G. Juarez, Carlos F. Jackson, and Vernnez Y. Rockett.

Part I

Historical and Conceptual Contexts of Depression in Primary Care Populations

The initial chapters of this volume place the topic of depression among primary care patients within a historical and conceptual context. The chapter by C. Clifford Attkisson and Jane M. Zich focuses on the emerging recognition that it is important to screen, diagnose, and treat primary care patients who suffer from depression and depressive symptoms. These patients comprise a large segment of clinical caseloads and the burdens and sequelae of depression rival those of many severe physical disorders. Paul S. Frame's chapter provides an overview of the trends and purposes of "screening" in primary care and specifies guidelines for determining whether screening for a particular disorder is warranted. Applying these screening desirability criteria to depression, Frame concludes that although depression fits a number of requisites for routine primary care screening, depression has not been demonstrated to meet all criteria. Frame's analysis highlights specific areas in need of research if depression screening is to become the state of practice in primary care.

In a companion chapter, Douglas B. Kamerow acknowledges the gaps in empirical support for routine depression screening in primary care. However, he argues that the potential value of instituting depression screening in primary care is substantial. Kamerow encourages further empirical investigation of the impact of screening procedures with special emphasis on studies that address screening issues of greatest concern to primary care practitioners.

Criterion validity is the most important unresolved research challenge at the current time. What exactly are we screening for when we screen for depression? How will we operationally define a "case" of depression in primary care? The complexity of the issue is illuminated by James Barrett. In his chapter, Barrett reviews the dominant nosological systems defining depression and notes that the defining characteristics of depressive disorders vary according to the diagnostic classificatory system used. In the course of delineating the historical context, particularly the goals behind the construction of each classification scheme, Barrett stresses the need for each clinician or researcher to define depression in a way that is theoretically and historically compatible with clinical or clinical research goals. A particularly thorny issue is the historical reality that the dominant psychiatric classification systems have been based on studies of mental health system populations. The value of strict application of such classificatory systems to primary care patients is questioned.

Wayne Katon and Michael Von Korff further explore the conceptual complexities of depression and depression screening in the primary care context. Katon and Von Korff review the relationships among depression and pain, medical disorders, and somatic complaints that may color the meaning and presentation of primary care patients with depressive disorders. Drawing parallels between two common medical disorders (hypertension and peptic ulcer disease) and depression, Katon and Von Korff argue for the importance of recognizing and treating "borderline" as well as severe cases of the depressive disorders. Like Barrett, Katon and Von Korff stress the need to investigate the assumption that what is pertinent and useful in the diagnosis and treatment of psychiatric clinic patients with depression applies equally well to primary care patients with depression.

1

Depression Screening In Primary Care: Clinical Needs And Research Challenges

C. Clifford Attkisson and Jane M. Zich

Psychological depression is a painful, distracting, inhibiting, costly, and often life-threatening disorder. Depression is typically reflected in disturbances in mood, affect, energy levels, and frequent fatigue. Irritability as well as sadness or despair may predominate. Other frequently associated vegetative symptoms and signs include changes in weight, appetite, sex drive, sleep patterns, headache and gastrointestinal distress. In its most disorganizing expression, depression can have psychotic and/or manic components. Social withdrawal, loss of interest in nearly all activities, a sense of worthlessness, or excessive guilt, self-doubt, and indecisiveness may also occur. Recurrent thoughts of death may take the form of somatic preoccupation and the suspicion that one has a serious, but as yet undiagnosed disease. Depressive disorders are also associated with increased risk of suicide and considerable psychic distress for family and friends as well as the individual afflicted. The effects of depression can be profound when viewed financially, interpersonally, and from the vocational perspective.

Antecedents of Depression

Psychological depression is often a correlate of physical illness or can be a direct response to illness. Depression can also be the result of changes in life circumstances, interpersonal discord or loss, and intrapsychic conflict. Three main causal pathways have been proposed. Antecedents of depression can include: (a) social experiences and life events as these interact with psychological structures, (b) biological and/or genetic causes that are not yet fully understood, and (c) medical conditions and their treatment (Jefferson & Marshall, 1981; Katerndahl, 1981; & Whitlock, 1982). Causality can be multiple and can reflect an interaction of social factors, biological predisposition, and occurrence of physical illness or incapacity.

Prevalence Of Depression

Depression ranks among the most prevalent mental disorders within the general population of the United States. During a given six month period, 3% of the population experiences a major depressive episode (Regier et al., 1988a). Lifetime prevalence rates, per 100 persons in the population, are reported at 5.8% for major depressive episode.

In contrast to prevalence in the general population, medical clinic patients are even more likely to suffer from depressive disorders and depressive symptoms (Barrett, Barrett, Oxman, & Gerber, 1988). In fact, depression is one of the most common disorders, medical or psychiatric, in primary care practice (Hoeper, Nycz, Cleary, Regier, & Goldberg, 1979; Katon, 1982; & Kessler et al., 1987). The prevalence of major depressive disorder among medical clinic patients has been estimated to be 6% (Hoeper et al., 1979), approximately double the rate reported for the general population (Regier et al., 1988a).

Co-occurrence with Medical Disorders

Most persons who are depressed are not seen by mental health specialists but are seen by their primary care physicians. In fact, visits to primary care physicians frequently increase coincident with depressive symptoms. Because of this, primary care physicians are in a uniquely strategic position for detecting and treating previously unrecognized depressed individuals. Furthermore, because the physician may also be caring for the depressed person's family, the physician may also have the opportunity to provide information, supportive counseling, symptom monitoring, treatment referrals, or preventive measures for family members genetically at risk for depression themselves.

The presence of a depressive disorder does not, of course, preclude the co-occurrence of medical disorders or the need to assess organic pathology that may underlie the depression. Given that medical clinic patients are distressed by pain, physical illness and disabilities, medication side effects, and health-related fears, the prevalence of depression in primary care practices is not surprising. Prompt detection and treatment of clinical depression, regardless of its etiology, however, may improve the patient's social and vocational functioning as well as his or her sense of well-being. It may also reduce the likelihood of drug abuse and suicide.

Response to Treatment

Early identification of persons suffering from depression can lead to treatments that can change the course of the disorder. Untreated, depression can become a progressively debilitating condition having costly consequences for the individual, family, and society (Billings, Cronkite, & Moos, 1983; Blumenthal & Dielman, 1975; Coryell, 1981; Paykel & Weissman, 1973; Sainsbury, 1986; Wells, 1985).

While certain therapeutic interventions, psychotherapy alone and/or combined with pharmacotherapy, have demonstrated clinical efficacy (National Institute of Mental Health [NIMH], 1983; Paykel, 1982; Weissman, 1979), most individuals with clinical depression do not consult mental health specialists. Reluctance to acknowledge psychological distress or seek treatment with a mental health specialist may lead individuals suffering from depression to seek relief in the services of a primary care physician—with whom patients may have an established, trusting relationship (Regier, Goldberg, & Taube, 1978). Limitations of health insurance coverage and benefits also restrict patient options. Consequently, when a patient is clinically depressed, there are compelling reasons for physicians to have the requisite clinical skills and diagnostic procedures to detect and diagnose the extent of these psychological conditions.

Depression and Primary Medical Care

Many studies report that the onset of depressive episodes is often associated with increased use of medical services (Kamerow, Pincus, & Macdonald, 1986; Richter, Barsky, & Hupp, 1983; Widmer & Cadoret, 1979). Changes in rate or pattern of medical visits may result when vegetative signs of depression (disturbances in energy, appetite, sleep, and libido) are interpreted by the patient as evidence of physical illness. For these reasons, the primary health care provider is in a crucial position to detect, treat, or refer, persons who are clinically depressed. Consequently, it is of great importance to enhance primary care physicians' capacity to recognize and respond effectively to depression. This objective is especially exemplified by the National Institute of Mental Health's Depression Awareness, Recognition, and Treatment (DART) Program (Regier et al., 1988b).

Although the physician may choose to refer patients with depression for psychiatric consultation rather than to take primary responsibility for the evaluation and treatment of the patient's depression, the physician's recognition of the presence of depressive disorder may, nonetheless, be an important factor in subsequent clinical decisions. Awareness that a patient is seriously depressed may indicate a need to change the patient's medication, due to the adverse mood altering effects of certain prescribed drugs, or may prompt the physician to address psychological and emotional aspects of the patient's clinical picture. Hopelessness and lack of interest in living, frequent symptoms in depressive disorders, may significantly interfere with a patient's ability or willingness to adhere to recommended medical treatments. These same factors may have highly detrimental effects on the patient's social adaptation and capacity to make important life decisions. In some patients with depression, social and role functioning is further compromised by abuse of alcohol and other substances—resulting in an even greater and more complex clinical challenge.

Indeed, there is compelling recent evidence that depression can have a profound impact on patient well-being and social functioning. Wells et al. (1989b) report that depression can be as debilitating and incapacitating as the various other chronic medical conditions that are associated with limitations in functional status. In a broad-based study of 11,242 primary care patients Wells et al. found that 22% reported symptoms of depression. Compared against patients with eight chronic health conditions (hypertension, diabetes, advanced coronary artery disease [ACAD], angina, arthritis, gastrointestinal problems, lung problems, and back problems), social functioning was worse for depressed patients. Patients with depression had significantly poorer health and role functioning than patients with chronic medical conditions (with the exception of angina and ACAD) and spent more days in bed than patients with chronic conditions other than lung problems and ACAD. Also, patients with depression reported more bodily pain than all other chronic conditions compared in the study (including patients with angina) except for arthritis. Finally, Wells et al. documented that the combination of depressive symptoms and other medical conditions has a compounding negative effect on social adaptation and functioning. For example, the combination of depressive symptoms and ACAD produces approximately twice the decrement in social functioning than is reported with either condition alone.

Detection of Depression in Primary Care

Since the prevalence of depression in primary care patients is high, and since there is a strong likelihood that medical patients with clinical depression will be seen by their physicians and not by mental health professionals, the ability of the primary care physician to detect and respond sensitively to clinically depressed medical patients may largely determine whether such patients are ever provided appropriate therapeutic interventions (Burns, Scott, Burke, & Kessler, 1983; Ficken et al., 1984; Jones, Badger, Ficken, Leeper, & Anderson, 1987; Regier et al., 1988b; Strain, Pincus, Houpt, Gise, & Taintor, 1985; Zung, George, Woodruff, & Mahorney, 1984). Wells et al. (1989a) report that primary care physicians do not detect depression in half of the patients who suffer from depressive disorders and that the level of detection may be even lower among physicians in prepaid health plans.

Clinical Needs and Research Challenges

How then can primary care physicians be alert to the possibility that a given patient may suffer from depressive symptoms or a depressive disorder? Various investigators have assessed physicians' ability to detect depression by comparing physician generated diagnoses against results of depression screening inventories completed by their patients. Numerous early studies in this line of research reported that physicians identify fewer patients as depressed than do depression screening instruments (Linn & Yager, 1982; Moore, Silimperi, & Bobula, 1978; Seller, Blascovich, & Lenkei, 1981; & Zung, Magill, Moore, & George, 1983). The research designs in these early depression screening studies, however, did not permit precise conclusions about: (a) whether physicians failed to detect clinical depressions in their patients, or (b) whether the screens misidentified as "depressed" those patients with depressive symptomatology who would not meet full criteria for an actual diagnosis of a depressive disorder.

More recent and methodologically stronger studies, have included rigorous criterion measures such as: (a) formal diagnostic evaluations by mental health specialists, (b) fixed-item rating scales like the Hamilton Depression Rating Scale (Hamilton, 1967), and (c) structured diagnostic interviews such as the Schedule for Affective Disorders and Schizophrenia (SADS) (Endicott & Spitzer, 1978) or the NIMH Diagnostic Interview Schedule (DIS) (Robins, Helzer, Croughan, & Ratcliff, 1981). These criterion measures were used by investigators to determine "hit" and "miss" rates for both the depression screening procedures and the opinions of primary care physicians. Results from these more sophisticated studies also indicate that physicians infrequently detect, or at least infrequently diagnose, depressive disorders (Jones et al., 1987; Nielsen & Williams, 1980; Schulberg et al., 1985).

Depression screening procedures, however, often yield far too many false positive findings to be efficient for routine use in primary care. Nondepressed medical clinic patients have been found to score higher on depression screening instruments than nondepressed persons in the general population (Schulberg et al., 1985). Consequently, when screens are used with medical populations, higher cut-off scores may be necessary (Zich, Attkisson, & Greenfield, 1990). Studies also suggest that the usefulness depression screening in primary care may be limited to certain demographic groups (for example, older males) whose depression is particularly likely to go undetected by physicians (Norris, Gallagher, Wilson, & Winograd, 1987; Shapiro, et al., 1987). Further complicating assessment of the utility of screening for depression is the fact that numerous depression screening instruments exist. Each has its specific strengths and weaknesses (Murphy, 1982), leading to the possibility that one screening instrument might prove more useful with medical patients than another.

Use of Depression Screening Procedures

An important consideration of the use of depression screening procedures is that the detection of depression takes time, something most physicians find is already stretched to the limit. Consequently, a theoretical argument for the value of screening for depression in primary care is likely to have little impact unless it is accompanied by a compelling argument that it is worth the time it takes. A case must be made that screening works well to identify patients who are depressed, that physicians feel capable of further evaluating, treating, or referring patients identified as depressed, and that the impact of these interventions is beneficial for patients and, preferably, also time-and cost-effective for the medical practice.

A second consideration involves the population being targeted. Primary care patients are apt to have medical illnesses with symptoms that overlap with presenting symptoms of depression, such as fatigue, weight change, headache, and alcohol or other substance abuse. Some illnesses, for example, thyroid disorders, may include clinical depression which resolves when the underlying medical disorder is corrected. Additionally, a number of medications prescribed for common medical disorders may cause or exacerbate depression. Finally, changes in health may be accompanied by a sense of loss, grief, and situation-appropriate depressive reactions. Looking for an underlying medical cause for the patient's presenting symptoms remains a focal concern for the primary care physician and for the patient.

The presence of medical illness does not rule out the co-occurrence of psychiatric disorder (or alcohol and other substance abuse disorder), however, any more than does the clear presence of psychiatric disorder refute the possibility of concomitant medical illness—although when one is discovered the other may be overlooked (Jefferson & Marshall, 1981; Katerndahl, 1981; Whitlock, 1982).

How is the primary care physician to go about detecting depression, given that: Presenting symptoms may be due to psychological conflict, or to an underlying medical illness, or to prescription drug side effects, or "normal" self-limiting adjustment to a significant life change, or an interaction of these factors, each of which may require a different type of intervention or support, and that assessment of each of these possibilities takes time?

One strategy that has received considerable recent attention is the use of fixed-item depression screening inventories with primary care clinic patients (Linn & Yager, 1982; Schulberg et al., 1985; Zich et al., 1990; Zung et al., 1983). Rucker et al. reported that use of such a depression screening procedure was viewed favorably by physicians in general medicine. Access to screening results not only increased physicians' recognition of patients with depression but also influenced physicians' subsequent treatment plans in 20% of the cases (Rucker, Frye, & Cygan, 1986). Findings in this area have been mixed, but are generally promising (Linn & Yager, 1982; Linn & Yager, 1984; Rand, Badger, & Coggins, 1988; Rucker et al., 1986; Shapiro et al., 1987). Ideally, such a fixed-item screening procedure would: (a) be acceptable to the patient population, (b) be relatively inexpensive in time and cost to the clinic and patient, (c) be highly effective in identifying clinically depressed patients in primary care, (d) be able to distinguish clinically depressed patients from patients without such a disorder, and (e) distinguish depressed patients apt to be responsive to one type of treatment versus another.

This volume examines the depression screening strategy in primary care and presents current knowledge about several important clinical and research questions: How is depression to be defined and identified in primary care? What screening instruments are being used to detect depressed patients, what are the limitations and advantages of these instruments, and how well have the instruments performed clinically in primary care settings? What is needed in order for depression screening to be valued and adopted by primary care physicians? What important methodological and instrumentation difficulties must be surmounted? What special population issues must be addressed in depression screening? The contributors to this volume have combined their expertise to synthesize current knowledge about these questions and to explicate what is reliably known as well as propose directions for future research.

References

Barrett, J.E., Barrett, J.A., Oxman, T.E., & Gerber, P.D. (1988). The prevalence of psychiatric disorders in a primary care practice. *Archives of General Psychiatry, 45,* 1100–1106.

Billings, A.G., Cronkite, R.C., & Moos, R.H. (1983). Social-environmental factors in unipolar depression: Comparisons of depressed patients and nondepressed control. *Journal of Abnormal Psychology, 92,* 119–133.

Blumenthal, M.D., & Dielman, T.E. (1975). Depressive symptomatology and role function in a general population. *Archives of General Psychiatry, 32,* 985–991.

Burns, B.J., Scott, J.E., Burke, J.D., & Kessler, L.G. (1983). Mental health training of primary care residents: A review of recent literature (1974–1981). *General Hospital Psychiatry, 7,* 157–169.

Coryell, W. (1981). Diagnosis-specific mortality: Primary unitary depression and Briquet's syndrome (somatization disorder). *Archives of General Psychiatry, 38,* 939–942.

Endicott, J., & Spitzer, R. (1978). A diagnostic interview—The Schedule for Affective Disorders and Schizophrenia. *Archives of General Psychiatry, 35,* 837–844.

Ficken, R.P., Milo, T., Badger, L.W., Leeper, J., Anderson, R.L., & Jones, L.R. (1984). Management of mental disorders by family practice residents. *Family Medicine, 16,* 170–174.

Hamilton, M. (1967). Development of a rating scale for primary depressive illness. *British Journal of Social and Clinical Psychology, 6,* 278–296.

Hoeper, E.W., Nycz, G.R., Cleary, P.D., Regier, D.A., & Goldberg, I.D. (1979). Estimated prevalence of RDC mental disorder in primary medical care. *International Journal of Mental Health, 8,* 6–15.

Jefferson, J., & Marshall, J. (1981). *Neuropsychiatric features of medical disorders.* New York: Plenum Publishing Corporation.

Jones, L.R., Badger, L.W., Ficken, R.P., Leeper, J.D., & Anderson, R.L. (1987). Inside the hidden mental health network: Examining mental health care delivery of primary care physicians. *General Hospital Psychiatry, 9,* 287–293.

Kamerow, D., Pincus, H., & Macdonald, D. (1986). Alcohol abuse, other drug abuse, and mental disorders in medical practice: Prevalence, costs, recognition, and treatment. *Journal of the American Medical Association, 255,* 2054–2057.

Katerndahl, D.A. (1981). Nonpsychiatric disorders associated with depression. *Journal of Family Practice, 13,* 619–624.

Katon, W. (1982). Depression: Somatic symptoms and medical disorders in primary care. *Comprehensive Psychiatry, 23,* 274–287.

Kessler, L.G., Burns, B.J., Shapiro, S., Tischler, G.L., George, L.K., Hough, R.L., Bodison, D., & Miller, R.H. (1987). Psychiatric diagnoses of medical service users: Evidence from the Epidemiologic Catchment Area Program. *American Journal of Public Health, 77,* 18–24.

Kupfer, D.J., Frank, E., & Perel, J.M. (1989). The advantage of early treatment intervention in recurrent depression. *Archives of General Psychiatry, 46,* 771–775.

Linn, L.S., & Yager, J. (1982). Screening of depression in relationship to subsequent patient and physician behavior. *Medical Care, 20,* 1233–1240.

Linn, L.S., & Yager J. (1984). Recognition of depression and anxiety by primary physicians. *Psychosomatics, 25,* 593–600.

Moore, J.T., Silimperi, D.R., & Bobula, J.A. (1978). Recognition of depression by family medicine residents: The impact of screening. *Journal of Family Medicine, 3,* 509–513.

Murphy, J.M. (1982). Psychiatric instrument development for primary care research: Patient self-report questionnaire. Manuscript for NIMH (NIMH Contract No. 80M014280101D).

Nielsen, A.C., & Williams, T.A. (1980). Depression in ambulatory medical patients; Prevalence by self-report questionnaire and recognition by nonpsychiatric physicians. *Archives of General Psychiatry, 37,* 999–1004.

NIMH Science Reports. (1983). Special report on depression research. DHHS Publication No. (ADM)83–1085.

Norris, J.T., Gallagher, D., Wilson, A., & Winograd, C.H. (1987). Assessment of depression in geriatric medical outpatients: The validity of two screening measures. *Journal of the American Geriatrics Society, 35,* 989–995.

Paykel, E.S. (ed.). (1982). *Handbook of affective disorders.* New York: Guilford Press.

Paykel, E.S., & Weissman M. (1973). Social adjustment and depression: A longitudinal study. *Archives of General Psychiatry, 28,* 659–663.

Rand, E.H., Badger, L.W., & Coggins, D.R. (1988). Toward a resolution of contradictions: Utility of feedback from the GHQ. *General Hospital Psychiatry, 10,* 189–196.

Regier, D., Boyd, J., Burke, J., Rae, D., Myers, J.K., Kramer, M., Robins, L.N., George, L.K., Karno, M., & Locke, B.Z. (1988a). One-month prevalence of mental disorders in the United States. *Archives of General Psychiatry, 45,* 977–986.

Regier, D.A., Goldberg, I.D., & Taube, C.A. (1978). The de facto US mental health services system: A public health prospective. *Archives of General Psychiatry, 35,* 685–693.

Regier, D.A., Hirschfeld, R.M., Goodwin, F.K., Burke, J.D., Lazar, J.B., & Judd, L.L. (1988b). The NIMH Depression Awareness, Recognition, and Treatment Program: Structure, aims, and scientific basis. *American Journal of Psychiatry, 145,* 1351–1357.

Richter, J.M., Barsky, A.J., & Hupp, J.A. (1983). The treatment of depression in elderly patients. *Journal of Family Practice, 17,* 43–47.

Robins, L.N., Helzer, J.E., Croughan, J., & Ratcliff, K.S. (1981). National Institute of Mental Health Diagnostic Interview Schedule: Its history, characteristics, and validity. *Archives of General Psychiatry, 38,* 381–389.

Rucker, L., Frye, E.B., & Cygan, R.W. (1986). Feasibility and usefulness of depression screening in medical outpatients. *Archives of Internal Medicine, 146,* 729–731.

Sainsbury, P. (1986). Depression, suicide, and suicide prevention. In A. Roy (ed.), *Suicide.* (pp. 73–88). Baltimore: Williams & Wilkens.

Schulberg, H.C., Saul, M., McClelland, M., Ganguli, M. Christy, W., & Frank, R. (1985). Assessing depression in primary medical and psychiatric practice. *Archives of General Psychiatry, 42,* 1164–1170.

Seller, R.H., Blascovich, J., & Lenkei, E. (1981). Influence of stereotypes in the diagnosis of depression by family practice residents. *Journal of Family Practice, 12,* 849–854.

Shapiro, S., German, P.S., Skinner, E.A., Von Korff, M., Turner, R.W., Klein, L.E., Teitelbaum, M.L., Kramer, M., Burke, J.D., & Burns, B.J. (1987). An experiment to change detection and management of mental morbidity in primary care. *Medical Care, 25,* 327.

Strain, J.J., Pincus, H.A., Houpt, J.L., Gise, L.H., & Taintor, Z. (1985). Models of mental health training for primary care physicians. *Psychosomatic Medicine, 47,* 95–110.

Weissman, M. (1979). The psychological treatment of depression— Evidence for the efficacy of psychotherapy alone, in comparison with, and in combination with pharmacotherapy. *Archives of General Psychiatry, 36,* 1261–1268.

Wells, K.B. (1985). *Depression as a tracer condition for the national study of medical care outcome: Background review.* The Rand Publication Series. Santa Monica: Rand.

Wells, K.B., Hays, R.D., Burnam, M.A., Rogers, W., Greenfield, S., & Ware, J.E. (1989a). Detection of depressive disorder for patients receiving prepaid or fee-for-service care: Results from the Medical Outcomes Study. *Journal of the American Medical Association, 262,* 3298–3302.

Wells, K.B., Stewart, A., Hays, R.D., Burnam, M.A., Rogers, W., Daniels, M., Berry, S., Greenfield, S., & Ware, J. (1989b). The functioning and well-being of depressed patients: Results from the Medical Outcomes Study. *Journal of the American Medical Association, 262,* 914–919.

Whitlock, F. (1982). *Symptomatic affective disorders: A study of depression and mania associated with physical disease and medication.* New York: Academic Press.

Widmer, R.B., & Cadoret, R.J. (1979). Depression in family practice: Changes in pattern of patient visits and complaints during subsequent developing depressions. *Journal of Family Practice, 9,* 1017–1021.

Zich, J.M., Attkisson, C.C., & Greenfield, T.K. (1990). Screening for depression in primary care clinics: The CES-D and the BDI. *International Journal of Psychiatry in Medicine,* in press.

Zung, W.W., Magill, M., Moore, J.T., & George, D.T. (1983). Recognition and treatment of depression in a family medicine practice. *Journal of Clinical Psychiatry, 44,* 3–6.

Zung, W.W., George, D.T., Woodruff, W.W., & Mahorney, S.L. (1984). Symptom perception by nonpsychiatric physicians in evaluating for depression. *Journal of Clinical Psychiatry, 45,* 26–28

2

Screening Procedures In Primary Care: History and Uses

Paul S. Frame

The primary care physician, in the role as caretaker for the whole patient, is constantly bombarded with recommendations from specialists, each of whom honestly believes his or her particular specialty is most important and deserves emphasis in day-to-day patient management. With all diseases, but especially with screening and prevention of disease, the primary care physician must analyze these recommendations and develop a cost-effective strategy to maximize patient benefit. This chapter describes the history and current status of office-based screening for disease in primary care with an emphasis on screening for depression.

The routine physical examination of otherwise healthy people is the predecessor of the concept of selective longitudinal health maintenance, the cornerstone of preventive medicine in primary care today. That physician examination could detect large amounts of occult disease was first appreciated in the early twentieth century as the result of examinations of military recruits and examinations performed by the life insurance industry.

After World War II, as medical preoccupation with infectious diseases subsided, the "routine, annual complete physical examination" became commonplace. Many companies started offering "executive" physicals for management personnel. In the 1950s the Kaiser health plan introduced the concept of multiphasic health screening, a method of offering multiple automated tests in a centralized location to decrease costs and increase the scope of preventive examinations.

Actually the "routine, annual complete physical examination" has never been routine, annual, or complete. Because of the high cost of such examinations, only affluent or particularly health conscious patients received them on a regular basis. Employers, if they paid for them at all, usually did so only for upper echelon employees. The majority of the population did not participate. Since there was never a standard definition of the content of the complete physical examination, it might vary from a half-hour history and physical to a three-day medical extravaganza complete with multiple tests, specialist evaluations, and in-depth psychosocial testing.

As early as 1945, Roemer suggested that preventive procedures should be selective and tailored to the age and situation of the individual patient. He proposed a program of screening procedures based on the individual's age and sex and specified intervals at which these procedures should be performed.

It was soon recognized that merely detecting disease does not make a screening program worthwhile. Detecting a disease for which there is no treatment does not benefit the patient, nor does detecting trivial disease or detecting disease that can just as well be treated after the appearance of symptoms. This knowledge led to the development in the 1960s of specific screening criteria that must be met before a disease is included in a rational health maintenance program (Hart, 1975). Table 2.1 outlines these criteria as used by Frame and Carlson (1975a, 1975b, 1975c, 1975d).

In 1975, Frame and Carlson published a series of articles, "A Critical Review of Periodic Health Screening Using Specific Screening Criteria," in which they analyzed thirty-six diseases to determine if they fulfilled screening criteria (Table 2.1). They then combined their recommendations into a practical health maintenance flow sheet for use by primary care physicians. This work was recently updated by Frame in 1986 (Frame, 1986a, 1986b, 1986c, 1986d) (Figure 2.1).

Breslow and Somers (1977) elaborated on this concept by looking at health maintenance in ten-year age groups and defining health maintenance goals for each age group as well as recommending specific procedures.

The Canadian Task Force on the Periodic Health Examination issued its landmark report in 1980. This report examined health maintenance procedures for all ages. Each recommendation was graded according to the quality of evidence supporting it. The report is remarkable both because of its comprehensive scope and because it was sponsored by the Canadian government. The task force continues to meet and periodically updates its recommendations (1984; 1986).

Healthy People: The Surgeon General's Report On Health Promotion and Disease Prevention was also published in 1979 (Public Health Service, 1979).

Table 2.1. Screening Criteria

1. The condition must have a significant effect on the quality of life.

2. Acceptable methods of treatment must be available.

3. The condition must have an asymptomatic period during which detection and treatment significantly reduce morbidity and/or mortality.

4. Treatment in the asymptomatic phase must yield a therapeutic result superior to that obtained by delaying treatment until symptoms appear.

5. Tests that are acceptable to patients must be available at reasonable cost to detect the condition in the asymptomatic period.

6. The incidence of the condition must be sufficient to justify the cost of screening.

AGES 18-49 YEARS

DATE																																
AGE	18	19	20	21	22	23	24	25	26	27	28	29	30	31	32	33	34	35	36	37	38	39	40	41	42	43	44	45	46	47	48	49
Blood Pressure	●		●		●		●		●		●		●		●		●		●		●		●		●		●		●		●	
Serum Cholesterol	●				●				●				●				●				●				●				●			
Hx of Tobacco Use	●		●										●										●									
Weight	●				●				●				●				●				●				●				●			
Td Booster							●										●										●					
Fecal Occult Blood																							●		●		●		●		●	
Pap Smear		●	●		●		●		●		●		●		●		●		●		●		●		●		●		●		●	
Breast Examination	●		●		●		●		●		●		●		●		●		●		●		●		●		●		●		●	
Eval Osteoporosis Risk																													●			
EDUCATION																																
Use of Seat Belts	●				●				●				●				●				●				●				●			
Self Examination of Skin, Oral Cavity, Testes	●				●				●				●				●				●				●				●			
Breast Self Examination	●				●				●				●				●				●				●				●			
Teach to Report Post Menopausal Bleeding																													●			

Figure 2.1. Adult Health Maintenance Flow Sheet

Figure 2.1. Continued

AGE	50	51	52	53	54	55	56	57	58	59	60	61	62	63	64	65	66	67	68	69	70	71	72	73	74	75	76	77	78	79	80	81
DATE																																
Blood Pressure	●	●	●		●		●		●		●		●		●		●		●		●		●		●		●	●	●	●	●	
Serum Cholesterol	●				●				●				●				●		●		●											
Weight	●				●				●				●				●											●				
Td Booster															●									●	●							
Fecal Occult Blood	●	●	●	●	●	●	●	●	●	●	●	●	●	●	●	●	●	●	●	●	●	●	●	●	●	●	●	●	●	●	●	●
Pap Smear	●	●	●	●	●		●						●				●		●													
Breast Examination	●	●	●	●	●	●	●	●	●	●	●	●	●	●	●	●	●	●	●	●	●	●	●	●	●	●	●	●	●	●	●	●
Mammogram	●	●	●	●	●	●	●	●	●	●	●	●	●	●	●	●	●	●	●	●	●	●	●	●	●	●	●	●	●	●	●	
Eval Osteoporosis Risk	●				●																											
EDUCATION																																
Use of Seat Belts	●				●				●				●				●				●				●				●			
Self Examination of Skin, Oral Cavity, Testes	●				●				●				●				●				●				●			●				
Breast Self Examination	●				●				●				●				●				●				●				●			
Teach to Report Post Menopausal Bleeding	●				●				●				●				●				●				●							

15

This document emphasizes the United States government's goals, priorities, and support of disease prevention. The American Cancer Society published its report on cancer screening recommendations in 1980.

All these reports endorse the concept of *selective longitudinal health mainte-nance*—"selective" because screening criteria similar to those in Table 2.1 must be fulfilled before a recommendation is made, and "longitudinal" because it is assumed the physician will be taking care of the patient over time and ideal frequencies for screening procedures must be specified. It is also assumed that recommendations are being made for a hypothetical totally asymptomatic person. It is recognized, of course, that many patients are not asymptomatic, and the physician will frequently individualize health maintenance to the particular patient.

Although most authorities agree on basic screening criteria, they may interpret the criteria differently, and many specific screening recommendations are contro-versial. There is, however, a basic core of agreement concerning screening for cardiovascular risk factors, preventing tobacco use, and screening for breast and cervical cancer. Unfortunately, the best screening protocol is useless unless it is implemented by practicing primary care physicians.

Health Maintenance In Primary Care Practice

The primary care physician ideally has a health maintenance plan that he or she tries to implement for all patients regardless of whether they have acute or chronic medical problems. Indeed, a major difference between primary and specialty care is that primary care physicians have a responsibility for the patient's well-being regardless of whether there are specific medical problems.

Usually the physician will try to establish a database of pertinent information about the patient when he or she is first seen. This is best done in the context of a "complete" physical examination. The questions asked may vary from a few questions about allergies and past medical problems to a comprehensive multipage questionnaire the patient completes and gives to the physician. Comprehensive questionnaires often include a functional assessment or depression screening instrument. It is perhaps surprising that very little research has been done to investigate which questions are important to ask on a database history.

In many cases the patient will be reluctant to spend the money for a complete physical examination, and the physician must "sneak" in database questions during the course of care for an acute problem. Obviously, in this situation a few key questions are better than a long list of marginal questions.

After the database is obtained, the manner in which screening procedures are incorporated into practice varies widely, ranging from the traditional annual physical to little health maintenance at all. This chapter will describe what is done at Tri-County Family Medicine (Steuben, Livingston, and Alleghany count-ies, New York) as an example of a busy family practice with an active health maintenance interest.

An attempt is made to obtain a database when the patient is first seen. This includes history questions and a head-to-toe physical but very little lab work, except a serum cholesterol, unless indicated by ongoing medical problems. A problem list is then formulated and strategies for dealing with ongoing problems are discussed. Only after acute concerns have been dealt with is it reasonable to discuss screening and health maintenance. The patient is given a handout with basic health maintenance guidelines on the front and a copy of the screening flow sheet (Figure 2.1) on the back.

A copy of the screening flow sheet is on the front cover of each patient's chart. The date is entered when screening procedures are done. A single slash (\) indicates procedures which were done and were normal. An X indicates procedures which were done and were abnormal. Abnormal problems are, of course, followed up in an appropriate manner. In the protocol described in Figure 2.1, healthy patients are instructed to return for a screening visit (not a complete physical examination) every two years until age 50 and every year thereafter.

Patients who would not otherwise be returning to the office for acute problems are sent a postcard reminder of their appointment at the appropriate time one or two years later. A few practices have developed computer technology to remind patients when health maintenance is due. Unfortunately, the majority of primary care practices have no reminder system or at best remind only women to return for Papanicolaou smears.

Lack of time is the major constraint on the provision of health maintenance services in primary care. A typical family physician will see thirty patients per day in the office or four to five patients per hour. In this hurried environment, acute problems are the priority, and screening is done only after other issues have been dealt with. The physicians must ask themselves at every patient visit, "Is the patient's health maintenance up to date?" Some mechanism such as a flow sheet must be available to allow instant appraisal of the patient's health maintenance status. In this context the rather simple program outlined in Figure 2.1 becomes a major commitment in time and effort. Before new procedures are included in the protocol, especially time consuming ones, their value must be firmly established.

The use of paramedical personnel is an increasingly attractive option in trying to provide preventive care as well as acute care. In this practice a full-time physician's assistant is the contact person and provides most care, including prevention, for a segment (in general, healthier and younger) of the practice. The group of six family physicians employs four physician's assistants. Preventive care can be coordinated by nurses and other office staff in addition to physician's assistants and nurse practitioners.

Screening For Depression

Neither the Canadian Task Force (1980) nor Frame (1986a, 1986b, 1986c, 1986d) recommends routine screening for depression in asymptomatic populations. Breslow and Somers (1977) recommend "professional counseling regarding nutrition, exercise, smoking, alcohol, marital, parental and other aspects of health-related behavior and lifestyle" (p. 603) without any statement as to how this should be done or evidence to support its value. The Canadian Task Force (1980) states: "There is fair justification for the recommendation that affective disorders and suicide be excluded from specific consideration in a routine health examination" (p. 47). In view of these negative recommendations it is useful to examine depression to determine why it fails screening criteria (Table 2.1).

Depression is a common illness with significant morbidity. Population-based studies have shown a lifetime prevalence of 3% men and 8% women (Robins et al., 1984). Within a given six months, 1.5% of men and 3% of women have had a major depressive episode (Myers et al., 1984). Morbidity from depression includes decreased quality of life, decreased productivity, and family and job disruption. The ultimate morbidity from depression is suicide, which occurs at a rate of 12 to 14 persons per 100,000 (Miller, Coombs, Leeper, & Barton, 1984). Risk factors for suicide, in addition to depression, include a previous suicide attempt, alcoholism, and being single or divorced (Pokormy, 1983).

Depression is defined by its symptoms and therefore cannot be truly asymptomatic. Nevertheless, depression is often unrecognized by medical practitioners (Magill & Zung, 1982). Several questionnaires, including the Beck Depression Inventory (Beck, Ward, Mendelson, Mack, & Erbargh, 1961), the Zung Self-Rating Depression Scale (SDS) (Zung, Magill, Moore, & George, 1983), the General Health Questionnaire (GHQ) (Johnstone & Goldberg, 1976), and others, have been introduced and validated for the diagnosis of depression. Short versions of most of these tests, suitable for screening, have also been developed.

Thus depression is a common disease with significant morbidity (criteria 1 and 6 on Table 2.1). Tests are available to detect it in the unrecognized if not asymptomatic phase (criterion 5). Furthermore, treatment of symptomatic depression by medication, counseling, and occasionally electroshock is effective (criterion 2). The problem is depression fails criterion 4: "Treatment in the asymptomatic phase must yield a therapeutic result superior to that obtained by delaying treatment until symptoms appear."

It is not clear that treating subtle unrecognized symptoms is better than waiting until more overt symptoms occur. Most of the studies of screening for depression have lacked adequate outcome analysis. Zung et al. (1983) report that patients with depression diagnosed by the SDS and treated with medication had improved SDS scores after four weeks compared with controls. Johnstone and Goldberg (1976), using the GHQ, found that patients diagnosed and treated for depression had fewer symptoms than did controls at the initial assessment, but at the end of one year the control subjects had also gotten better and there was no significant difference between the two groups. Thus, although screening tests can increase the recognition of depression and perhaps affect short-term outcome, there is no evidence that recognition results in long-term benefit to the patient.

Efforts to prevent suicide have also been disappointing. No test has been developed with adequate sensitivity and specificity to predict which patients will attempt suicide (Pokormy, 1983; Murphy, 1983). The proliferation of suicide prevention centers has not resulted in a significant decrease in suicide rates (Hudgens, 1983). Miller et al. (1984) report that only among women aged less than 24 has the presence of suicide prevention centers seemed to decrease rates of suicide.

This analysis points to several areas where further research is needed before screening for depression is included in routine health maintenance programs. Most important is proving that the detection of occult depression, by whatever method, benefits the patient. Next, it is important to determine which of the many available screening tools is most efficient for use in primary care. Finally, the question "Does the whole population, or just a subset of the population need to be screened?" should be analyzed.

References

American Cancer Society (1980). ACS report on the cancer related health checkup. *Ca-A Journal for Clinicians, 30,* 194–240.

Beck, A. T., Ward, C., Mendelson, M., Mack, J., & Erbaugh, J. (1961). An inventory for measuring depression. *Archives of General Psychiatry, 4,* 561–571.

Breslow, L., & Somers, A. R. (1977). The lifetime health monitoring program: A practical approach to preventive medicine. *New England Journal of Medicine, 296,* 601–608.

Canadian Task Force on the Periodic Health Examination (1979). The periodic health examination. *Canadian Medical Association Journal, 121,* 1194–1254.

Canadian Task Force on the Periodic Health Examination (1980). *Periodic health examination monograph* (Catalogue No. H39–3/1980E). Hull, Quebec, Canada: Canadian Government Publishing Centre.

Canadian Task Force on the Periodic Health Examination (1984). The periodic health examination: 2. 1984 update. *Canadian Medical Association Journal, 130,* 1278–1285.

Canadian Task Force on the Periodic Health Examination (1986). The periodic health examination: 2. 1985 update. *Canadian Medical Association Journal, 134,* 724–729.

Frame, P. S. (1986a). A critical review of adult health maintenance: Part 1. Prevention of atherosclerotic diseases. *The Journal of Family Practice, 22,* 341–346.

Frame, P. S. (1986b). A critical review of adult health maintenance: Part 2. Prevention of infectious diseases. *The Journal of Family Practice, 22,* 417–422.

Frame, P. S. (1986c). A critical review of adult health maintenance: Part 3. Prevention of cancer. *The Journal of Family Practice, 22,* 511–520.

Frame, P. S. (1986d). A critical review of adult health maintenance: Part 4. Prevention of metabolic, behavioral and miscellaneous conditions. *The Journal of Family Practice, 23,* 29–39.

Frame, P. S., & Carlson, S. J. (1975a). A critical review of periodic health screening using specific screening criteria: Part 1. Selected diseases of respiratory, cardiovascular, and central nervous system. *The Journal of Family Practice, 2,* 29–36.

Frame, P. S., & Carlson, S. J. (1975b). A critical review of periodic health screening using specific screening criteria: Part 2. Selected endocrine, metabolic, and gastrointestinal diseases. *The Journal of Family Practice, 2,* 123–129.

Frame, P. S., & Carlson, S. J. (1975c). A critical review of periodic health screening using specific screening criteria: Part 3. Selected diseases of the genitourinary system. *The Journal of Family Practice, 2,* 189–194.

Frame, P. S., & Carlson, S. J. (1975d). A critical review of periodic health screening using specific screening criteria: Part 4. Selected miscellaneous diseases. *The Journal of Family Practice, 2,* 189–194.

Hart, C. R. (1975). The history of screening. In C. R. Hart (ed.), *Screening in general practice,* (pp. 12–13). Edenbourough: Churchill Livingstone.

Hudgens, R. W. (1983). Preventing suicide. *The New England Journal of Medicine, 308,* 897–898.

Johnstone, A., & Goldberg, D. (1976). Psychiatric screening in general practice; a controlled trial. *Lancet, 1,* 605–608.

Magill, M. K., & Zung, W. W. K. (1982). Clinical decisions about diagnosis and treatment for depression identified by screening. *The Journal of Family Practice, 14,* 1144–1149.

Miller, H. L., Coombs, D. W., Leeper, J. D., & Barton, S. N. (1984). An analysis of the effects of suicide prevention facilities on suicide rates in the United States. *American Journal of Public Health, 74,* 340–343.

Murphy, G. E. (1983). On suicide prediction and prevention. *Archives of General Psychiatry, 40,* 343–344.

Myers, J. K., Weissman, M. M., Tischler, G. L., Holzer, C. E., Leaf, P. J., Orvaschel, H., Anthony, J. C., Boyd, J. H., Burke, J. D., & Kramer, M. (1984). Six-month prevalence of psychiatric disorders in three communities, 1980—1982. *Archives of General Psychiatry, 41,* 959–967.

Pokormy A. D. (1983). Prediction of suicide in psychiatric patients. *Archives of General Psychiatry, 40,* 249–257.

Public Health Service (1979). *Healthy people; the surgeon general's report on health promotion and disease prevention* (DHEW Publication No. 79–55071). Washington, D.C.: U.S. Government Printing Office.

Robins, L. N., Helzer, J. E., Weissman, M. M., Orvaschel, H., Gruenberg, E., Burke, J. D., & Regier, D. A. (1984). Lifetime prevalence of specific psychiatric disorders in three sites. *Archives of General Psychiatry, 41,* 949–958.

Roemer, M. I. (1945). A program of preventive medicine for the individual. *Milbank Memorial Fund Quarterly, 23,* 209–226.

Zung, W. W. K., Magill, M., Moore, J. T., & George, D. T. (1983). Recognition and treatment of depression in a family medicine practice. *Journal of Clinical Psychiatry, 44,* 3–6.

3

Is Screening For Depression Worthwhile in Primary Care? Screening Criteria and the Current State of Depression Research

Douglas B. Kamerow

Screening questionnaires and antidepressants are cheap, and depressive illnesses can be long-lasting and cause great suffering; the case for a more active approach seems unanswerable.

Thus concludes a 1986 editorial in *The Lancet* on the subject of screening for depression in medical settings (Anonymous, 1986).[1] In contrast, Frame (1986), in a critical review of adult health maintenance, stated that "screening for depression is not indicated because there is no evidence that early diagnosis of unrecognized symptoms results in net benefit to the patient" (p. 33). Is screening for depression worthwhile in primary care?

Many authors have proposed criteria for screening asymptomatic persons for disease. Frame (1986) requires that six separate criteria be met before any screening test is recommended. These criteria may be summarized as follows: The condition must have a significant effect on the quality or quantity of life, and must have an asymptomatic phase during which treatment makes a difference. It must be a treatable condition and be common enough to justify the cost of screening. In addition, there must be an acceptable screening test available for the condition at a reasonable cost.

Less stringent criteria are proposed by Rucker, Frye, and Cygan (1986). They require that the screening test discover new, actual disease; that it be found useful by the physician as a clinical tool; that the information from the screen alter physician behavior (test-ordering, decision-making); and, finally, that patient outcome be changed. Similar criteria for screening in medical settings have been published by Sackett, Haynes, and Tugwell (1985) and the World Health Organization (Wilson & Jungner, 1968).

This chapter actually discusses case-finding (Sackett & Holland, 1975) rather than true screening, although the latter term will continue to be used. That is, rather than testing healthy volunteers in the community or those who are called in by the practitioner for the purpose of screening, in case-finding patients are

---

[1]Adapted with permission from the *Journal of Family Practice*, 1987, *25*, 181–184.

tested when presenting for an unrelated complaint. It can be argued that case-finding requires less stringent criteria for use, in that there is not the implicit guarantee of benefit necessary in population- or practice-wide screening programs (Williams, 1986). This chapter will evaluate the evidence for "screening" primary care patients for depression, examining both the condition itself and the screening tests available for it.

Depression in Primary Care

There is ample documentation that depression is a serious disorder that is very costly in terms of deaths, morbidity, and health care utilization (Kamerow, Pincus, & Macdonald, 1986). In 1985, there were 28,620 suicides in the United States (National Center for Health Statistics, 1986), and it has been shown that approximately half of all persons committing suicide are suffering from major depressive illness (Sainsbury, 1986). Direct and indirect costs incurred by persons with depression exceed $16 billion a year (Stoudemire, Frank, Hedemark, Kamlet, & Blazer, 1986).

Mental disorders are commonly seen in primary care. The prevalence of patients with mental disorder in general medical settings has been shown to be between 20% and 30% and more than half of these patients probably have depression (Hoeper, Nycz, Cleary, Regier, & Goldberg, 1979; Kessler et al., 1987; Shepherd, Cooper, Brown, & Kalton, 1966). Research has shown that the majority of patients with depression is not recognized as such by their physicians (Nielsen & Williams, 1980; Schulberg et al., 1985). Efficacious treatments are certainly available for major depressive disorders, comprising either drugs or psychotherapy or both (Paykel, 1982), although the vast majority of treatment trials has been done in the specialty mental health sector, not primary care.

Since depression is currently diagnosed only by symptoms and history, it is impossible to make a diagnosis at a truly asymptomatic stage in the course of the illness. Instead, the question should be whether intervention early in the course of depression has been shown to make a difference. Studies in the so-called "cost-offset" literature imply that early treatment of patients with mental disorders is associated with decreased costs (and presumably risks) of medical visits and procedures (Jones & Vischi, 1979; Mumford, Schlesinger, Glass, Patrick, & Cuerdon, 1984). Some clinical trials of treatment of depression have shown that early treatment leads to early improvement (Zung, Magill, Moore, & George, 1983), and positive results of the first prevention trials of depression are starting to appear (Muñoz, Ying, Armas, Chan, & Gurza, 1987).

Available Screening Tests

Specific, short screening questionnaires have been tested and validated for depression. (Other, more general but equally valid instruments, such as the

General Health Questionnaire [Goldberg, 1972] and the Hopkins Symptom Checklist [Derogatis, Lipman, Rickels, & Covi, 1974] will not be examined here.) Numerous studies have documented the acceptability and validity of these instruments. A thirteen-item version of the Beck Depression Inventory (BDI) was developed in 1972 for use in primary care settings (Beck & Beck, 1972), and it has been used in many studies (Nielsen & Williams, 1980; Rucker et al., 1986). The twenty-item National Institute of Mental Health (NIMH) Center for Epidemiologic Studies Depression Scale (CES-D), first published in 1977 as a population screen (Radloff, 1977), subsequently has been used extensively in general medical settings (Hough, Landsverk, Stone, Jacobson, & McGranahan, 1982; Muñoz et al., 1987; Schulberg et al., 1985). The Zung (1965) Self-Rating Depression Scale (SDS), which also has twenty questions, is the best known and most utilized depression scale in primary care (Linn & Yager, 1980; Moore, Silimperi, & Bobula, 1978; Zung et al., 1983).

Benefits of Screening Tests

Outcome of the use of screening instruments in primary care can be measured in different ways. Increased physician recognition of mental disorders with screening test feedback (as measured by chart notation, for example) is the simplest outcome measure, and these tests seem to accomplish that (Moore et al., 1978; Linn & Yager, 1980). The next level of outcome analysis is evaluating change in what physicians *do;* that is, do doctors increase prescrip tions, counseling, or referrals if given positive screening test results? Fewer studies have evaluated outcome at this level. Rucker, et al. (1986) found that physicians felt that feedback of the BDI result had been useful for 58% of 375 patients and that it altered their treatment plan in 21%.

The ultimate gold standard for screening outcome is, of course, improvement in patient outcome. Do controlled trials indicate that patients live longer or better if a screening test for mental disorder is used? Zung et al. (1983) found that significantly more screened patients who were treated with antidepressants improved after four weeks compared with untreated controls. Preliminary results of a current trial of SDS score feedback to physicians show that depressed patients whose scores were known to physicians improved sooner than those whose scores were not known (W. W. K. Zung, personal communication, 1987).

Thus, although many of the necessary criteria for adopting a screening test for depression are satisfied, all of them are not. Depression is a common, important disorder, seen frequently in primary care, and there is no question that the use of currently available questionnaires will result in more cases being identified. Gaps exist, however, in demonstrating that early intervention in primary care patients with depression makes a difference and in rigorously documenting that the use of screening questionnaires can change patient outcome.

These screening tests may have other important (and as yet unproven) uses in the clinical setting that deserve mention. Some physicians may wish to use a depression questionnaire when they are uncertain of the diagnosis, as in a patient with multiple somatic complaints. A positive screening test in such circumstances could help make a diagnosis. Another possible use is as a confirmatory "lab test" to show to a patient who is denying his or her illness. A score of 16 on the BDI, for instance, could be presented to a patient complaining of frequent headaches and backaches to help focus discussion on psychological issues and improve compliance with antidepressive medication.

It may be that these screening tests are best used only on patients at high risk for the disorders in question. Such "selective screening" is a well-established practice for other diseases (Schechter, Miller, Baines, & Howe, 1986), and risk factors as varied as a family history of mental illness, high utilization of health services, and a recent death in the family might select a patient for such screening. Currently, a study of the outcome of psychiatric consultation for such patients is being undertaken (W. Katon, personal communication, 1987).

Conclusions

In conclusion, the current answer to the question "Is screening for depression worthwhile?" is only a less than resounding "probably." More research is needed about the nature and course of this illness in primary care as well as on treatment and outcome (Kamerow, 1986). If as many resources had been applied to evaluating screening for mental disorders as have been used to test screening for cancer or heart disease, more answers would be available today.

Specifically, long-term studies that follow physician training or screening interventions through patient recognition to treatment or referral and finally to patient outcome over time must be done. The optimal relationship between primary care physicians and their colleagues in the specialty mental health sector also needs to be defined (Kamerow & Burns, 1987). Depression is one of the disorders to be evaluated in the National Study of Medical Care Outcomes, a longitudinal research project examining health care costs and outcomes of a number of chronic illnesses (Wells, 1985; see also ch. 8 in this volume). Studies such as this one will provide the underlying information needed for definitive research to be done answering the questions discussed here.

Screening tests for depression undoubtedly can uncover undiagnosed illnesses. While they may not fully satisfy all required criteria for inclusion in routine health maintenance schedules for all adults, they may be usefully employed selectively to assist primary care physicians in diagnosing and treating their patients with mental health problems.

References

Anonymous (1986). Treatment of depression in medical patients. *Lancet, 1,* 949–950.

Beck, A. T., & Beck, R. W. (1972). Screening depressed patients in family practice: A rapid technique. *Postgraduate Medicine, 58,* 81–85.

Derogatis, L. R., Lipman, R. S., Rickels, K., & Covi, L. (1974). The Hopkins Symptom Checklist: A self-report symptom inventory. *Behavioral Science, 19,* 1–15.

Frame, P. S. (1987). A critical review of adult health maintenance: Part 4. Prevention of metabolic, behavioral, and miscellaneous conditions. *Journal of Family Practice, 23,* 29–39.

Goldberg, D. P. (1972). *The detection of psychiatric illness by questionnaire.* London: Oxford University Press.

Hoeper, E. W., Nycz, G. R., Cleary, P. D., Regier, D. A., & Goldberg, I. D. (1979). Estimated prevalence of RDC mental disorder in primary medical care. *International Journal of Mental Health, 8,* 6–15.

Hough, R. L., Landsverk, J. A., Stone, J. D., Jacobson, G. F., & McGranahan, C. (1982). *Comparison of psychiatric screening questionnaires for primary care patients* (Final Report of NIMH Contract No. 278–81–0036[DB]). Rockville, MD: National Institute of Mental Health.

Jones, K. R., & Vischi, T. R. (1979). Impact of alcohol, drug abuse and mental health treatment on medical care utilization. *Medical Care, 17* (supplement), ii–82.

Kamerow, D. B. (1986). Research on mental disorders in primary care settings: Rationale, topics, and support. *Family Practice Research Journal, 6,* 5–11.

Kamerow, D. B., & Burns, B. J. (1987). The effectiveness of mental health consultation and referral in ambulatory primary care: A research lacuna. *General Hospital Psychiatry, 9,* 111–117

Kamerow, D. B., Pincus, H. A., & Macdonald, D. I. (1986). Alcohol abuse, other drug abuse, and mental disorders in medical practice: Prevalence, costs, recognition, and treatment. *Journal of the American Medical Association, 255,* 2054–2057.

Kessler, L. G., Burns, B. J., Shapiro, S., Tischler, G. L., George, L. K., Hough, R. L., Bodison, D., & Miller, R. H. (1987). Psychiatric diagnoses of medical service users: Evidence from the Epidemiologic Catchment Area Program. *American Journal of Public Health, 77,* 18–24.

Linn, L. S., & Yager, J. (1980). The effect of screening, sensitization, and feedback on notation of depression. *Journal of Medical Education, 55,* 942–949.

Moore, J. T., Silimperi, D. R., & Bobula, J. A. (1978). Recognition of depression by family medicine residents: The impact of screening. *Journal of Family Practice, 7,* 509–513.

Mumford, E., Schlesinger, H. J., Glass, G. V., Patrick, C., & Cuerdon, T. (1984). A new look at evidence about reduced cost of medical utilization following mental health treatment. *American Journal of Psychiatry, 141,* 1145–1158.

Muñoz, R. F., Ying, Y. W., Armas, R., Chan, F., & Gurza, R. (1987). The San Francisco depression prevention research project: A randomized trial with medical outpatients. In R. F. Muñoz (ed.), *Depression prevention: Research directions* (pp. 199–216). Washington, D.C.: Hemisphere.

National Center for Health Statistics (1986). Annual summary of births, marriages, divorces and deaths, U.S., 1985. In *Monthly Vital Statistics Reports* (Vol. 34, No. 13) (DHHS publication No. PHS 86–1120). Hyattsville, MD: Public Health Service.

Nielsen, A. C., & Williams, T. A. (1980). Depression in ambulatory medical patients: Prevalence by self-report questionnaire and recognition by nonpsychiatric physicians. *Archives of General Psychiatry, 37,* 999–1004.

Paykel, E. S. (ed.) (1982). *Handbook of affective disorders.* New York: Guilford.

Radloff, L. S. (1977). The CES-D Scale: A self-report depression scale for research in the general population. *Applied Psychological Measurement, 1,* 385–401.

Rucker, L., Frye, E. B., & Cygan, R. W. (1986). Feasibility and usefulness of depression screening in medical outpatients. *Archives of Internal Medicine, 146,* 729–731.

Sackett, D. L., Haynes, R. B., & Tugwell, P. (1985). *Clinical epidemiology: A basic science for clinical medicine*. Boston: Little, Brown.

Sackett, D. L., & Holland, W. W. (1975). Controversy in the detection of disease. *Lancet, 2,* 357–359.

Sainsbury, P. (1986). Depression, suicide, and suicide prevention. In A. Roy (ed.), *Suicide* (pp. 73–88). Baltimore: Williams & Wilkens.

Schechter, M. T., Miller, A. B., Baines, C. J., & Howe, G. R. (1986). Selection of women at high risk of breast cancer for initial screening. *Journal of Chronic Disease, 39,* 253–260.

Schulberg, H. C., Saul, M., McClelland, M., Ganguli, M., Christy, W., & Frank, R. (1985). Assessing depression in primary medical and psychiatric practices. *Archives of General Psychiatry, 42,* 1164–1170.

Shepherd, M., Cooper, B., Brown, A. C., & Kalton, G. (1966). *Psychiatric illness in general practice*. London: Oxford University Press.

Stoudemire, A., Frank, R., Hedemark, N., Kamlet, M., & Blazer, D. (1986). The economic burden of depression. *General Hospital Psychiatry, 8,* 387–394.

Wells, K. B. (1985). *Depression as a tracer condition for the national study of medical care outcomes* (Rand Publication No. R-3293-RWJ/HJK). Santa Monica, CA: Rand Corporation.

Williams, P. (1986). Mental illness and primary care: Screening. In M. Shepherd, G. Wilkinson, & P. Williams (eds.), *Mental illness in primary care settings* (pp. 57–67). London: Tavistock.

Wilson, J. M. G., & Jungner, G. (1968). *The principles and practice of screening for disease*. Geneva: World Health Organization.

Zung, W. W. K. (1965). A self-rating depression scale. *Archives of General Psychiatry, 12,* 63–70.

Zung, W. W. K., Magill, M., Moore, J. T., & George, D. T. (1983). Recognition and treatment of depression in a family medicine practice. *Journal of Clinical Psychiatry, 44,* 3–6

4

Issues of Criterion Validity For Screening Measures for Depressive Disorders in Primary Care

James Barrett

In recent usage, *criterion validity,* or *predictive validity,* has two different, although related, meanings.[1] One meaning concerns whether a score on a screening device predicts the presence of a particular disorder, as response to a skin test predicts who has tuberculosis. The theme of this book is screening for depression in primary care, which implies one clear criterion: Does a score on a screening scale identify those with depressive disorders? Case identification is the criterion by which the screen is assessed.

Another meaning of "predictive validity," discussed by Bruce and Barbara Dohrenwend in an article examining issues of validity in field studies of psychological disorder, is the ability to predict outcome, such as admission to treatment, future psychiatric condition, or social functioning (Dohrenwend & Dohrenwend, 1965). The criterion is not diagnosis itself, whether or not a screen predicts who has a disorder; rather, it is the ultimate utility of the diagnostic category, the disorder identified by the screen, particularly in reference to outcome or functioning. Robert Kendell, in discussing validity for psychiatric disorders, commented that reliability is concerned with the defining characteristics of a diagnostic category, whereas validity is concerned with the correlates of that category (Kendell, 1975, ch. 3); this is the sense in which the Dohrenwends used "predictive validity". Applying it to screening for depression, the criterion for a screening device becomes: Are there useful correlates for those who are screened positive? Does the screening score predict who will benefit from a particular intervention, or some other relevant outcome?

In these initial remarks I am introducing two criteria by which to assess screening for depression: (a) screening for case identification and (b) screening to identify persons with particular outcomes or correlates, such as response to treatment. The link between these two criteria is the classification system used;

[1]Some of the material reported in the chapter came from research supported by Grant No. MH-37582 from the National Institute of Mental Health. I also wish to acknowledge the family, physicians, and general internists associated with Dartmouth Medical School and its Department of Community and Family Medicine, for their interest, support, and constructive discussions.

27

if categories in the classification system relate directly to outcome, then these criteria become essentially the same. However, the fact is that classification systems, as well as the individual categories in them, have different purposes. There will be several recurrent themes in my remarks, and one of them is that classification systems have different goals, and it is important, indeed vital, to be clear about those goals. A related theme is that when used to identify cases, screening measures relate to particular classification systems, and here too it is essential to be clear about the purposes of the categories of a particular system. Were those categories conceptualized to relate to outcome, as emphasized by the Dohrenwends, or did they have some other purpose?

Purpose of Classification Systems and of Individual Diagnostic Categories

Classification systems can be grouped according to their primary purpose or goal. Statistical classification is one such purpose. Comprehensive systems such as ICD–9 and DSM-III are examples; their principal purpose is to classify and count, usually for planning purposes, all disorders present in a given unit, be it mental health center, state, or country. A requirement of such a system is that it must be comprehensive—all disorders are to be included. Another is that all people involved in treating patients will use it. In other words, the principal requirements of a statistical classification system are complete coverage and acceptance or compliance. Such a system typically evolves by gathering together individuals with different points of view, to be sure that all possible categories are included, and then arriving at a consensus, both about which categories to include and how to define them. At the category level, then, it tends to be a heterogeneous system, with categories included for various reasons and purposes. Ideally, such a classification system is also concerned with the reliability and validity of its categories, but in practice the method of arriving at the categories and their definitions is through committee work and consensus. Such a system is usually atheoretical, for it must encompass all points of view in the region or country concerned. Often its categories are used for planning purposes.

A second group of classifications has research as its primary goal. The principal concern of a research classification system is validity for each category; the categories must be useful in some way for research purposes, whatever that research may be. Since validation is a primary concern, reliability is essential for the categories. One way to increase reliability is to limit coverage; thus, in a research nosology an "other" category is often used as a place to put heterogeneous groups or for those unrelated to the research involved. An example of such a classification system is the Research Diagnostic Criteria (RDC) (Spitzer, Endicott, & Robins, 1978). In the RDC classification, the underlying validation principle was clinical course. Based on existing data from clinical follow-up studies, categories that were internally consistent, descriptively clear, and related to course were chosen. Of necessity, in this system there was a large "Other Psychiatric Disorder" category, as a repository for individuals who seemed to have something wrong with them but who did not fit the full criteria for any of the defined disorders in the nosology. It is important to note that, as a classification system, a research nosology does not need to be accepted by everyone, although it is desirable to have acceptance by the research community working in the same research area.

A third type of classification system is one that exists primarily for clinical purposes. Its principal concern is clinical utility, that its categories relate directly to particular treatment or management. It must predict who will respond favorably to what treatment, or, if there are no treatments, it must accurately predict the course of the disorder. Reliability of categories is certainly desirable and often assumed, but it is not the principal guiding criterion in arriving at the classification categories. As with classification systems for research purposes, coverage need not be complete. An "other" category can be used for those conditions for which response to treatment is uncertain, or for which outcome is highly variable. What is important is the inclusion as specific categories of all disorders for which there is a known treatment that is efficacious or whose course without treatment are relatively invariant. A related goal is to have as separate categories conditions that relate to particular management strategies, even though that management may not yet be established as efficacious.

In presenting these three types of classification systems, let me quickly acknowledge that their differing purposes need not lead to different categories in each system. There can be, and often is, considerable overlap among the three types of systems. In an ideal world, there would be complete overlap. There would be a statistical classification system in which each and every category would be clinically precise and reliable and would have meaningful correlates— clinical, biochemical, familial, or any other abstraction felt to be relevant for the category involved. This ideal classification would have complete coverage. All disorders would have a place, and everyone would agree about the necessity and reasonableness of their inclusion. The categories would have proven usefulness established by carefully designed basic research and clinical research studies. Each category would relate to a specific treatment or management program. Such a system would be intrinsically so desirable that everyone would wish to comply with it.

Needless to say, we are not yet at such a happy state. Not only do classification schemes have different purposes, but, within a comprehensive statistical classification system such as DSM-III, different categories relate to different purposes in an analogous fashion. Some categories, such as bipolar disorder and major depressive disorder, relate to established effective treatments. In practice, a category such as bipolar disorder usually began at an early stage as a descriptive category, but then evolved over time, through basic research and clinical outcome studies, into a category with a direct relationship to a specific treatment, lithium salts. Other categories, such as antisocial personality, also evolved from careful descriptive studies with follow-up, but unfortunately do not relate directly to any proven treatment. At present, antisocial personality is thus primarily a category for research purposes, both applied (establishing treatment efficacy and planning for desired services) and basic (discovering etiology). One hope for research categories is that eventually they will lead to the discovery of a specific treatment. DSM-III also includes categories such as "Pathological Gambling Disorder." Since there are few established treatments for gambling and because validation data to establish the utility of the category are currently sparse, I would characterize the category as one existing in an early descriptive stage, primarily for statistical classification purposes, something to monitor, and possibly to use as an indicator for need for services.

Screening in Primary Care: Screening for What?

Reviewing the varying purposes of diagnostic categories raises a central question: What should be the principal purpose for screening in primary care and in particular for screening for depression? Should it be to develop new knowledge about proposed categories (a research purpose), or should it be to guide management and treatment? If a goal of such screening is case identification, what should be the primary focus of the "case" classification categories for depression used by clinicians in primary care?

The primary focus of classification categories in primary care, those to be used by primary care providers, should be utility for clinical management. The categories should relate directly to known treatments of proven efficacy, as for example, in the use of anti-depressants in major depression, or of lithium in bipolar illness. When there is no clearly established effective treatment, the categories should relate to those management techniques hypothesized to be helpful, techniques that are either recommended but not yet established interventions, such as group therapy for alcohol dependence, or nonspecific interventions, such as marital counselling. As Clare and Blacker (1986) remark, "From the point of view of the general practitioner who finds himself responsible for the management of a considerable amount of psychiatric morbidity in the general population. . . classification which is developed will have to be reliable, quick to use, and relevant to that population as a whole" (p. 22). Relevant to their clinical needs is implied, which in primary care has two management possibilities: treatment by the practitioner or referral to some other treatment resource.

These remarks should not be taken to mean that there is no place for other classification purposes for categories in primary care. Clearly there is a need for new knowledge, but such groupings, which would be research categories since their goal would be new knowledge, should also have management implications.

With relation to outcome, the evolution of a category in psychiatry has typically begun with careful clinical description, often related to a describable clinical course. The category then is subjected to research efforts, both basic and applied, which further modify it, or, in some cases, cause it to disappear if there are no useful correlates, such as established etiology or response to treatment. This evolutionary process thus proceeds from a descriptive, heuristic phase to one of increasing specificity of prediction of outcome, of management, and, one hopes, of etiology. Unfortunately, in psychiatry many categories are not at this advanced stage, and there is also considerable diversity of treatments—psychosocial, behavioral, and pharmacologic—with no clear superiority of a particular treatment for many conditions. Thus, systems that focus on problems, rather than specific disorders, potentially have a place, if, by identifying those problems, direction for future research is established or appropriate referrals can be made.

To repeat my point, which is central to my approach to criterion validity in primary care: Classification categories in primary care, and related screening for them, should relate to clinical management. If such management is not clearly established, categories and associated screening should relate to hypothesized management methods so that needs can be highlighted and new, treatment-related knowledge potentially advanced.

The Problem With Diagnosis as a Guide to Management

DSM-III: A Multipurpose System. In primary care the principal use of screening for depression has been case identification: Who has a particular disorder? If DSM-III disorders are the "cases" identified, i.e. are the criteria against which a screen is validated, how do they relate to treatment specificity? I begin with the categories of DSM-III because it provides the official psychiatric nomenclature of the United States. In most of the research on depression in primary care, DSM-III categories are the ones used. For example, they are frequently used to assess the diagnostic skills of primary care physicians at recognizing depression. How useful are its categories, keeping management in mind as criterion?

DSM-III is a heterogeneous system. It contains categories at different stages of development. Some categories, such as major depression, currently relate to specific treatment; they have clear clinical utility. Other categories exist for research and planning purposes; these categories indicate where treatment is desirable but no clearly effective treatments yet exist. Examples would include dysthymic disorder and various character disorders such as histrionic, dependent, or borderline character.

Other DSM-III categories are at an early descriptive stage; they are felt to be disorders, but they may not require treatment. An example could be the "adjustment disorders" group, described recently by Fabrega, Mezzich, and Mezzich (1987) as a "transitional illness category," which includes categories with relatively mild symptomatology and impairment. Specificity of treatment for these categories is not established, and some may remit spontaneously without treatment. "Pathological gambling," which I mentioned earlier, is another category still at an early descriptive stage. It serves to define a group of people to follow, but etiologic or treatment related correlates have yet to be established.

DSM-III categories evolved from the study of hospital-based patients, and, more recently, of psychiatric outpatients. The categories thus reflect the psychopathology of patients in the specialty sector, which may be different from that in the general population or in related primary care patient populations. Included may be categories of little relevance to what presents in primary care, and, conversely, categories of possible importance in primary care may be omitted. How useful have DSM-III categories been as criteria in primary care?

DSM-III Categories as a Guide to Management or Need. Our research group recently conducted a study to determine the prevalence of specific psychiatric disorders in a primary care practice. With respect to DSM-III depressive disorders, we found that 2.8% of patients had major depressive disorder, either treated or untreated. Another 2.1% had dysthymic disorder, and 2.4% had adjustment disorders with depression. Another 2.3% had other depressive disorders, principally histrionic or explosive character. Taking these categories together, 10% of these primary care patients had a specific DSM-III disorder.

An unexpected finding in this study was that many patients with significant depressive symptoms did not fit into any of these specific DSM-III depressive disorder categories. In our study we simultaneously categorized patients by the RDC system, which permits an "Other Psychiatric Disorder" category for those patients who do not meet the criteria for specific disorders. Another 10% of patients with significant depression fit in this "Other Psychiatric Disorder" category. On clinical grounds, we separated this category into two subgroups: masked/suspected depression (6% of patients) and mixed anxiety depression (4% of patients). Many of these patients were called depressed by their primary care physicians, who did feel something was wrong.

Several points can be made regarding our findings. One is that, in general, the specific DSM-III categories were useful as far as they went. All the patients whom we diagnosed as exhibiting signs of major depression were seen as depressed by their physicians, and in most cases appropriate treatment had been initiated. For the other specific depressive categories, about 75% of the time the physicians also saw the patients as depressed, although there was uncertainty about how to manage each case, particularly dysthymic disorder and histrionic character. The DSM-III categories thus seemed appropriate as descriptors of certain patients, although of varying utility as guides to management.

Approximately 50% of the patients we believed to be depressed did not fit into a specific DSM-III depressive disorder category. If our primary care physicians had been using only DSM-III categories to classify depressives, these physicians would appear to have "missed" the depression 50% of the time, when significant depressive symptoms were indicated using the psychiatrist RDC diagnoses as criterion. Similarly, had we been using a depression screen scale score as a criterion to identify a case, approximately 50% of the time the physicians would appear to have missed a diagnosis of depression if only DSM-III specific depress-ive disorder categories had been available to them. That general medical physi-cians fail to diagnose depression a significant proportion of the time when it is present, as determined by a screening inventory is widely quoted in services research literature (Nielsen & Williams, 1980; Schulberg et al., 1985). One wonders if some of these results reflect the classification system used as criterion, in contrast to a failure of physicians to detect depression.

Other findings that raise questions similar to those raised in our findings come from the Epidemiologic Catchment Area (ECA) Project data. In the ECA study, DSM-III diagnostic categories were used as a unit of analysis to relate to need. That project, with systematic data gathered on over 15,000 community residents of five separate U.S. communities (Eaton et al., 1984; Regier et al., 1984), is truly a unique data resource. With its focus on who provided treatment for psychiatric disorders, it highlighted the importance of the primary care sector in treating psychiatric disorders. The ECA study used the Diagnostic Interview Schedule (DIS) (Robins, Helzer, Crougham, & Ratcliff, 1981) as a case identifi-cation instrument. This standardized interview is capable of providing DSM-III diagnoses for 31 diagnostic categories, although not all the categories were used at all sites. One finding was that "a majority of persons in virtually all recent DIS disorder categories do not see any provider for mental health reasons during a six month period" (Shapiro et al., 1984, p. 978). A related finding was that persons classified as having no DIS disorder accounted for about one-third of all the people who see a provider for a mental or emotional problem. The authors of this report, which was addressing utilization of health and mental health services, go on to conclude that these findings indicate "that any effort to estimate the burden of mental or emotional problems on the health care system will need to go beyond those with a DIS disorder" (Shapiro et al., 1984, p. 978). Again, can these findings be partially explained by the fact that some DIS categories do not relate to treatment? If so, the fact that sizable numbers of individuals with DIS disorders did not seek treatment in a six month period is not surprising. Conversely, that there were no DSM-III categories for some individuals with significant symptoms, as was the case in our study, could partially explain the finding that many individuals with no DSM-III disorder do see providers for mental or emotional problems.

Earlier I emphasized the importance of the different purposes behind the individual diagnostic categories within DSM-III. Notice what happened in the interpretation of data from the ECA study. There was a shift from one goal—to determine how many DSM-III disorders were present in the community—to another: to determine what was the need for services, with DSM-III categories now the criteria for need. The problem of heterogeneity of purposes within DSM-III categories reemerges. Some DSM-III categories relate well to need for services. Other categories relate poorly to specific services, although the need for something to be done is clear enough. Some may not relate to need at all and can be considered analogous to the "common cold" in psychiatry. Finally, it is likely that there may be individuals with "need" for services who are not captured by existing DSM-III categories, as we found in our study in primary care. In recent papers from the ECA study, there is implicit acknowledgement that DIS diagnosis alone is not an adequate indicator of need for services; in those reports a DIS diagnosis was only one of three required criteria selected to serve as indicators of need (Shapiro, Skinner, Kramer, German, & Romanoski, 1986).

Let me be very clear that it is not my intent to criticize the DSM-III harshly or to condemn the ECA Project. DSM-III is highly useful for certain purposes, as is the wealth of data from the ECA Project. Rather, my intent is to highlight the problems that arise when particular screening goals, such as determining need for treatment, are mediated through case identification of particular categories that are at different stages of development or evolved for different purposes.

Summarizing, and returning specifically to depression, I think the evidence is that DSM-III categories as a group have serious shortcomings in primary care as criteria for treatment or management and the related issue of need for services. What other systems have been used or suggested?

Problem-Oriented Approaches in Primary Care as Criteria for Management

Classification systems other than traditional medical categories have been recommended for use in primary care. Many of these follow a problem-oriented approach, in which patient complaints or needs are coded into problem categories, and these in turn relate to interventions. For example, "conflicts with spouse" might be a problem category, with "referral for family therapy" a possible intervention. Such systems frequently follow an axial approach, with a separate axis for physical, psychological, or social problems. A partial listing of such problem-oriented systems would include the Reason for Visit Classification (RVC) developed by the National Center for Health Statistics (Schneider, Appleton, & McLemore, 1979); the International Classification of Health Problems in Primary Care (World Organization of National Colleges, Academies, and Academic Association of General Practitioners/Family Physicians, 1979), or ICHPPC-2, (it is now in its second version); the tri-axial system developed by NIMH (the National Institute of Mental Health) and WHO (World Health Organization) (Lipkin & Kupka, 1982); the General Practice Research Unit classification developed in the United Kingdom (Fitzgerald, 1978); and the various problem-oriented medical record systems in use in many medical facilities in the United States. In this discussion, with its focus on criteria against which to assess screening, I will take up in more detail the problem-oriented system reported by Longabaugh and the tri-axial system developed by WHO.

Problem-Oriented Records. In the 1970s Longabaugh and his associates were instrumental in introducing problem-oriented records as part of hospital requirements for record keeping at certain Rhode Island hospitals. Coding was required for both patient problems and treatment interventions. There were many problem categories, over 4,000, which could be grouped into three broad areas: physiologic, psychologic, and social. Treatments were grouped as physical, psychological, social, "life tasks," and "cultural" (Longabaugh, Stout, Kriebel, McCullough, & Bishop, 1986). For a series of patients admitted during 1981–1982, Longabaugh examined the relationship of categorization of the patient to treatment interventions, comparing categorization by DSM-III categories with categorization by problem categories. He found that DSM-III categories did well in predicting various medical treatments—use of lithium, neuroleptics, and antidepressants—which was reassuring. The problem categories also did well in predicting medical treatments, and the two combined gave improved treatment predictability, indicating that each system provided information not present in the other. For both systems the degree of intervention predictability was less overall for the psychosocial interventions, and for some interventions—psychotherapies and behavioral interventions—problem categories were better predictors than diagnostic categories. For other interventions—social-system and life-task interventions—diagnoses were virtually irrelevant, but problem categories continued to show some predictability.

The Longabaugh study was done on hospital inpatients, not primary care patients, but the results and methodology have implications for diagnostic systems in primary care. Of particular importance is the finding that some problem categorizations related as well to medication use as did DSM-III diagnostic categories, and that problem categories related better than DSM-III diagnoses to psychosocial interventions. One would expect these trends to be even more pronounced in a primary care population, in which disorders are less severe and the appropriateness of medication use is more problematic. If management— treatment by the practitioner or appropriate referral—is to be a principal criterion for primary care classification, studies using a methodology similar to Longabaugh's need to be done, in which psychiatric diagnosis is put in a horse race against problem categorization to determine which relates best to management interventions. Even better would be studies that used outcome, not intervention, as the prediction criterion.

The Tri-Axial System. In 1979, under the auspices of WHO, an international conference took place in Bellagio, Italy, to address classification needs in primary care. There was consensus that the present systems were inadequate as guides to management and as indicators of need in primary care, and a work group was formed to devise appropriate categories for use in primary care settings. In 1981, the group proposed a tri-axial system of recording. The first axis was to be classification of physical problems and disorders according to systems currently in use, such as the International Classification of Diseases, ninth revision (ICD–9). Two additional axes were added: a psychological problem axis and a social problem axis. With respect to depression, the psychological problem axis included such items as feeling depressed, crying excessively, feeling hopeless, and various other "problems" indicative of a depressive mood. There were some 18 psychological problem categories; individual symptoms in the first 9 could be symptoms of depressive illness as well as of other conditions. The social problem axis included 11 categories; examples included housing problems, financial problems, or problems within a family.

This system went through subsequent revisions with input from both developed and developing countries about the content of the various problem categories. The most current revision was adopted by the Division of Mental Health of the World Health Organization, and, under the auspices of WHO, was to undergo extensive field trials to assess its utility. For various reasons, primarily lack of funding, this field testing has not been carried out. I mention the system because it had broad input in its conceptualization and was specifically designed to potentially relate to management interventions in primary care. Also, the categories of the psychological and the social axes were utilized in two of the chapters, chapter P and chapter V, of ICHPPC-2, the detailed classification system designed as a descriptor of all possible reasons for a visit to a primary care provider (World Organization of National Colleges, Academies, & Academic Associations of General Practitioners/Family Physicians, 1979). The primary goal of ICHPPC-2 was statistical classification, to capture what presents in primary care independent of management, although one of the descriptive goals for its use was to determine what interventions are currently being utilized for which problems by primary care providers. A large pilot study has been carried out, using primary care patients from eight nations. Results of this effort are not yet in the public domain, and thus I cannot comment further except to point out that the tri-axial psychological and social problem axes are currently in use, at least in this pilot fashion.

In this brief summary of problem-oriented systems, I have considered all categories, not just those that relate to depression, the topic of this book. I did so because in primary care the issues that relate to screening for depression are similar to those that relate to other conditions. Do particular depressive disorder diagnoses guide treatment better than depressive symptoms coupled with other symptoms, as advocated by the problem-oriented approach? One would hope so for categories such as major depression. But what about other depressive disorder categories found from research studies to be common in primary care—adjustment disorder with depression, for example? There is suggestive evidence that a problem-oriented approach would be a better guide to intervention for the less severe and often mixed conditions, but at this point such evidence must remain speculative, since definitive studies remain to be done.

Whether all behavioral conditions are being considered or just those where significant depression is present the criterion validation issue is the same: categorization for what purpose?

Screening as Identification of Depressive
Diagnostic Categories in Primary Care

One proposed use of screens by primary care practitioners is to identify people who will respond to treatment, and thus a common criterion to evaluate the screen is diagnosis—how well it identifies those individuals with depressive disorders from those with other conditions. Setting aside for a moment the question of the varying relationship of the individual disorder categories to treatment and outcome, how effective are the screens as case identifiers at separating those with depressive disorders from those with other, or no, psychiatric condition? In this discussion I am not going to review in detail screening devices that have been used. Instead, in order to illustrate some of the criterion validity issues I have raised, I will examine one study, by William Zung and his associates, which was designed to screen for depression in a primary care practice with a focus on treatment and management (Zung, Magill, Moore, & George, 1983). They used the Zung Symptoms of Depression Scale (SDS) (Zung, 1965) to identify individuals with significant clinical depression. The screening goal here was clear: to identify those with a depressive disorder for whom treatment with an antidepressant was appropriate. SDS scales were administered to patients in the practice, and those above a cut score of 55, 13.2% of patients, were considered as having depressive disorders, "clinically significant symptoms of depression," for which use of antidepressants was appropriate treatment. In the study the effect of notifying the physician that a patient was above cut-score was also assessed, with use of anti-depressants as the outcome variable.

There are at least two shortcomings of a screen used in this fashion in primary care. The screen scale score itself has now become the criterion for treatment, but this is only because that score is assumed to identify correctly all those with depressive disorders that will respond to antidepressants. Indications for use of this medication seem most clear for major depressive disorder, less so for dysthymic disorder, and even less so for histrionic character or adjustment reaction with depression, although individuals with these disorders also score high on the SDS scale. One problem is that, even if the screen were perfectly sensitive and specific for all depressive disorders, it would not be specific at the disorder level; whatever SDS score was chosen as criterion would not be specific for major depression. Included above that cut score would be depressive disorder categories for which antidepressant treatment is not established as effective. A second problem is that the screen does not have adequate sensitivity and specificity to be used as an identifier of all those with a depressive disorder. If a low cut score is used to give adequate sensitivity, then specificity is lacking; there are too many false positives. Conversely, if a high screen score is used, giving reasonable specificity for any depressive disorder, such a score is relatively insensitive; there would be too many false negatives. Any reasonably sensitive cut score selected would include above it sizable numbers of individuals for whom use of antidepressants would be questionable treatment, and it is also likely that some with a treatable disorder would be excluded. Many investigators (Myers & Weissman, 1980; Roberts & Vernon, 1981; Schulberg et al., 1985) have commented on the inefficiency of depression scales for clinical purposes, which I maintain should be the principal purpose for a screen in primary care. According to Myers and Weissman (1980), "The group defined as 'cases' by such instruments also includes many people with other diagnoses or with no diagnoses at all" (p. 1083).

The issue here is that the SDS was developed not to identify individuals with a particular disorder, but as a thermometer of depressive symptomatology. Thus, a scale developed for one purpose—a research purpose, a nonspecific indicator of level of depression—is now being used for another purpose for which it was not designed—the identification of a particular disorder, major depression, which relates directly to a specific treatment.

Screening for Depression in Primary Care: Possible Current Roles and Related Criteria

The Alerting Function of Screening in Primary Care. I now turn to the principal focus of this book, screening for depression in primary care. To review my earlier remarks, I outlined three separate goals or purposes for screening in primary care: (a) screening to identify cases for management, either treatment by the practitioner or referral; (b) screening to assist planning for services; and (c) screening for basic research, to develop new knowledge about particular disorders. I indicated that screening for basic research goals, although highly appropriate for researchers, was inappropriate as a routine for physician practitioners; that screening for management was highly appropriate, a first priority; and that screening for planning was a second priority. I briefly reviewed one experience with screening for identifying cases for specific treatments and concluded that screening for this purpose had serious shortcomings, related to the use of diagnostic DSM-III categories as criteria.

There is another treatment/management function for screening in primary care, and that is as an alerting device, as a means to enable a busy practitioner to think of conditions that he or she might otherwise miss. Through the use of a screening scale, such as the SDS, the practitioner can be alerted to the possibility that a treatable depressive disorder may be present, leading to further investigation of the depressive symptomatology elicited by the screen; appropriate depressive disorder diagnoses can then be made and appropriate treatment initiated. I suggest that this alerting function of existing scales is more important at present than any specific case identification function because of the relatively poor sensitivity and specificity of these scales for identifying specific treatable disorders. When one is considering criterion validity, these different functions must be kept separate. In case identification, a screen would be evaluated by its ability to identify specific disorders against some gold standard. In the alerting function, a screen would be evaluated by the degree to which it enables a given physician to be more sensitive to the presence of treatable depression when it is present. Criterion validity for this latter goal would be how often a given primary care provider identified treatable depression using the screen, compared to how often that provider identified treatable depression when not using the screen. The study discussed earlier, by Zung and associates (Zung et al., 1983), could be seen as an example of using the SDS as an alerting device, except that in that study the investigators equated a particular SDS score with treatable depression. There was no attempt to assess the ability of the practitioner to accurately identify a depressive disorder when one was present using other gold standard criteria.

Use of a problem-oriented approach, such as the tri-axial system, also could be seen as providing an "alerting" function with treatment/management implications. Here the use of the psychological and social problem categories, with the practitioner reminded of them at each patient encounter, can be seen as a screening device in the sense of this "alerting function." In fact, this was a purpose planned for the tri-axial system; use of the categories was expected to increase practitioner awareness of psychosocial factors involved in a particular patient visit, with the implication that appropriate management interventions would then be taken. In theory, those interventions are problem specific, with some outcome measure, as improved functioning, or reduction of dysphoric symptomatology, the appropriate criterion against which to assess the efficacy of the psychological and social axes as management related screens.

The Services Planning Function of Screening in Primary Care. In the earlier description of the tri-axial system, I indicated that a second planning purpose was to identify frequently occurring problem areas for patients in primary care, with the expectation that this identification would serve as a stimulus to develop programs or interventions which did not previously exist for those problems. This would be a services planning role, mentioned as a secondary, but important, role for screening in primary care. It is a role similar to that played by epidemiologic studies, such as the ECA project. Problem areas are identified, which then serve to guide planning for services. Paul Williams (1979), in an article about "deciding how to treat," outlined several benefits of including a problem-oriented approach in primary care. Those benefits included: treatment is closely related and directly relevant to the problem; problems with reliability and validity of diagnostic categories do not arise; the clinical team is reminded of the patient's total situation; and different conceptual models of illness can be adapted for different problems within the same patient. Williams advocates using a problem-oriented approach as an extension, not a replacement, of diagnosis.

There indeed appears a possible role for screening in primary care for at least two management related functions: alerting practitioners to the possible presence of treatment specific disorders, and, as part of routine practice, identifying problem areas for which there exist appropriate referral and services. This latter function would also serve to identify problem areas where services are needed but are not available.

Summary and Suggestions for Research

Let me summarize this discussion of criterion validity for screening for depression in primary care. First, such criteria should be management related, relevant to clinical needs, as implied by Clare and Blacker (1986). Second, using screening as case identifiers for categories of comprehensive systems such as DSM-III has relatively poor utility for treatment/management purposes because of the varying purposes underlying the categories of those nosological systems. Third, problem-oriented approaches appear to have management utility in primary care. They can be viewed both as a classification system and as a screening device. The criterion against which their screening function should be assessed is patient outcome.

These summary statements suggest the following areas as suitable for research:

1. Research to improve the use of existing depressive disorder categories in primary care, as a guide to management. For example, of the existing DSM-III categories, which should be kept separate, and which might be combined into a broader category, with treatment outcome as criterion? The existing classification system should be packaged so that it relates directly to treatment related outcomes, and screens for these categories should be developed.

2. Research to develop new disorder categories, of direct relevance to management, which relate to clinical presentation in primary care. Is "masked depression" a real clinical entity? Can defining criteria be developed for it, so that outcome related research, such as response to antidepressants, can be carried out on it? The same can be done for other syndromes. The need here is to move away from the specialty-based categories, to develop new ones of utility to management in primary care, and then in turn to develop screens for them.

3. There is a clear need for continuing longitudinal research on the issue of what constitutes a true disorder requiring intervention. To use an analogy from general medicine, a common cold is a clear disorder, with a known pathology and with impairment. It is also a condition that recovers spontaneously and for which treatment, if any, is aimed at symptom relief for a brief period. What are the common colds in psychiatry? Particularly for primary care, we need to establish which depressive disorders require treatment and which disorders recover spontaneously, with no lasting morbidity, given minimal or no intervention. With such knowledge, it follows that better screens for disorders that require treatment can be developed.

4. Further research on the utility of problem-oriented systems is recommended. These systems appear to have value as alerting devices. A problem list of manageable size, one whose categories would be used by practitioners and would show a relationship to outcome, needs to be developed. The tri-axial

system is a step in that direction, but I suspect that its goal of having categories of relevance to all cultures severely limits its acceptance and its utility for specific management in a given culture. For each country, can a short category list be developed, with clarity of the categories, and with utility for management? These are reasonable questions, and such work needs to be done.

With respect to criteria for screening for depression in primary care, I conclude by repeating that there is clearly a need for additional work on the depression categories used as criteria for the primary care clinician. We need to get away from applying specialty-based diagnoses to the outpatients that present in primary care and to develop instead categories that relate to depressive disorders as seen by the treating practitioner. It is a tedious process to develop operational criteria for such categories, but it is only through such a process that knowledge can progress, both about whether a category is a true separate entity, and, if it is, whether effective treatments or management techniques can be developed. It is only then that we can begin to develop and assess screening devices with clear management implications.

References

Clare, A. W., & Blacker, R. (1986). Some problems affecting the diagnosis and classification of depressive disorders in primary care. In M. Shepherd, G. Wilkinson, & P. Williams (eds.), *Mental illness in primary care settings* (pp. 7–26). London: Tavistock.

Dohrenwend, B. P., & Dohrenwend, B. S. (1965). The problem of validity in field studies of psychological disorder. *Journal of Abnormal Psychology, 70,* 52–69.

Eaton, W. W., Holzer III, C. E., Von Korff, M., Anthony, J. C., Helzer, J. E., George, L., Burnam, M. A., Boyd, J. H., Kessler, L. G., & Locke, B. Z. (1984). The design of the epidemiologic catchment area surveys. *Archives of General Psychiatry, 41*(10), 942–948.

Fabrega, H., Jr., Mezzich, J. E., & Mezzich, A. C. (1987). Adjustment disorder as a marginal or transitional illness category in DSM-III. *Archives of General Psychiatry, 44,* 567–572.

Fitzgerald, R. (1978). The classification and recording of social problems. *Social Science and Medicine, 12,* 255–263.

Kendell, R. E. (1975). *The role of diagnosis in psychiatry.* Oxford: Blackwell.

Lipkin M., Jr., & Kupka, K. (1982). A classification of psychological symptoms and social problems for inclusion in a triaxial classification of health problems. In M. Lipkin, Jr., and K. Kupka (eds.), *Psychosocial factors affecting health* (pp. 329–333). New York: Praeger.

Longabaugh, R., Stout, R., Kriebel, G. W., Jr., McCullough, L., & Bishop, D. (1986). DSM-III and clinically identified problems as a guide to treatment. *Archives of General Psychiatry, 43,* 1097–1103.

Myers, J. K., & Weissman, M. M. (1980). Use of a self-report symptom scale to detect depression in a community sample. *American Journal of Psychiatry, 137* (9), 1081–1084.

Nielsen, A. C., & Williams, A. (1980). Depression in ambulatory medical patients: Prevalence by self-report questionnaire and recognition by nonpsychiatric physicians. *Archives of General Psychiatry, 37,* 999–1004.

Regier, D. A., Myers, J. K., Kramer, M., Robins, L. N., Blazer, D. G., Hough, R. L., Eaton, W.

W., & Locke, B. Z. (1984). The NIMH epidemiologic catchment area program. *Archives of General Psychiatry, 41*(10), 934–941.

Roberts, R. E., & Vernon, S. W. (1983). The center for epidemiologic studies depression scale: Its use in a community sample. *American Journal of Psychiatry, 140,* 41–46.

Robins, L. N., Helzer, J. E., Crougham, J., & Ratcliff, K. S. (1981). National Institute of Mental Health diagnostic interview schedule: Its history, characteristics, and validity. *Archives of General Psychiatry, 38,* 381–389.

Schneider, D., Appleton, L., & McLemore, T. (1979). *A reason for visit classification for ambulatory care.* (DHEW Publication No. PHS 79–1352). Hyattsville, MD: U.S. National Center for Health Statistics.

Schulberg, H. C., Saul, M., McClelland, M., Ganguli, M., Christy, W., & Frank, R. (1985). Assessing depression in primary medical and psychiatric practices. *Archives of General Psychiatry, 42,* 1164–1170.

Shapiro, S., Skinner, E. A., Kessler, L. G., Von Korff, M., German, P. S., Tischler, G. L., Leaf, P. J., Benham, L., Cottler, L., & Regier, D. A. (1984). Utilization of health and mental health services. Three epidemiologic catchment area sites. *Archives of General Psychiatry, 41,* 971–978.

Shapiro, S., Skinner, E. A., Kramer, M., German, P. S., & Romanoski, A. (1986). Need and demand for mental health services in an urban community: An exploration based on household interviews. In J. E. Barrett & R. M. Rose (eds.), *Mental disorders in the community* (pp. 307–320). New York: Guilford Press.

Spitzer, R. L. Endicott, J., & Robins, E. (1978). Research diagnostic criteria: Rationale and reliability. *Archives of General Psychiatry, 35,* 773–782.

World Organization of National Colleges, Academies, and Academic Associations of General Practitioners/Family Physicians (1979). *International classification of health problems in primary care* (2nd ed.). Chicago: American Hospital Association.

Williams, P. (1979). Deciding how to treat—the relevance of psychiatric diagnosis. *Psychological Medicine, 9,* 179–186.

Zung, W. W. K. (1965). A self-rating depression scale. *Archives of General Psychiatry, 12,* 63–70.

Zung, W. W. K., Magill, M., Moore, J. T., & George, D. T. (1983). Recognition and treatment of depression in a family medicine practice. *Journal of Clinical Psychiatry, 44,* 3–6.

5

Caseness Criteria for Major Depression: The Primary Care Clinician and the Psychiatric Epidemiologist

Wayne Katon and Michael Von Korff

The purpose of this chapter is to describe factors that make accurate recognition of "caseness" of major depression difficult for both the primary care physician and the mental disorder epidemiologist. The major points of emphasis are:

1. Depression and chronic medical illness frequently occur together. Depression often exacerbates disability and the subjective dimensions of illness.

2. Patients with depression frequently amplify physical sensations, which impedes the ability of physicians to accurately diagnose major depression.

3. Primary care patients with depression typically have lower levels of severity of their affective illness compared to psychiatric patients. They are often borderline cases on usual research diagnostic categories.

4. About one-third of all primary care patients has significant psychiatric symptoms. Physicians are constantly faced with the challenge of distinguishing transient emotional distress from syndromes requiring substantial treatment.

5. Few treatment studies assess the effectiveness of tricyclic antidepressants and psychotherapy in primary care patients with depression and limited empirical basis for recommendations regarding the specific treatment protocols.

6. None of the studies thus far has evaluated the economic impact of treatment on social parameters of affective illness such as medical utilization, family life, job absenteeism, and disability.

In the face of these difficulties and gaps in knowledge, the response of psychiatric researchers has often been to highlight the shortcomings of the primary care physician in case recognition, in overuse of certain psychoactive medications, and in prescribing subtherapeutic dosages of others. These six factors and the differing perspectives and "tensions" of the primary care clinician and mental disorder epidemiologist will be considered by comparing research on the diagnosis and treatment of two medical conditions, peptic ulcer disease and hypertension, to major depression.

Somatization

Epidemiologic studies in the community have demonstrated that 3 to 4% of adults suffer from major depression, but only about one-third receives specific mental health treatment (Myers et al., 1984; Weissman, Myers, & Thompson, 1981). These untreated adults with major depression average significantly more visits to their primary care physicians over a one-year period than comparable controls who are not depressed (Weissman et al., 1981). Thus, many studies have documented that patients with depression are over-represented in medical clinics. Studies utilizing depression rating scales have documented a 12 to 25% rate of clinically significant depression in primary care clinics (Barnes & Prosen, 1984; Hankin & Locke, 1982; Katon, Berg, Robins, & Risse, 1986; Nielson & Williams, 1980; Salkind, 1969; Seller, Blaskovich, & Lenke, 1981; Zung, Magill, Moore, & George, 1983). Although these scales are sensitive and pick up most patients with depression, they are not very specific in their ability to distinguish major depression from other psychiatric illnesses. Studies utilizing structured psychiatric interviews such as the Diagnostic Interview Schedule (DIS) (Robins, Helzer, Croughan, & Ratcliff, 1981) or Schedule for Affective Disorders and Schizophrenia (SADS) (Endicott & Spitzer, 1978) and Research Diagnostic Criteria (RDC) (Spitzer, Endicott, & Robins, 1978) and DSM-III (American Psychiatric Association [APA], 1980) have found that 6 to 10% of adult primary care outpatients meet criteria for major depression (Hoeper, Nyczi, Cleary, Regier, & Goldberg, 1979; Schulberg et al., 1985).

Despite the high prevalence of depression in primary care outpatients, multiple studies have documented poor recognition of this affective illness by primary care physicians. These studies have determined that 50 to 82% of patients with depression were not accurately diagnosed (Hoeper et al., 1979; Katon et al., 1986; Nielson & Williams, 1980; Seller et al., 1981; Schulberg et al., 1985; Zung et al., 1983).

Reasons for Misdiagnosis

Before we are too critical of the primary care physician, it is essential to recognize that there are differences in phenomenology among patients with depression in the community, in primary care, and in psychiatric systems. Yet most descriptions of major depression, as well as treatment studies, are based on highly selected psychiatric patients with moderate to severe depression. A recent community study of major depression emphasized the highly selected patients that the psychiatrist sees compared to the primary care physician. Tansella, Williams, Balestrieri, Bellantuaro, and Martini (1986) found that for every 100 psychiatric contacts at the primary care level for affective illness, ten patients will be referred for outpatient psychiatric care and one will be admitted for inpatient psychiatric care. As depicted in Figure 5.1, psychiatric patients with

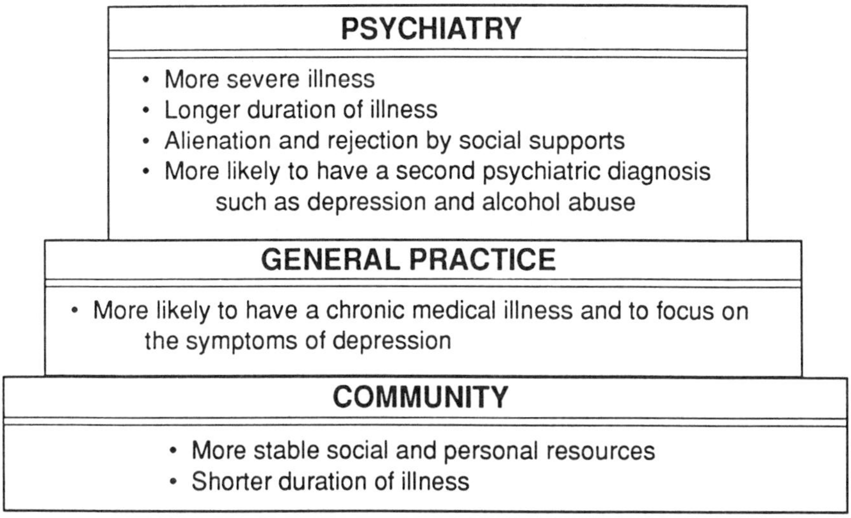

PSYCHIATRY
• More severe illness • Longer duration of illness • Alienation and rejection by social supports • More likely to have a second psychiatric diagnosis   such as depression and alcohol abuse

GENERAL PRACTICE
• More likely to have a chronic medical illness and to focus on   the symptoms of depression

COMMUNITY
• More stable social and personal resources • Shorter duration of illness

Figure 5.1. Differences in Patients with Affective Illness According to Setting.

affective illness are likely to have: a longer duration of illness; more severe symptoms; increased alienation from social support systems; and multiple psychiatric diagnoses. Thus, descriptions of the phenomenology, natural history, and treatment of affective illness in psychiatric patients may not be entirely generalizable to affective illness in medical patients or in the community.

Copeland (1981) has pointed out the erroneous view, still pervasive in medicine, that diseases are entities in themselves, rather than "the result of an interaction, the manifestations which will vary according to the variations in the agent, host and environment" (p. 10). As every clinician knows from experience, few patients' illnesses fit classical textbook descriptions of disease. Depression is often precipitated by major life changes (death of a close family member, divorce) that lead to somatic, cognitive, and affective symptoms and a tendency to amplify minor physical aches and pains. Patients may selectively focus on one component of the syndrome, and what it is will depend on their individual, family, and vocational circumstances as well as cultural factors affecting the interpretation, perception, and presentation of illness (Katon, Kleinman, & Rosen, 1982a).

The stigma of mental illness in Western society results in a common perception that patients with depression are morally culpable and weak as a result of their conditions. This stigma influences reporting of symptoms to both clinicians and epidemiologists. Thus, Cannel, Oksenburg, and Converse (1977), summarizing results of interviews with respondents with known medical and psychological conditions, found that 71% of asthma sufferers and 60% of those with heart disease reported their condition at interview, compared to 25% of respondents with mental illness and 22% with genito-urinary disease.

Primary care patients with depression are more likely to selectively focus on and amplify the somatic components of depression or present the emotional components as secondary to chronic medical illness. Patients who visit a psychiatrist are more likely to present and amplify the psychologic and cognitive features of depression. Thus two recent studies have demonstrated that 50 to 70% of patients with mental illness in general and depression specifically complained initially to their physician about somatic systems (Bridges & Goldberg, 1985; Schurman, Kramer, & Mitchell, 1985). About one-fourth to one-third of primary care patients with depression has one or more chronic medical illnesses, and these patients often present with amplification of complaints about their chronic medical illness and distract the physician from the emotional illness. Bridges and Goldberg (1985) have reported that 96% of patients who openly complain to primary care physicians about affective symptoms are accurately diagnosed, but among patients with depression who focus on somatic complaints and/or chronic medical illness, the diagnostic accuracy falls to 50%. Freeling, Rao, Paykel, Sireling, and Burton (1985) have also found that primary care patients with unrecognized depression had: (a) less overt depressive symptoms, mood, and appearance, (b) more chronic medical illnesses, (c) less insight, and (d) increased likelihood of having depression secondary to a physical illness.

A consequence of the lack of diagnostic accuracy is that patients utilize more visits to the primary care physician and have significantly more medical evaluations, many of which may be unnecessary. Our unit has studied this problem by prospective study of primary care patients with and without depression (Katon et al., 1986). Patients were screened using the Beck Depression Inventory (Beck & Beamesderfer, 1974) and the Zung Depression Self-Rating Scale (Zung, 1965), and a sample of depressives were interviewed with the SADS (Endicott & Spitzer, 1978). Physicians were not notified of the diagnosis of depression and the patients with depression were compared to nondepressed patients over one year of usual care. Over a one-year period, primary care outpatients with depression made significantly more visits and telephone calls to their primary care physician and had more medical evaluations (lab tests, x-rays, etc.) than primary care patients who were not depressed. The depressed patients were also significantly more likely to complain of nonspecific, psychophysiologic, and pain symptoms compared to controls.

There are two major factors in the tendency of patients with depression to focus on somatic symptoms. One of these factors is an "internal" factor based on the physiologic changes secondary to the illness; the other is an "external" or systems factor based on the tendency of the patient's environment to shape or modify the perception and presentation of illness. Two components of the "internal" factor are: the tendency of depression and anxiety to increase internal monitoring of symptoms, lowering the threshold of perception of physiologic symptoms; and the tendency of depression and anxiety to lead to increased autonomic arousal and abnormal sleep-wake cycles, resulting in a wide variety of physiologic symptoms (headache, fatigue, epigastric pain) (Lipscomb & Katon, 1987).

A recent study of high frequency consulters of medical care presents data and a conceptual model that helps explicate the "internal" physiologic mechanism by which depression leads to increased somatic complaints. Robinson and Granfield (1986) compared 40 frequent consulters (20 or more visits in one year) of primary care clinics to 40 less frequent attenders. They found that frequent consulters reported more symptoms, particularly more upper respiratory, gastrointestinal, and back troubles. They took more psychoactive medicines and more vitamin pills and were less inclined to ignore symptoms. They were more inclined to negative moods (depression, boredom, irritation/anger, and sleeplessness). Although they had slightly fewer stressful life events, they coped less well with them, perhaps because they had less satis factory family and social support.

Robinson and Granfield (1986), developed a model based on their research to explain the frequent consulter. The model is illustrated in Figure 5.2. A represents a state of total comfort that rarely occurs physiologically. Diary studies of patients have demonstrated that the average patient has a new symptom every 5 to 7 days, few of which are brought to the attention of a physician (Demers, Altamore, Mustin, Kleinman, & Leonardi, 1980). Tendencies toward discomfort that are subthreshold events stemming from internal organs, joints, muscles and so on are represented by bumps of various heights on the surface. The height represents the seriousness of the tendency in terms of its becoming consciously felt. During emotional upset, this surface will become more bumpy due to autonomic nervous system arousal leading to psychophysiologic symptoms, i.e., insomnia, headache, peptic ulcer, and fatigue.

Surface B represents a threshold on the vertical dimension above which a discomfort becomes consciously felt. This surface is driven up or down by mood state, anxiety, stress, direction of attention, and so on. Robinson and Granfield characterize the frequent consulter as having a low threshold surface, easily allowing symptom discomfort into the conscious life.

Depression and anxiety seem to be two of the major emotional states that cause an amplification of minor physiologic symptoms. Two recent studies have demonstrated that when patients with major depression are compared to nondepressed controls on a medical review of systems, depressives complain of significantly more symptoms (Mathews, Weinman, & Mirafi, 1981; Waxman, McCreary, Weinrit, & Carner, 1985). In the first study, 51 depressives were compared to 51 controls. The depressives averaged 12.3 ($\pm$ 5.4) symptoms versus 3.6 ($\pm$ 2.8) in controls (Mathews et al., 1981). In the second study, 127 community elderly volunteers were assessed with the Geriatric Depression Scale (Yesavage et al., 1983) and a portion of the Cornell Medical Index (Brodman, Erdmann, Lorge, & Wolff, 1951). Patients with low depression scores averaged 3.6 complaints, middle depression participants had a mean of 6.0 complaints,

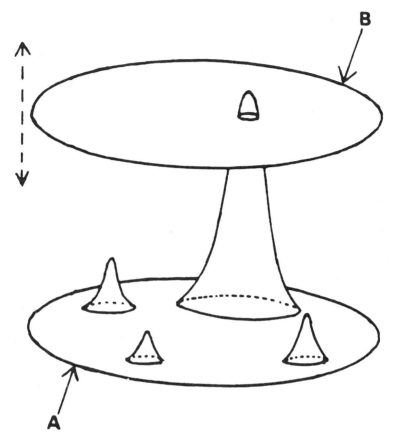

Figure 5.2. A Model of Symptoms.
Reprinted with permission from the *Journal of Psychosomatic Research*, 5,
(p. 598) Robinson and A. J. Granfield, "The Frequent Consulter in Primary
Medical Care," 1 Pergamon Press.

and high depression participants had a mean of 12.1 complaints (Waxman et al.,
1985). Depressives had more respiratory, cardiovascular, musculoskeletal, and
nervous system complaints. In this study, depressed participants were not much
more likely than nondepressed participants to report the presence of a chronic
medical illness.

Pain complaints seem especially common in patients with major depression.
Thus, patients with chronic pain complaints such as headache (Garvey, Schaffer,
& Tuason, 1983), abdominal pain (Young, Alpers, Norland, & Woodruff, 1976),
back pain (Katon, Egan, & Miller, 1985; Krishman et al., 1985), diabetic neuropathy (Turkington, 1980), chest pain (Clouse & Lustman, 1983; Katon et al.,
1988), and pelvic pain (Walker, Katon, Harrop-Griffith, Russo, & Hickok, 1987)

have all been reported to have high prevalence rates of depression. Patients selected for major depression have also been found to have high rates of pain complaints. Thus, Von Knorring, Perris, Eisemann, Eriksson, and Perris (1983) determined that 57% of psychiatric patients with major depression had one or more pain complaints for a minimal duration of three months.

It is unclear from these studies whether pain causes depression or depression causes pain. Probably both are true, and one author has advocated the pragmatic clinical use of the term *pain depression syndrome* to suggest that the two problems frequently present together, and have a similar treatment response to tricyclic antidepressants. They also note that which problem presented first is an academic question that is not as important to the clinician (Lindsay & Wyckoff, 1981).

In our unit, we have begun to study the psychiatric illnesses associated with a wide variety of chronic pain complaints as well as other nonspecific complaints believed to be associated with psychiatric illness. Table 5.1 demonstrates that each specialty in medicine has a large number of patients with a subgroup of symptoms in which specific organ pathology does not psychologically explain the extent of symptoms. We have used the National Institute of Mental Health (NIMH) Diagnostic Interview Schedule (Robins et al., 1981) interview to determine the lifetime psychiatric illnesses associated with each of these syndromes. Table 5.2 demonstrates a remarkable similarity in each of these studies: (a) a high prevalence rate of current and lifetime major depressive episodes and (b) a high median number of depressive episodes that demonstrates that a large number of these patients has a history of recurrent depression. In fact, in each of these studies, most patients with lifetime episodes of depression were found to have one or more of their episodes antedating the start of the chronic pain (Katon et al., 1985; Katon, Vitalliano, Russo, Jones, & Anderson 1987; Walker et al., 1987), tinnitus (Harrop-Griffiths, Katon, Dobie, Sakai, & Russo, 1987), or chronic fatigue syndrome (Katon, Gold, Riggs, Corey, & Russo, 1988). An attractive hypothesis from these data is that depression causes amplification of nociceptive physiologic input by increasing autonomic arousal, increasing the

Table 5.1. Medical Specialists and Their Problem Patients

Orthopedics	Low back pain
OB/Gyn	Chronic pelvic pain, PMS
ENT	Tinnitus
Neurology	Headache, dizziness
Cardiology	Atypical Chest pain
Pulmonary	Hyperventilation syndrome
Rheumatology	Fibromyalgia
Gastroenterology	Irritable bowel syndrome
Dentistry	Temporalmandibular joint pain
Medicine (Virology)	Chronic EBV infection

Table 5.2. Relationship of Affective Illness to Chronic Pain and Other Aversive Symptoms

	Current Major Depression	Lifetime Major Depression	Number of Episodes	Associated Psychiatric and/or Medical
Back Pain	33%	57%	3	Alcoholism
Chest Pain vs. Controls	35% vs. 3%	64% vs. 16%	5	Panic Disorder
Pelvic Pain vs. Controls	34% vs. 10%	66% vs. 16%	5	Substance Abuse Sexual Abuse
Tinnitus vs. Controls	60% vs. 7%	75% vs. 15%	3.5	Mild Sensorineural Hearing Loss
Chronic fatigue vs. Controls	41% vs. 0%	69.6% vs. 17%	2.5	

number and severity of symptoms, and as in the Robinson and Granfield (1986) model, lowering the threshold at which symptoms are perceived. This hypothesis is supported by an epidemiologic survey of chronic pain recently completed in Seattle by Dworkin, Von Korff, and LeResche (1987) as well as a study of patients with irritable bowel syndrome (IBS) by Drossman, McKee, and Sandler (1987). Using an algorithm applied to symptom checklist data, Dworkin and colleagues found that persons with a single pain condition had the same prevalence of major depression as persons with no pain complaints—about 2%. However, after adjustment for age and sex, persons with two pain symptoms had a prevalence rate of depression four times greater, and persons with three or more pain symptoms had a six-fold increased prevalence of depression compared to persons without multiple pain complaints.

Drossman and colleagues (1987), in a recent study of patients with irritable bowel syndrome, compared 73 IBS patients who sought medical care for their symptoms to 82 persons with IBS who did not. They found that the IBS patients visiting physicians had higher scores on psychological tests of depression and other neurotic subscales measuring anxiety and somatization. They concluded that psychosocial features such as depression and anxiety play a large role in symptom reporting and healthcare seeking behavior of IBS patients.

A second major factor in the selective focus on somatic complaints is the environment of the patient. Patient perception of depression occurs, not in a vacuum, but in the plural contexts of his or her social environment (Katon, Kleinman, & Rosen, 1982b). People are influenced by feedback from the settings in which they live, including their family, the work environment, the health care system, and other settings. Depression frequently results from long-standing difficulties in one's family and job coupled with acute life stress (Brown, Bifulco, & Harris, 1986). The somatic symptoms of depression may enable the patient to have leverage in social systems where they felt powerless to change long-term difficulties and unhappiness (Kleinman, 1986). Thus, for a housewife with little education and many children to care for, a somatic illness may induce increased support and caring from a husband who was formerly distant and unhelpful, or at least support and caring from her larger social system. A somatic illness may likewise provide an honorable way out for an aging logger with little education who can no longer keep up with his coworkers in their strenuous physical vocation. In each of these cases, the emotional and cognitive symptoms of depression would lead to little social advantage and in fact might lead to further critical behavior of spouse or colleagues.

As a result of their medical training, physicians in the medical system are also likely to preferentially focus on somatic aspects of illness. Many physicians tend to value physical illness and feel helpless about treating mental illness. Patients expect their physician to diagnose accurately or exclude relatively uncommon life-threatening physical diseases that may be producing nonspecific physical symptoms. The difficulty of correctly differentiating physical disease and mental disorder under these circumstances should not be underestimated.

One of the seminal reasons for recognizing depression in primary care is to provide accurate diagnosis and treatment of troublesome somatic symptoms that patients bring to their physicians. Our data suggest that not only is a current episode of major depression associated with chronic pain and other troublesome somatic symptoms, but also a lifetime history of recurrent episodes of depression is associated with these somatic symptoms. These patients do not meet "caseness" criteria for a current depression but often have subclinical symptoms. Wells, Stewart, and Burnam (1987) have also found that patients with depressive symptoms who do not meet criteria for major depression still have marked impairment in their social, vocational, and family lives equal to patients with major depression (Wells, Stewart, & Burnam, 1987). Moreover, both depressive symptoms and major depression had large and significant effects on perceived general and mental health status, social role, physical functioning, and pain. These effects were similar to or larger than the associations between these health variables and seven medical conditions—namely hypertension, diabetes, advanced coronary artery disease, back problems, chronic obstructive and restrictive lung disease, and chronic gastrointestinal disorders.

If both major depression and depressive symptoms are associated with patient amplification of symptoms, high utilization of medical clinics, and a perception of poor physical health status, then it is essential for treatment studies to begin to intervene with patients with varying levels of severity of depressive symptoms and to measure results of treatment on health perception and social and vocational parameters of disability.

Analogies to Medical Illness

How can we begin to establish a more secure empirical foundation for diagnosis and therapy of major depression and depressive symptoms in primary care? It may be helpful to examine how similar problems have been solved for physical disease. The first analogy is to peptic ulcer disease. As Table 5.3 shows, both depression and peptic ulcer disease are influenced by genetic factors that cause a vulnerability to illness, both diseases often run an episodic course and both can be precipitated by stressful life events (Akiskal & McKinney, 1975; Brown et al., 1986; Hendrix, 1972). Yet, when these illnesses develop, they tend to "have a life of their own" and may continue long past the resolution of the precipitating stressful life event. Both may decrease the patient's ability to cope with stress once they are present. For instance, patients with peptic ulcer disease often develop epigastric pain in situations that they would have coped with quite well in the past. Patients with depression often suffer from maladaptive cognitive interpretations of their ability to cope with environmental stress, thereby undermining confidence and increasing passivity (Beck, Rush, Shaw, & Emery, 1979). Both illnesses cause changes in the patients' biologic rhythms such as sleep and appetite. Each illness typically resolves well with biologic treatments, but has a high relapse rate once treatment is withdrawn (Akiskal & McKinney, 1975; Thomas & Misiewicz, 1984).

The issue of what is a case of depression or peptic ulcer disease raises vexing problems for the clinician and epidemiologist. Prior to fiberoptic endoscopic

Table 5.3. Comparison of Major Depression to Peptic Ulcer Disorder

Major Depression		Peptic Ulcer Disease	
1)	Genetic factors	1)	Genetic factors
2)	Course-episodic, relapsing remitting disorder	2)	Course-episodic, relapsing remitting disorder
3)	Often precipitated by stressful life events	3)	Often precipitated by stressful life events
4)	Severe disease marked by measurable biologic changes (abnormal dexamethasone suppression test, sleep EEG markers)	4)	Severe disease marked by mucosal lesion
5)	Pharmacologic treatment effective, but high relapse rate when medication withdrawn	5)	Pharmacological treatment effective, but high relapse rate when medication withdrawn
6)	Changes in biologic rhythms such as sleep and appetite	6)	Changes in biologic rhythms such as sleep or appetite
7)	May effect coping mechanisms adversely	7)	Adverse effect on coping mechanisms

techniques, peptic ulcer disease was defined by a clinical description of symptoms. For instance, patients with peptic ulcer disease had pain described as heartburn, a gnawing epigastric sensation, and found relief of discomfort through ingestion of food or alkali; they also remarked on the presence of pain at night and its absence in the early morning. Later, as endoscopy developed, patients in treatment studies were also required to have a mucosal lesion. However, several treatment studies found that pain relief did not correlate well with mucosal lesion healing (Peterson et al., 1977). In fact, in one widely cited study as many patients had persistent pain in the active medication group with a higher amount of complete mucosal healing as in the placebo group where mucosal lesion healing was significantly lower (Peterson et al., 1977). Thus, does research diagnostic criteria for peptic ulcer disease excluding patients without mucosal lesions leave out a significant group of patients with milder illness who still have significant suffering? For the clinician, the typical description of ulcer symptoms and concurrent suffering of the patient will lead to treatment. Thus studies of both short-term and long-term usage of the H_2-antagonists (the mainstay of treatment of peptic ulcer disease) have found that these medications are prescribed based on the results of clinical impression with half of the patients receiving either no evaluation or negative results of objective studies (Cocco & Cocco, 1981; Ulaszek, Seabloom, Samplinger, & Jones, 1984). This usage of H_2-antagonists should not be viewed necessarily as inappropriate because studies have shown that symptomatic patients who lack a demonstrable ulcer may have nonulcer dyspepsia and histologic evidence of gastroduodenitis and perhaps benefit from a short course of H_2-antagonist therapy (Greenlaw et al., 1980).

The epidemiologist or clinical researcher wishes to identify more clearly defined cases with both typical history and mucosal lesions, resulting in a more restricted and severe spectrum of disease and more measurable treatment results. Conversely, as a result of diagnosing cases earlier in the disease process, having a better placebo effect due to the stronger therapeutic alliance with a known patient rather than a research subject, and seeing cases with less severity, the primary care physician may experience more favorable outcomes with more conservative therapy.

Depression cases in primary care share many of the same characteristics as peptic ulcer disease and lead to the same dilemmas about caseness. To the researcher, it is important to select cases of depression with a high level of specificity so that studies of etiology, course, and treatment efficacy pertain to a relatively homogeneous set of patients. This requires establishing a significant level of severity so that there is a high level of agreement among researchers on "caseness." In the case of the researcher evaluating medications, a high level of severity is believed more likely to ensure success of active versus placebo treatments. As a result, caseness criteria have usually been tested initially on psychiatric populations with high levels of illness severity.

The primary care clinician, on the other hand, is faced with a large group of patients with psychological distress. Most of these patients present that distress in a somatic idiom and frequently have overlapping chronic medical illnesses (Bridges & Goldberg, 1985). Thus the clinician must establish whether the symptoms are caused by medical illness, medications the patient has been prescribed, concurrent medical and psychiatric illness, or psychiatric illness alone. Upon diagnosis of a primary care patient with depression, studies have then shown that the physician is usually faced with a less severely ill patient than seen in the psychiatric outpatient setting (Fahy, 1974; Johnson & Mellor, 1977; Sireling, Paykel, Freeling, Rao, & Patel, 1985). Sireling and colleagues (1985) found that, compared to a matched group of psychiatric outpatients, primary care depressives scored significantly lower on 18 out of 36 depressive symptoms on the Clinical Interview for Depression (Paykel, 1987), and only 36% of the patients that the primary care physicians treated with a tricyclic antidepressant and 14% of the primary care depressives who received other psychological or medication treatments scored 17 or greater on the Hamilton Depression Scale (Sireling, Freeling, Paykel, & Rao, 1985). Among psychiatric patients diagnosed as having major depression, 86% met this criteria (17 is a common inclusion criteria for outpatient drug trials).

Unlike the epidemiologist or clinical researcher, the clinician is apt to decide upon treatment based on the extent of patient suffering, how well the patient is coping with the illness, and how confident the clinician is in administering a variety of treatment modalities (antidepressants, anti-anxiety agents, and psychotherapy). In the Sireling study, the clinicians were significantly more likely to choose tricyclic antidepressants for more severely ill depressives and anti-anxiety and other psychotherapy treatments in depressives who had milder forms of depression that were often accompanied by anxiety disorders and other psychiatric diagnoses (Paykel, Hollyman, Freeling, & Sedgwick, 1988; Sireling et al., 1985; Sireling, Paykel et al., 1985). Several recent studies suggest that this differentiation of treatment by the primary care physician depending on severity of depression may be quite rational. Studies comparing Alprazolam to a tricyclic antidepressant have found comparable efficacy in outpatients with mild to moderate depression (Feighner, Aden, Fabre, Rickels, & Smith, 1983), whereas in severe depressives selected for the treatment study by a biologic abnormality (abnormal sleep EEG characteristic of depression), the tricyclic antidepressant was clearly superior to Alprazolam (Rush, Erman, & Schlesser, 1985). The recent NIMH collaborative treatment study of depression in ambulatory outpatients also found high rates of placebo response in mild to moderate depressives such that active treatments with tricyclic antidepressants and psychotherapy did not differ from the placebo-treated group (Klerman & Weissman, 1987; Pilkonis, 1987). On the other hand, patients with severe depression responded significantly better than the placebo-treated group when treated with antidepressant medication and interpersonal psychotherapy but not cognitive-behavioral therapy (Klerman & Weissman, 1987; Pilkonis, 1987).

The clinician well trained in primary care will, in theory, have a high level of sensitivity but a low level of specificity to a diagnosis of depression based on DSM-III (APA, 1980) or RDC (Spitzer et al., 1978) criteria. In fact, studies have demonstrated that for the average primary care clinician (with little psychiatric training), both sensitivity and specificity are poor. Thus Schulberg et al. (1985), in a study of 294 primary care patients who were screened for depression with the DIS, recently found that primary care clinicians correctly diagnosed only 7 of 27 cases of depression as identified by the DIS and DSM-III and also identified 5 additional cases of depression that were not diagnosed by the DIS and DSM-III.

In the Sireling, Paykel, et al. study (1985), the clinicians were found to diagnose and treat depression in many cases that would be borderline or probable on the DSM-III or RDC. Many of the cases met mood criteria but fell short on the number of vegetative and cognitive symptoms needed. These "borderline cases" may be analogous to the cases of peptic ulcer disease by history where no mucosal lesion is found. Although these borderline cases may be unimportant to the clinical researcher studying the effect of a new antidepressant, the clinician is still faced with a suffering patient who frequently is amplifying somatic complaints, and he or she feels obligated to make a specific diagnosis and treatment plan. These "borderline" cases have received renewed research attention from Brown and colleagues (1986), who demonstrated that these patients are three times as likely to develop a major depression given a severe life event as patients who do not meet criteria for borderline caseness. Also, Keller, Shapiro, Lavori, and Wolfe (1982) have demonstrated that a large group of patients who develop major depression has "double depression"; i.e., a major depressive disorder develops in a patient with chronic depressive symptoms. Patients with double depression have a significantly higher relapse rate. Thus these borderline states do not appear to be clinically insignificant. They not only cause suffering, but are predictors of subsequent caseness as well as relapse with treatment. Also, both Wells and colleagues (1987) and our data suggest that these borderline cases are associated with hypochondriacal complaints and a perception of poor health status. Our own unit's studies of panic disorder (which is frequently associated with major depression) in primary care have found similar results. A large subgroup of patients was found who did not meet severity criteria for panic disorder, but had infrequent panic attacks (Katon et al., 1986). Compared to normals, these patients had significantly more social phobias and resultant avoidance behavior, a higher lifetime risk of major depression, and higher scores on psychological indices of anxiety, depression, and somatization. They were as likely as patients with panic disorder to be hypochondriacal.

The key point is the lack of treatment studies aimed at patients who meet criteria for "borderline cases." There are only three published placebo controlled studies utilizing tricyclic antidepressants in primary care patients with depression (Blashki, Mowbray, & Davies, 1971; Rickels et al., 1973; Thompson et al.,

1982), and all three have demonstrated that the tricyclic antidepressants were significantly more effective than placebo. However, these studies have been either in the more severe spectrum of general practice depressives or in samples not well characterized, and no attempts were made to distinguish characteristics of those who show the drug-placebo differences. What are needed are treatment studies (of both pharmacologic and psychotherapeutic modalities) aimed at both definite cases by DSM-III or RDC as well as borderline cases. At this time we do not know empirically what represents a borderline case versus a definite case if evaluated by efficacy of treatment.

Preliminary results of a study by Paykel and colleagues (1988) are the first data to appear in this area. In this double blind controlled trial of amitriptyline versus placebo in a heterogenous sample of general practice depressives, particular emphasis was placed on classification of severity of the affective illness as well as on the effect of stress, demographic, and historical variables on outcome. One hundred and forty-one general practice depressives were treated for six weeks with amitriptyline versus placebo. Drug was superior to placebo in virtually all groups, the exception being depressives fitting only criteria for RDC minor depression rather than major depression and those with a lower initial severity, below 13 on the 17-item Hamilton Scale for depression.

Another useful analogy in the treatment of depression in primary care is the change in caseness criteria for hypertension that has developed over twenty years of careful empirical research on the natural history of hypertension and the effectiveness of treatment on differing levels of caseness. In the 1950s, initial screening for hypertension in the general population demonstrated a lack of accurate detection and poor treatment once it was detected. The problem was severalfold:

1. Physicians were poorly educated about detection of hypertension and its treatment.

2. Physicians were poorly motivated to undertake treatment since treatment trials had not been completed, especially in less severe forms of hypertension.

3. The public was not educated about the importance of early detection and diagnosis, and patients often resisted diagnosis.

The change began with the large collaborative Veterans Administration Hospitals (VAH) study that demonstrated that diagnosis of hypertension with diastolic blood pressure of more that 120 mm Hg decreased the occurrence of stroke and myocardial infarction (Veterans Administration Cooperative Study on Antihypertensive Agents, 1967). Subsequently, it was shown that treatment of diastolic hypertension between 90 and 120 mm Hg was associated with a significant decrease in morbidity and mortality. Hypertension caseness criteria were established by the demonstration of benefits of treatment at varying levels of severity through randomized controlled trials. At that point, treatment effectiveness was established and practical approaches to implementation in primary care developed. Education of physicians and patients became markedly more effective.

For major depression, DSM-III criteria have arbitrarily put case thresholds at two weeks of dysphoric mood and four or more vegetative and cognitive symptoms. At six months to one year follow-up, one-third to one-half of the patients with depression in primary care no longer meet these caseness criteria (Hankin & Locke, 1982; Mann, Jenkins, & Belsey, 1981). Only a small percentage of cases per year go to inpatient psychiatric care or to suicide, although utilization of medical care, divorce, work, disability, effects on young children, and secondary drug and alcohol abuse are high in many studies. Studies that establish the utility of diagnosing depression at each level of severity of depressive illness are needed. The assumption that treatment protocols evaluated in the psychiatric clinic represent the standards of care in the primary care clinic needs to be tested empirically. If the evaluations of diagnostic criteria and the effectiveness of treatment protocols remain within the confines of the psychiatric clinic, it is likely that the benefits of those treatments will too frequently be confined to psychiatric clinics as well.

Conclusion

Copeland (1981), in his provocative chapter "What is a Case? A Case for What?" states:

> Cases are not entities any more than are the illnesses from which they suffer, and they cannot be defined in vacuo. The division of subjects into cases and non-cases is a classification, and like all classifications it is man-made and not in nature. It is a concept and is useful only in so far as it serves that purpose. (p. 10)

The purposes of the primary care clinician and the psychiatric researcher in defining a case are not the same, and this has often led to criticism of the primary care physicians' diagnostic acumen. The primary care physician frequently has the challenge of sorting out a psychiatric illness from a myriad of somatic symptoms, chronic medical illnesses, and psychological symptoms. Unlike the fifty minutes that the psychiatrist often has for a patient interview, the primary care physician has ten-twelve-minute appointments. Add to this the current medical-legal atmosphere that raises physician anxiety about missing a medical illness, the lack of training about mental illness in primary care training programs, as well as the prevalence of somatization and stigmatization of mental illness in our society, and it is apparent that rates of misdiagnosis and lack of accurate diagnoses of mental illness will be quite high.

The purpose of diagnosing depression for the primary care physician is to redefine patient symptoms, which are often somatic, so that patients can see their symptoms as a part of a wider syndrome (Goldberg, 1982). The clinician diagnoses for the purpose of defining treatment and prognosis. Thus, the diagnosis of depression is followed by an explanation to patients of the cause of their symptoms, a treatment plan and prognosis. In primary care the treatment plan is often limited by factors like patient biases about specific treatments (many patients will accept medication, but not psychotherapy) and physician expertise (the physician may be uncomfortable with the use of tricyclic antidepressants or psychotherapy).

We clearly need to add to our knowledge base about the level of severity of depressive symptomatology that leads to high utilization of primary care, maladaptive illness behavior, as well as interference with the patient's social, vocational, and family functioning. Studies like the recent ones by Sireling and colleagues from Great Britain (Sireling et al., 1985; Sireling, Paykel et al., 1985) and the NIMH collaborative study (Klerman & Weissman, 1987; Pilkonis, 1987) have begun to add to our knowledge base about the treatment modalities that are most effective in varying levels of severity of depression. Measurements of treatment effectiveness must take into account social as well as psychological parameters. Brown and colleagues (1986) have amply demonstrated that depression is invariably precipitated by social changes and the expanding somatization literature has demonstrated significant effects on the depressed person's vocational, family, and social life as well as the perception of health status.

The development of these data in the primary care management of depression should then enable researchers and clinicians to develop sound recommendations to primary care clinicians about diagnosis and treatment of affective illness at varying levels of severity much like what has occurred in medical illnesses such as peptic ulcer disease and hypertension.

References

Akiskal, H., McKinney, W. T. (1975). Overview of recent research in depression. *Archives of General Psychiatry, 32,* 285–305.

American Psychiatric Association (1980). *Diagnostic and statistical manual of mental disorders* (3rd ed.). Washington, D.C.: Author.

Barnes, G. E., & Prosen, H. (1984). Depression in Canadian general practice attendees. *Canadian Journal of Psychiatry, 29,* 2–10.

Beck, A. T., & Beamesderfer, A. (1974). Assessment of depression: The depression inventory, modern problems in pharmacopsychiatry. *Modern Problems of Pharmacopsychiatry, 7,* 151–169.

Beck, A. T., Rush, J. A., Shaw, B. F., & Emery, G. (1979). *Cognitive therapy of depression.* New York: Guilford Press.

Blashki, T. G., Mowbray, R., & Davies, B. (1971). Controlled trial of amitriptyline in general practice. *British Medicine Journal, 1,* 133–138.

Bridges, K. W., & Goldberg, D. P. (1985). Somatic presentation of DSM-III psychiatric disorders in primary care. *Journal of Psychosomatic Research, 29,* 563–569.

Brodman, K., Erdmann, A. J. Lorge, I., & Wolff, H. G. (1951). The Cornell Medical Index-Health Questionnaire II as a diagnostic instrument. *Journal of the American Medical Association, 142,* 152–157.

Brown, G. W., Bifulco, A., & Harris, T. (1986). Life stress, chronic subclinical symptoms and vulnerability to clinical depression. *Journal of Affective Disorders, 11,* 1–19.

Cannel, C., Oksenburg, L., & Converse, J. (1977). *Experiments in interviewing techniques: Field experiments in health reporting, 1971–1977.* Hyattsville, MD: U.S. Dept. of Health, Education and Welfare. Public Health Service, Health Resources Administration, National Center for Health Services Research.

Clouse, R. E., & Lustman, P. J. (1983). Psychiatric illness and contraction abnormalities of the esophagus. *New England Journal of Medicine, 309,* 1339–1342.

Cocco, A. E., & Cocco, D. V. (1981). A survey of cimetadine prescribing. *New England Journal of Medicine, 304,* 1281–1285.

Copeland, J. (1981). What is a case? A case for what? In J. K. Wing, P. Bebbington, & L. N. Robins (eds.), *What is a Case: The problem of definition in psychiatric community surveys* (pp. 9–11). London: Grant McIntyre.

Demers, R. Y., Altamore, R., Mustin, H., Kleinman, A., & Leonardi, D. (1980). An exploration of the dimensions of illness behavior. *Journal of Family Practice, 11,* 1085–1091.

Drossman, D., McKee, D. C., & Sandler, R. S. (June, 1987). Psychosocial factors in irritable bowel syndrome. Paper presented at Mental Disorders in General Health Care Settings: A Research Conference, Seattle.

Dworkin, S. F., Von Korff, M., & LeResche, L. (1987). Pain co-morbidity, depression and somatization. Paper presented at Mental Disorders in General Health Care Settings: A Research Conference, Seattle.

Endicott, J., & Spitzer, R. L. (1978). A diagnostic interview: The schedule for affective disorders and schizophrenia. *Archives of General Psychiatry, 35,* 837–844.

Fahy, T. J. (1974). Depression in hospital and general practice: A direct clinical comparison. *British Journal of Psychiatry, 124,* 231–242.

Feighner, J. P., Aden, G. C., Fabre, L. F., Rickels, R., & Smith, W. T. (1983). Comparison of alprazolam, imipramine and placebo in the treatment of depression. *JAMA, 249,* 3057–3064.

Freeling, P., Rao, B. M., Paykel, E. S., Sireling, L. I., & Burton, R. H. (1985). Unrecognized depression in general practice. *British Medical Journal, 290,* 1880–1883.

Garvey, M. J., Schaffer, C. B., & Tuason, V. B., (1983). Relationship of headaches to depression. *British Journal of Psychiatry, 143,* 544–547.

Goldberg, D. (1982). The concept of a psychiatric "case" in general practice. *Social Psychiatry, 17,* 61–65.

Greenlaw, R., Sheahan, D. C., Deluca, V., Miller, D., Myerson, D., & Myerson, P. (1980). Gastroduodenitis—a broader concept of peptic ulcer disease. *Digestive Disease Science, 25,* 660–672.

Hankin, J. R., & Locke, B. Z. (1982). The persistence of depressive symptomatology among prepaid group practice enrollees: An exploratory study. *American Journal of Public Health, 72,* 1000–1009.

Harrop-Griffith, J., Katon, W., Dobie, R., Sakai, C., & Russo, J. (1987). Chronic tinnitus: Association with psychiatric diagnoses. *Journal of Psychosomatic Research, 31,* 613–622.

Hendrix, T. R. (1972). Peptic ulcer and dyspepsia. In A. M. Harvey, R. J. Jones, A. H. Owens, &

R. S. Ross, (eds.), *The principles and practice of medicine* (18th ed.) (pp. 711–720). New York: Appleton-Century-Crofts.

Hoeper, E. W., Nyczi, G. P., Cleary, P. D., Regier, D., & Goldberg, I. (1979). Estimated prevalence of RDC mental disorder in primary care. *International Journal of Mental Health, 8,* 6–15.

Johnson, D. A. W., & Mellor, V. (1977). The severity of depression in patients treated in general practice. *Journal of Royal Colleges of General Practice, 27,* 419–422.

Katon, W., Berg, A., Robins, A. J., & Risse, S. (1986). Depression: Medical utilization and somatization. *Western Journal of Medicine, 144,* 564–568.

Katon, W., Egan, K., & Miller, D. (1985). Chronic pain: Lifetime psychiatric diagnoses and family history. *American Journal of Psychiatry, 142,* 1156–1160

Katon, W., Gold, D., Riggs, R., Corey, L., & Russo, J. (1988). Chronic Fatigue Syndrome: A collaborative virologic, immunologic, and psychiatric study. Paper presented at the American Psychiatric Association Meeting, Montreal.

Katon, W., Hall, M. P., Russo, J., Cormier, L., Hollifield, M., Vitaliano, P. P., & Beitman, B. D. (1988). Chest pain: The relationship of psychiatric illness to coronary arteriography results. *American Journal of Medicine, 84,* 1–9.

Katon, W., Kleinman, A., & Rosen, G. (1982a). Depression and somatization: A review, part I. *American Journal of Medicine, 72,* 127–135.

Katon, W., Kleinman, A., & Rosen, G. (1982b). Depression and somatization: A review, part II. *American Journal of Medicine, 72,* 241–247.

Katon, W., Vitalliano, P. P., Russo, J., Jones, M. L., & Anderson, K. (1987). Panic disorder: Spectrum of severity and somatization. *Journal of Nervous and Mental Disease, 175,* 12–19.

Keller, M. B., Shapiro, R. W., Lavori, P. W., & Wolfe, N. (1982). Relapse in major depressive disorder: Analysis with the life table. *Archives of General Psychiatry, 39,* 911–915.

Kleinman, A. (1986). *Social origins of distress and disease: Depression, neurasthenia and pain in modern China.* New Haven: Yale University Press.

Klerman, G. L. & Weissman, M. M., (1987). Interpersonal psychotherapy (IPT) and drugs in the treatment of depression. *Pharmacopsychiatry, 20,* 3–7.

Krishman, K. R. R., France, R. D., Pelton, S., McCann, U. D., Davidson, J., & Urban, B. J. (1985). Chronic pain and depression. I. Classification of depression in chronic low back pain patients. *Pain, 22,* 279–287.

Lindsay, P. G., & Wyckoff, M. (1981). The depression-pain syndrome and its response to antidepressants. *Psychosomatics, 22,* 571–577.

Lipscomb, P., & Katon, W. (1987). Depression and somatization. In O. G. Cameron (ed.), *Presentations of depression: Depression in medical and other psychiatric disorders* (pp. 185–212). New York: John Wiley & Sons.

Mann, A. H., Jenkins, R., & Belsey, E. (1981). The twelve-month outcome of patients with neurotic illness in general practice. *Psychological Medicine, 11,* 535–550.

Mathews, R. J., Weinman, M. L., & Mirafi, M. (1981). Physical symptoms of depression. *British Journal of Psychiatry, 139,* 293–296.

Myers, J. K., Weissman, M. M., Tischler, G. E., Holzer, C. E., Leaf, P. J., Orvaschel, H., Anthony, J. C., Boyd, J. H., Burke, J. D., Kramer, M., & Stolzman, R. (1984). Six-month prevalence of psychiatric disorders in three communities. *Archives of General Psychiatry, 41,* 959–970.

Nielson, A. C., & Williams, T. A. (1980). Depression in ambulatory medical patients. *Archives of General Psychiatry, 37,* 999–1004.

Paykel, E. S., Hollyman, J. A., Freeling, P., Sedgwick, P. (1988). Predictors of therapeutic benefit from amitriptyline in mild depression: A general practice placebo-controlled trial. *Journal of Affective Disorders, 14,* 83–95.

Paykel, E. S. (1985). The clinical interview for depression: Development, reliability and validity. *Journal of Affective Disorders, 9,* 85–96.

Peterson, W. L., Sturdevant, R. A. L., Frankl, H. D., Richardson, C. T., Isenberg, J. I., Elashoff, J. D., Jones, J. Q., Gross, R. A., McCallum, R. W., & Fordtran, J. S. (1977). Healing of duodenal ulcer with antacid regimen. *New England Journal of Medicine, 297,* 341–345.

Pilkonis, P. A. (May, 1987). Acute treatment and changes in social functioning among depressives. Paper resented at the American Psychiatric Association Meeting, Chicago.

Rickels, K., Gordon, P. E., Jenkins, B. W., Perloff, M., Sachs, T., & Stepansky, W. (1970). Drug treatment in depressive illness (amitriptyline and chlordiazepoxide in two neurotic populations). *Diseases of the Nervous System, 31,* 30–42.

Robins, L. N., Helzer, J. E., Croughan, J., & Ratcliff, K. S. (1981). National Institute of Mental Health Diagnostic Interview Schedule: Its history, characteristics and validity. *Archives of General Psychiatry, 38,* 381–389.

Robinson, J. O., & Granfield, A. J. (1986). The frequent consulter in primary medical care. *Journal of Psychosomatic Research, 30,* 589–600.

Rush, A. J., Erman, M. K., & Schlesser, M. A. (1985). Alprazolam vs. amitriptyline in depressions with reduced REM latencies. *Archives of General Psychiatry, 42,* 1154–1159.

Salkind, M. R. (1969). Beck Depression Inventory in general practice. *Journal of Colleges of General Practice, 18,* 267–273.

Schulberg, H. C., Saul, M., McClelland, M., Gangali, M., Christy, W., & Frank, R. (1985). Assessing depression in primary medical and psychiatric practices. *Archives of General Psychiatry, 12,* 1164–1170.

Schurman, R. A., Kramer, P. D., & Mitchell, J. B. (1985). The hidden mental health network: Treatment of mental illness by nonpsychiatrist physicians. *Archives of General Psychiatry, 42,* 89–94.

Seller, R. H., Blaskovich, J., & Lenke, E. (1981). Influences of stereotypes in the diagnosis of depression by family practice residents. *Journal of Family Practice, 12,* 849–854.

Sireling, L. I., Freeling, P., Paykel, E. S., & Rao, B. M. (1985). Depression in general practice: Clinical features and comparison with out-patients. *British Journal of Psychiatry, 147,* 119–126.

Sireling, L. I., Paykel, E. S., Freeling, P., Rao, B. M., & Patel, S. P. (1985). Depression in general practice: Case thresholds and diagnosis. *British Journal of Psychiatry, 147,* 113–119.

Spitzer, R. L., Endicott, J., & Robins, E. (1978). Research diagnostic criteria: Rationale and reliability. *Archives of General Psychiatry, 35,* 773–782.

Tansella, M., Williams, P., Balestrieri, M., Bellantuaro, C., & Martini, V. (1986). The management of affective disorders in the community. *Journal of Affective Disorder, 11,* 73–79.

Thomas, J. M., & Misiewicz, G. (1984). Histamine H_2-receptor antagonism in the short- and long-term treatment of duodenal ulcer. *Clinical Gastroenterology, 13,* 501–541.

Thompson, J., Rankin, H., Ascroff, G. W., Yates, C. M., McQueen, J. K., & Cummins, S. W. (1982). The treatment of depression in general practice: A comparison of L-tryptophan, amitriptyline and a combination of L-tryptophan and amitriptyline with placebo. *Psychological Medicine, 12,* 741–751.

Turkington, R. W. (1980). Depression masquerading as diabetic neuropathy. *Journal of the American Medical Association, 243*, 1147–1150.

Ulaszek, K. M., Seabloom, K. D., Samplinger, R. D., & Jones, W. N. (1984). Appropriateness of long-term cimetadine prescribing. *Drug Intelligence and Clinical Pharmacology, 18*, 623–625.

Veterans Administration Cooperative Study Group on Antihypertensive Agents (1967). Effects of treatment on morbidity in hypertension. *JAMA, 202*, 116–130.

Von Knorring, L., Perris, C., Eisemann, M., Eriksson, U., & Perris, H. (1983). Pain as a symptom in depressive disorders I. Relationship to diagnostic subgroup and depressive symptomatology. *Pain, 15*, 19–26.

Walker, E. W., Katon, W., Harrop-Griffiths, J., Russo,J., & Hickok, L. (1988). Chronic pelvic pain: The relationship to psychiatric diagnoses and childhood sexual abuse. *American Journal of Psychiatry, 145*, 75–80.

Waxman, H. M., McCreary, G., Weinrit, R. M., & Carner, E. A. (1985). A comparison of somatic complaints among depressed and nondepressed older persons. *The Gerontologist, 25*, 501–507.

Weissman, M. M., Myers, J. K., & Thompson, W. D. (1981). Depression and its treatment in a U.S. urban community 1975–1976. *Archives of General Psychiatry, 38*, 417–421.

Wells, K. B., Stewart, A., & Burnam, M. A. (1987). Profiles of health and functioning for depressed and nondepressed adult outpatients of mental health and medical clinicians. Paper presented at the American Psychiatric Association Meeting, Chicago.

Yesavage, J. A., Rose, T. L., Lum, O., Huang, V., Adey, M., & Leirer, V. O. (1983). Development and validation of a geriatric depression screening scale: A preliminary report. *Journal of Psychosomatic Research, 17*, 37–49.

Young, S. J., Alpers, D. H., Norland, C. C., & Woodruff, R. A. (1976). Psychiatric illness and the irritable bowel syndrome: Practical implications for the primary physician. *Gastroenterology, 70*, 162–166.

Zung, W. W. K. (1965). A self-rating depression scale. *Archives of General Psychiatry, 12*, 263–275.

Zung, W. W. K., Magill, M., Moore, J. T., & George, D. (1983). Recognition and treatment of depression in a family medicine practice. *Journal of Clinical Psychiatry, 44*, 3–9.

Part II

Depression Screening Procedures: Methodological Considerations and Empirical Findings

In the ideal case, depression screening is most efficiently accomplished by a standardized cost-efficient screening inventory easily understood by medical patients and readily completed by them. The efficient screening procedure would correctly identify virtually all patients with depression (i.e., have high "sensitivity" for depression) and hardly ever misidentify a nondepressed patient as depressed (i.e., have high "specificity" for depression).

There are a number of brief, standardized depression screening inventories available for clinical evaluation and research. Jane M. Murphy reviews a number of these inventories, assesses the reliability and validity of available instruments, and discusses the implications of their various formats and item content for detecting clinical depression in medical patients. In addition to a review of the structure and clinical performance of these scales, Murphy offers an alternative to predetermined cutoff scores in assessing the utility of a given inventory. Murphy argues for Receiver Operating Characteristics (ROC) curve analysis and illustrates the advantages of this method over the use of standard cutoff scores.

Given the availability of reliable and valid screening measures for detecting depression, when is it cost-effective to employ such measures? Taking the perspective of a statistician, Patrick E. Shrout illustrates situations in which the use of a relatively effective screening instrument has little, if any, advantage over doing a full-scale evaluation of each patient's depression. By contrast, Shrout presents situations that do argue for preliminary screening before undertaking a more thorough and costly evaluation. Recognizing that it is unlikely that any diagnostic system, screening inventory, or methodology for detecting depression in medical patients will be optimal for all studies, Shrout emphasizes the need to fit our depression measures and methodologies to our research and clinical goals.

Among the strategies Shrout illustrates is a two-stage method for detecting depression. This method begins with an initial screening of all patients, or potential study participants, for depression. Those who screen positive for depression are then assessed thoroughly to see if they meet diagnostic criteria. In their paper, M. Audrey Burnam and Kenneth B. Wells describe such a two-stage case-defining methodology they applied in the National Medical Outcomes Study.

Faced with the task of identifying the depressed patients among 25,000 study participants, the investigators opted for a two-stage procedure designed to maximize depression detection accuracy while minimizing expense, an equation of concern to researchers and clinicians alike. In the course of describing the development of their methodology, Burnam and Wells highlight some of the critical issues in depression screening.

Three empirical chapters follow. In the first of these, Joel Yager and Lawrence S. Linn present the results from a series of investigations designed to assess the impact of providing depression screening feedback to primary care physicians on subsequent patient care utilization, chart notations, and physician behavior. In the chapter by Richard L. Hough, John A. Landsverk, and Gerald F. Jacobson, three psychiatric screening instruments are compared for their effectiveness in detecting depressed patients, with special attention to the demographic variables influencing their effectiveness. William W. K. Zung, Kathryn Magruder-Habib, and John R. Feussner present results from an intervention study with a sample of medical patients at a Veterans Administration Hospital. The investigators report a relationship between depression and anxiety in medical patients and a relationship between depression and physical health status. These findings are discussed in relationship to treatment priorities and diagnostic complications introduced by comorbidity.

In the final paper of this section, Paul D. Cleary highlights some of the methodological issues raised in research on depression in medical patients. He cautions that the trend in the field to find an optimal screening instrument is too restrictive. Cleary argues that more attention should be paid to the broader issues of determining an appropriate "gold standard" for depression in primary care. Cleary also advocates more focus on empirical demonstrations of the efficacy of treatments for depressed medical patients; and points out the need to address administrative, educational, and fiscal constraints limiting the likelihood that depressed medical patients will be detected and offered appropriate care.

6

Depression Screening Instruments: History and Issues

Jane M. Murphy

The purpose of this chapter is to review some aspects of the history of psychiatric screening instruments as background for discussing current issues relevant to the use of a depression screener in primary care.[1] The points to be made derive from three endeavors: one is a review of seven screening instruments carried out for the Primary Care Research Branch of the National Institute of Mental Health (Murphy, 1981); another is experience in using one of these instruments in an epidemiologic study of a general population, the Stirling County Study (Murphy, 1980); and the third is a project concerned with the application of decision analytic methods to improve the performance of depression screeners (Murphy et al., 1987).

The seven screening instruments on which I will focus do not comprehend the universe of such instruments but they illustrate salient features of history. They offer a general overview of effort to separate populations into those who are probably ill and those who are probably well by asking persons to respond to questions about moods, feelings, and symptoms.

In the order of the years in which they were first described in the literature, the seven instruments include:

CMI   Cornell Medical Index (Brodman, Erdmann, & Wolff, 1949)

HSCL   Hopkins Symptom Checklist (Parloff, Kelman, & Frank, 1954),

HOS   Health Opinion Survey (Macmillan, 1957),

[1] The work on which this paper is based has been supported by the National Institute of Mental Health Contract Number 80M014280101D and grants MH 39576 and MH 40076 as well as National Health Research and Development project 6603-1154-44, Department of Health and Welfare of Canada, and the Sandoz Foundation.

Figures 6.2 to 6.5 appeared originally in Murphy, J. M., Berwick, D. M., Weinstein, M. C., Borus, J. F., Budman, S. H., & Klerman, G. L. (1987). Performance of screening and diagnostic tests: Application of receiver operating characteristics (ROC) analysis. *Archives of General Psychiatry, 44,* 550–555. Permission to reproduce them here has been granted by the American Medical Association, copyright 1987.

BDI   Beck Depression Inventory (Beck, Ward, Mendelson, Mock, & Erbaugh, 1961),

22IS   Twenty-Two Item Scale (Langner, 1962),

GHQ   General Health Questionnaire (Goldberg, 1972), and

CES-D Center for Epidemiologic Studies—Depression Scale (Radloff, 1977).

These seven borrowed liberally from each other in terms of the selection and design of items, and many have been compared to each other. In addition, they drew items from a number of other instruments, among them the Minnesota Multiphasic Personality Inventory (Dahlstrom, Welsh, & Dahlstrom, 1972), the Maudsley Personality Inventory (Eysenck, 1947), and the U.S. Army's Neuropsychiatric Screening Adjunct (Star, 1950). Each of the seven has undergone investigation of validity. In the early years this often meant that screened subjects were later assessed by clinical psychiatrists. In recent years it has become customary to use structured interviews for this purpose. The main validators have been the Standardized Psychiatric Interview (SPI), which was designed by members of the General Practice Research Unit of the Maudsley Hospital (Goldberg, Cooper, Eastwood, Kedward, & Shepard, 1970), the Present State Examination (PSE) (Wing, Cooper, & Sartorius, 1974), the series of schedules leading to the Schedule for Affective Disorders and Schizophrenia (SADS) (Endicott & Spitzer, 1978; Spitzer, Endicott, Fleiss, & Cohen, 1970; Spitzer, Fleiss, Endicott, & Cohen, 1967), and the National Institute of Mental Health's (NIMH) Diagnostic Interview Schedule (Robins, Helzer, Croughan, & Ratcliff, 1981).

Of the seven screeners, only the CMI and the GHQ were designed specifically for primary care, but almost all of them have now been used in such studies as well as in general population epidemiology. All have also been administered to psychiatric patients, at least for validation purposes and sometimes to follow the course of illness while the patient was being treated.

This extended and somewhat inbred family of instruments has more than a forty-year history that dates back to World War II. The CMI, for example, was a direct outgrowth of an instrument called the Cornell Selectee Index (Weider, Mittelmann, Wechsler, & Wolff, 1944). From the psychometric point of view, these screeners had initial and sustained achievement in regard to internal consistency. There has, however, been an increase of factor analytic studies. As far as I was able to determine, the CMI is the only one of these instruments that has not been factor analyzed. Some of the others, especially the HSCL and GHQ, have undergone such analyses many times (Derogatis, Lipman, Covi, & Rickels, 1972; Derogatis, Lipman, Rickels, Uhlenhuth, & Covi, 1974; Goldberg, 1972; Goldberg & Hillier, 1979; Lipman, Rickels, Covi, Derogatis, & Uhlenhuth, 1969; Mattsson, Williams, Rickels, Lipman, & Uhlenhuth, 1969; Williams et al., 1968; Worsley, Walters, & Wood, 1978). This work has clarified the dimensional content of the instruments.

There has also been an increasing amount of attention paid over the years to response styles and their control. Many of the modern instruments are well balanced in terms of both negative and positive responses being pathological indicators (Goldberg, 1972; Radloff, 1977). Virtually every recent instrument uses at least four response categories as an aid to reducing the pitfalls of yea-and-nay-saying and middle category preference.

Another historical change is a shift away from asking respondents for lifetime generalizations about symptomatology, as in the CMI, HOS, and 22IS, and toward asking about the current clinical state as in the HSCL, BDI, GHQ, and CES-D. This is best illustrated by comparing the CMI and the GHQ. The CMI wants symptoms to be "usual" ones; the GHQ wants them to be those recent "unusual" ones that represent a break from the individual's normal state. Measuring the current clinical status was obviously necessary for instruments such as the HSCL and BDI, which were initially designed to *monitor* the course of illness during treatment (Kelman & Parloff, 1957; Little & McPhail, 1973). But the emphasis on the present state spread to other instruments as well, and all the recent screeners have a short time frame and instruct the respondent to focus on "today," the "recent week," or the "recent few weeks."

The almost universal focus on the current clinical state has, however, had repercussions on test-retest reliability (Duncan-Jones & Henderson, 1978). Unless care is taken to assure that respondents can be considered to be in the same clinical state at both administrations, test-retest shows more fluctuation than was true of the older lifetime-oriented instruments. It bears reflection that these older instruments grew from effort to *predict* which soldiers would in the future become psychiatrically disabled, not which among them was ill at the time of being screened (Star, 1950). The test-retest stability of these older instruments suggests that they may have been especially good at detecting those chronic tendencies and long-standing traits that often lead to the development of full blown episodes.

Chronicity and episodicity are important issues for the screening of depression in primary care. When episodicity is put in the forefront, depression tends to be viewed as a time-limited, albeit recurrent, illness that is often a reaction to life circumstances. There is increasing evidence, however, that persons may suffer depression over fairly long durations. The CES-D, for example, is a typical modern instrument in having a short time frame, and its test-retest correlations tend to fluctuate (Radloff, 1977). At the same time, if we study the number of persons who continue to report above a cutting-point over the administrations— both in the general population and in primary care—we learn that a sizeable proportion can be thought of as chronic (Hankin & Locke, 1979; Hornstra & Klassen, 1977;). The work leading to the concept of *double depression* among psychiatric patients emphasizes both chronicity and episodicity (Keller & Shapiro, 1982). It suggests that a major depression often resolves into dysthymia, and that dysthymic, patients then continue to be at risk for another major episode.

It seems self-evident that a depression screener in primary care must measure the current clinical state. But questions remain as to whether and how best it can also measure chronic conditions. One aspect of this is that "current" symptoms are not necessarily "*un*usual" symptoms. While not minimizing the many psychometric advances represented in the GHQ, a backward look on history suggests that the GHQ swung too far away from the CMI in its requirement that the current state consist in symptoms that have recently caused a departure from the usual state. The GHQ is the only modern screener that has this feature, and it is a feature that seems to have engendered a proclivity for GHQ symptoms to rise and fall quickly.

If we accept that "current" is simply "current," a methodologic issue is whether innovative ways can be designed to gather information about the duration of symptomatology within the framework of a screener. For example, the Diagnostic Interview Schedule accomplishes the blending of past and present by asking subjects if they *ever* had a given collection of symptoms and then by bringing the discourse up to the present state (Robins et al., 1981). Where a short screener is concerned, it might be useful to experiment with the opposite approach—that is, to ask about the present symptoms and then to trace back to their onset.

Turning to another topic, it will not have gone unnoticed that the titles "Cornell Medical Index" and "General Health Questionnaire" do not reveal that these instruments are concerned with psychiatric illness. The CMI and the GHQ are not alone in this feature since "symptom checklist" and "health opinion" are key phrases in other titles. There has been a historical trend toward greater willingness to identify the content of the questions in the screener's title, with the BDI and CES-D, for examples, specifically using the word "depression." The movement away from euphemism probably relates in part to the more open attitudes about mental illness in society at large. There is also, however, a scientific yield in that, when the title is explicit, research peers and potential users know what an instrument is intended to screen.

Despite the fact that the names of the instruments do not convey their similarities in content, this family of instruments has a high level of shared characteristics. At a minimum, the seven instruments ask questions about depressive mood and some of the "vital," "vegetative," or physiologic concomitants of depression. With the exception of those named as depression scales, all of them also ask questions about generalized anxiety. None has questions about hallucinations, delusions, cognitive deficit, or alcohol and drug use. Except in the longest versions of the HSCL, even the more rare anxiety disorders, such as phobias and obsessive-compulsive disorders, are also weakly represented (Derogatis & Cleary, 1977). Thus the content that most clearly holds this family together is depression, or depression and generalized anxiety.

Against this background of similar content, an intriguing feature of history is how very different were the concepts of mental illness that the originators of these instruments thought they were measuring. In Figure 6.1, the concepts are

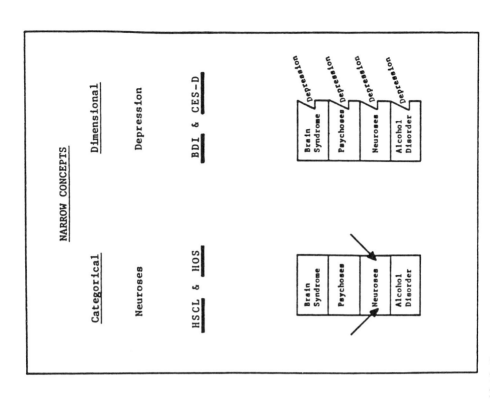

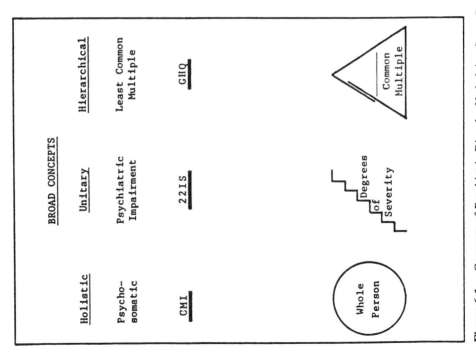

Figure 6.1. Concepts of Psychiatric Disorder Underlying Seven Psychiatric Screeners.

69

divided as to whether they appear to be broad or narrow. The broad concepts can be called "holistic," "unitary," and "hierarchical."

The originators of the CMI were particularly interested in psychosomatic medicine, and thus the CMI was affiliated with a focus on the whole person in terms of the way in which emotional states influence physical disabilities and viceversa (Brodman, Erdmann, Lorge, Deutschberger, & Wolff, 1954). The 22IS was affiliated with the Midtown Manhattan Study, which in various ways subscribed to the unitary concept of mental illness put forth by Menninger and others (Menninger, 1959; Srole, Langner, Michael, Opler, & Rennie, 1962). This concept suggests that mental illnesses vary more in degree than in kind, and thus the 22IS was thought of as measuring degrees of severity or levels of impairment. The concept of psychiatric disorders with which the GHQ came to be identified is a hierarchical one. The depression and anxiety indicators on which the GHQ concentrates often coexist with disorders higher in the hierarchy. At the same time, they constitute the broad base of the hierarchy where there is sometimes a fine line between normal and pathologic responses (Goldberg, 1979).

Another broad concept with which nearly all of these instruments have now been affiliated is *demoralization* (Dohrenwend & Dohrenwend, 1982; Dohrenwend, Shrout, Egri, & Mendelsohn, 1980; Frank, 1974; Link & Dohrenwend, 1980). Demoralization is thought of as a state of mind that sometimes mixes with true psychopathology and other times is a normal response to stressful life events. While the association between these instruments and demoralization has attracted attention, it is also a controversial issue. An argument has been made that screening results do not fit well the paradigmatic attributes of the concept (Murphy, 1986).

The narrower concepts in Figure 6.1 can be described as categorical and dimensional. The HSCL and HOS were presented as dealing mainly with the category known in pre—DSM-III days as neurotic disorders (American Psychiatric Association, 1980). On the other hand the BDI and CES-D can be affiliated with the dimensional approach. They are concerned, implicitly or explicitly, with depressive symptomatology, which, as a dimension of psychopathology, might figure in multiple types of disorder.

The fact that these seven instruments were presented as measuring different conceptualizations of mental illnesses probably obfuscated their many similarities and may have retarded the growth of the field. Yet some of the problems that these different concepts emphasize remain unresolved. For example, specifying the kind or type of disorder to be screened appears to be a better approach than adhering to the unitary concept of psychiatric illness. Nevertheless, differentiating degrees of severity so that a depression screener tells its users whether the case is mild, moderate, or severe is a goal that has not yet been completely accomplished. Given its orientation to severity, the 22IS was one of the few instruments that was published with two recommended cutpoints for demarcations along these lines. It seems probable that multiple thresholds continue to need consideration as avenues for measuring severity.

The fundamental problem that the other concepts of mental illness reveal is the issue of comorbidity. The possibility of comorbidity involving physical disorders and psychiatric disorders was responsible for the holistic orientation of the CMI. Comorbidity is also involved in the hierarchical orientation in that a hierarchy cannot be implemented without excluding one type of morbidity in favor of another. Even the dimensional orientation involves comorbidity since it recognizes that depression, for example, can be a feature of many types of psychopathology.

A continuing problem about screening for depression is the likelihood that depression will have a comorbid relationship with something else. The fact that a considerable amount of comorbidity exists is probably the reason these screeners have done as well as they have in identifying diagnostically mixed groups of psychiatric patients in validation studies. While none of the instruments has been found to identify all types of psychiatric disorders equally well, many studies have shown that they sometimes identify patients diagnosed as schizophrenic, for example (Goldberg, 1972; Schwartz, Myers, & Astrachan, 1973). This is probably due to the fact that depression and anxiety symptoms are sometimes comorbid features of such other types of psychiatric disorders. Without using the lengthy diagnostic schedules that make it possible to *exclude* organic brain disorders and schizophrenia, for example, it is very likely that any screener for depression will sometimes pick up cases from these higher order categories. Thus a serious issue is whether a screener that focuses with *clarity on depression* can be considered acceptable even though it does not necessarily identify *only depression*.

An even more troublesome aspect of comorbidity concerns the frequent alliance of depression and its lower order category of anxiety. This type of comorbidity is especially characteristic of the neurotic category. It bears note that when this history began, the prominence of anxiety in psychoanalytic formulations of psychiatric disorders meant that depression, at least neurotic depression, was thought of as an epiphenomenon to anxiety. Depression was, in other words, considered to be a reaction to the more basic and underlying anxiety (Derogatis, Klerman, & Lipman, 1972).

The HSCL and HOS illustrate the emphasis on anxiety at that period of history. Both instruments were concerned with identifying neurotic disorders and both were designed in the 1950s when DSM-I indicated that anxiety was the hallmark of all types of neuroses (American Psychiatric Association, 1952). Most of the persons identified in the early HSCL work were called anxious neurotics, and most of the patients used in the HOS calibration study were diagnosed as having chronic generalized anxiety states (Macmillan, 1954; Williams et al., 1968). Both of these instruments were changed in various ways to cover depression, but their changes were simply a microcosmic reflection of the historical change that brought us to a period in which depression is given much more attention than anxiety. The reasons for this change are multifaceted and beyond the scope of this chapter. The likelihood of comorbidity between depression and anxiety, however, is another continuing issue for depression screeners in primary care.

Depression and anxiety are so often adhesive to each other that the closeness of these two syndromes cannot be ignored. Despite numerous attempts to bring about separation of the two types of symptomatology, screeners for depression have almost always been found to correlate to some degree with screeners for anxiety, and screeners that involve both depression and anxiety regularly achieve high marks for internal consistency even when they have been shown to display a factorial structure that clearly differentiates depression and anxiety (Dinning & Evans, 1977; Radloff, 1977; Weissman, Sholomskas, Pottenger, Prusoff, & Locke, 1977). In view of this degree of affiliation, it might be advisable in primary care research to measure both depression and anxiety on the assumption that they are distinct even if often found together.

Given that numerous depression screeners already exist, an important question concerns whether the best possible screener is now available and, if so, how to be sure it is the best. Traditionally, in this field concurrent criterion validity has been taken as the most valuable means of indicating whether a screener is good or bad. Major progress has been made by the development of criterion validators that are structured and explicit such as the Standard Psychiatric Interview (SPI), PSE, SADS, and DIS. That there are multiple validators to choose from is, however, almost as much a problem as the multiplicity of screeners. The GHQ, for example, has been compared to all these validators (Finlay-Jones & Murphy, 1979; Goldberg & Blackwell, 1970; Hoeper, Nycz, Cleary, Regier, & Goldberg, 1979; Kessler et al., 1987). Its best validity results, both sensitivity and specificity being above 90%, for example, have usually been the same as those of the SPI. This is not a surprising result when one considers that both the screener and the validator were outgrowths of work at the Maudsley General Practice Research Unit. It seems reasonable to suggest, therefore, that the results were good partly because the SPI validator embodies the concept of psychiatric disorder that the GHQ screener was intended to measure.

Validators that use a somewhat different definition of disorder from that of the screener obviously put that screener at risk for poor performance. Validators that involve lifetime diagnoses put short time frame screeners at risk. Validators that are administered after a lapse of time that outreaches the short time-frame of a screener also increase the likelihood that the screener will perform poorly, as do the validity designs that test the ability of the screener to identify all types of psychiatric disorders, in contrast to those in which depression and anxiety are dominant features.

The designs of validation studies used for these instruments have shown considerable variation in these regards. Nevertheless, it is interesting that the larger the number of validation studies carried out for a given screener, the greater the *range* of performance shown. That all of these instruments have demonstrated both good and bad results suggests that improved standards for the quality and design of validation studies are needed. If we are to know which depression screener is the best, good validity results need to be demonstrated over several replications of a high-quality validation design.

Criterion validity stands on the shoulders not only of reliability but also of other antecedent forms of validity such as content validity. The availability of operational criteria for depression in DSM-III means that the questions asked in a given screener can be compared to the symptomatic profile of the depression syndrome in the diagnostic manual to determine if the content coverage is adequate or not (American Psychiatric Association, 1980). Several of the existing screeners pass this test quite well. It seems fair to suggest that at the present time we seem to know which symptoms need to be queried, and we have learned much about the importance of incorporating these symptoms in questions that are formulated in understandable and unambiguous language.

Methods of scoring could well be further explored. If there is one generalization about the history of screening that holds up to rigorous scrutiny, it is, I suggest, that some form of the "count and cut" method has been used. Sometimes this is solely a matter of counting the number of pathological responses and applying a cutpoint, as in the CMI and GHQ. More often it is a matter of weighing the number of pathological responses in terms of the respondents judgment about the frequency, bothersomeness, or intensity of each symptom as in the HSCL and CES-D. One way or the other, a given cutpoint on a given score range is the attribute of a screener that is foremost when a concurrent criterion validation study begins. Based on this cutpoint, it is now routine procedure to calculate sensitivity, specificity, kappa, and increasingly predictive values as well. Changing the cutpoint upward or downward has been the most traditional approach to improving the performance of a screener vis-a-vis a validator. However, once a given cutpoint has been determined as the best, it is often thought of as a fixed attribute of the screener. Sometimes this is disadvantageous to the screener.

Recently, a more comprehensive means for assessing screener performance has begun to be incorporated among evaluation techniques. Especially useful is receiver operating characteristic (ROC) curve analysis, an approach that has entered medical decision analysis after having been used in engineering (Metz, 1978; Swets & Pickett, 1982; Weinstein et al., 1980). ROC curves provide information about all possible sensitivity and specificity values. The full range of scores can be taken into account as a basis for comparing different screeners or different scoring systems for a single screener.

Figure 6.2 shows ROC curves for hypothetical tests A and B. The pairs of possible sensitivity and specificity values are joined into one curve by plotting the true-positive rates (sensitivity) on the vertical axis and the false-positive rates (one minus specificity) on the horizontal axis. If a screener has no discriminating power for the presence and absence of a disorder as defined by a validator, the

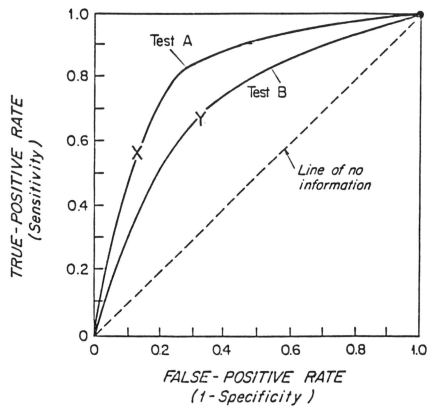

Figure 6.2. Receiver Operating Characteristic (ROC) Curves for Two Hypothesized Tests (A and B).

curve tracks along the diagonal. The diagonal is known as the *line of no informa-tion*. The more clearly the test is able to make the discrimination between cases and noncases the farther will its ROC curve deviate toward the left upper corner of the graph.

Statistical methods have been developed for fitting ROC curves to categorical data and for measuring the *area under the curve* (Hanley & McNeil, 1982, 1983). The *area under the curve* (AUC) may be interpreted as an estimate of the probability that a randomly chosen subject with the disorder will have a higher score at each cutpoint than a randomly chosen subject who does not have the disorder. If a screener lacks information content and its ROC curve lies on the line of no information, the AUC probability is 0.50. A perfect screener with an AUC value of 1.00 has an ROC curve that follows the left and upper boundary of the square that demarcates the graph.

In Figure 6.2, X shows the recommended cutpoint for Test A, which gives a sensitivity of 58% and specificity of 88%. The cutpoint for Test B, shown as Y, gives a higher sensitivity (68%) but lower specificity (76%). Yet, throughout the range of scores, Test A has a more favorable performance than B. Further, a cutpoint for A could be shown—one closer to the corner—that would increase sensitivity to about 75% without serious loss of specificity.

The utility of ROC analysis for assessing psychiatric instruments has recently been demonstrated by evaluating different scoring systems for the HOS (Murphy et al., 1987). We used data from the Stirling County Study in which responses to the HOS had been read along with other materials by psychiatrists to make decisions regarding which subjects in this general population study appeared to suffer from depression and anxiety disorders and which did not (Leighton, Harding, Macklin, Macmillan, & Leighton, 1963). Since the psychiatrists based these judgments partly on the HOS responses, the demonstration does not provide validity evidence in the strict sense of being derived from a completely independent source. Nevertheless, the standard serves to show how psychiatrists evaluate responses about symptoms.

One purpose was to see if scoring the HOS by a simple count of symptoms was markedly different from scoring it in Likert fashion as a frequency-weighted score (Likert, 1932). While these two types of procedures are commonly used for screeners, we hypothesized that a frequency-weighted score would perform better because it uses more information given by the subjects. The HOS has twenty questions to which the subjects are asked to respond "often," "sometimes," or "never" in regard to the frequency with which they are bothered by the symptom.

For a simple count of the symptoms, "often" and "sometimes" responses were grouped as "symptom present" and "never" as "symptom absent." As shown in Figure 6.3, the ROC curve for this dichotomous symptom enumeration score begins in the upper right-hand corner with a score of 2, where sensitivity is perfect and specificity nearly imperfect, and then sweeps to the left and down where, with a score of 19, specificity and sensitivity have reversed themselves. Nevertheless, in overall terms the performance is good since the AUC value of .90 is significantly different ($p < .001$) from the line of no information.

Using the frequency-weighted score that is customary for the HOS, Figure 6.4 shows its ROC curve. This curve is very similar in shape to the previous one, and its AUC value of .91 is also similar. There is no statistical difference between the two curves. While frequency-weighing of this type cannot damage the performance of the HOS, in this case it also does not improve it.

The results of this experiment with the HOS are rather similar to those for the GHQ, an instrument that has four response categories that have often been collapsed into two. It was found that dichotomous and Likert scoring did not make much difference to the validity of the GHQ (Goldberg, 1972). While this was not shown by means of ROC analysis, the similarity in results raises some questions about response categories. If a large number of response categories for

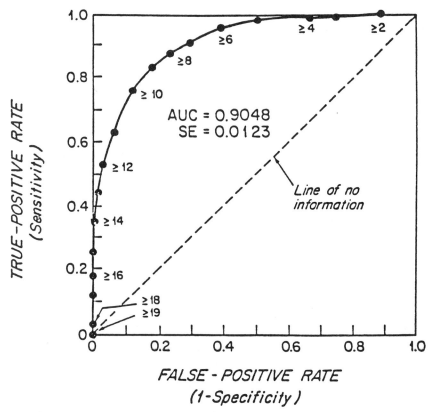

Figure 6.3. Receiver Operating Characteristic (ROC) Curve for Dichotomous Symption Enumeration Score Using Health Opinion Survey. Points on curve are cutpoint thresholds. AUC indicates area under curve.

frequency or intensity are found in other studies to have little relevance to validity, it can be interpreted that their main purpose is to control response bias. Furthermore, it is possible that this latter goal could be achieved in less cumbersome ways.

Finally, I would like to suggest it may be timely to consider that the numerous depression screeners that seem to pass the tests of reliability and content validity well have reached the ceiling of their performance by virtue of using "count and cut" methods. I raise this issue because simple "count and cut" methods cannot distinguish between the *essential features* and *associated symptoms* of depression that are fundamental to perceiving the pattern of symptomatology that makes up the depression syndrome in DSM-III.

Suppose a cutpoint for the CES-D were set at four or more positive responses. Even though the CES-D has good coverage of both the essential mood symptoms

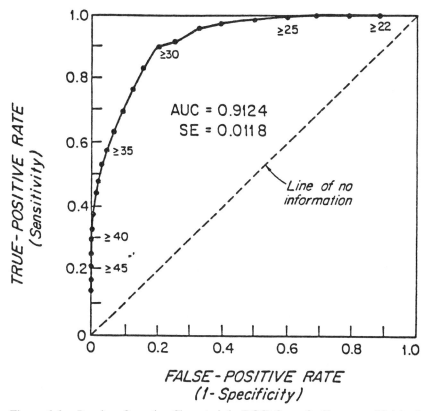

Figure 6.4. Receiver Operating Characteristic (ROC) Curve for Frequency-Weighted Symptom Enumeration Score Using Health Opinion Survey. AUC indicates area under curve.

and the associated vital symptoms of depression, it would be easy for a subject to screen positive without endorsing a single feature of depressed mood. The requirement for four symptoms could be met by positive responses to questions about feeling tired, poor appetite, trouble sleeping, everything being an effort, and generally being bothered by things. While these items form a factor named "somatic and retarded activity," their meaning is difficult to interpret in the absence of depressed mood (Radloff, 1977).

If the scoring of screeners were to follow the pattern of a diagnostic algorithm, such as used in the computer program for the DIS or in the PSE's CATEGO program, it is possible that performance could be improved (Robins et al., 1981; Wing et al., 1974). Since personal computers, which could accomplish such scoring, will probably soon be as common in primary care settings as stethoscopes, within a few moments after the patient completed the screener, the physician would have access to information about whether the evidence met the full criteria for depression, was borderline, or was negative.

For the Stirling County Study, we decided that trying to develop a diagnostic computer program might take us out of what we perceived to be the quagmire of "count and cut" methods (Murphy, Neff, Sobol, Rice, & Oliver, 1985). A program was designed for the HOS and was named DPAX; the DP stands for depression, and the AX stands for anxiety. The first step divides the subjects into those who are entirely well, and those who have any conceivable evidence of depression and anxiety. This division derives from the application of linear coefficients from discriminant function analyses. The second step establishes that there is sufficient psychological symptomatology reported and identifies those who reach the next higher level of probability in regard to having a disorder. The third step applies criteria for impairment in one's ordinary work role and its duration, and it thereby identifies a borderline category. The fourth establishes that the symptomatology meets preestablished levels of intensity.

Following these steps, the DPAX program carries out an algorithm that is specifically concerned with diagnostic differentiation between depression and anxiety, and it catalogues whether the subject meets criteria for both or only one of the syndromes. Again, it is useful to describe the diagnostic component of the program as having four steps. In regard to depression, for example, the first step concerns essential features and is a requirement for a positive response to a question about being in poor spirits; the second, for associated symptomatology, has two parts in that positive evidence is required for three clusters of symptoms—disturbances of sleep, appetite, and energy—and then over and above this require-ment a threshold on a frequency-weighted score is applied; the third requires evidence of at least mild impairment in one's ordinary work role; and the fourth requires a minimum duration of one month. From eight to ten subjects identified by the program either volunteer that they are bothered by nerves or answer positively to a question about nervous breakdown. These features of "nervous-ness" can be thought of as a colloquial way for subjects to convey a general orientation to depression or anxiety even though this orientation does not serve to differentiate between the two syndromes.

In regard to ROC analysis, we constructed a curve by applying the first four steps of the DPAX program sequentially, aggregating depression and anxiety together. In figure 6.5 the first step is represented by the right-most point; the performance of the complete algorithm, including all four steps, is represented by the left-most point. This curve is very different from those using simple-counting methods. Each step has a true-positive rate above 90%, and the curve is composed mainly of differences in the false-positive rates. The AUC value is .97, and this curve is significantly better than the previous two ($p < .001$). While the HOS is an instrument of an earlier vintage than those that would be considered for screening depression in current primary care studies, the DPAX program can

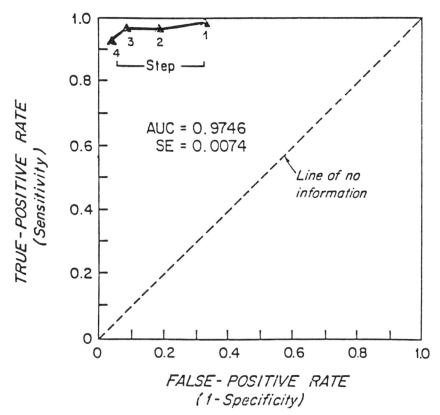

Figure 6.5. Receiver Operating Characteristic (ROC) Curve for Scoring Health Opinion Survey by Diagnostic Algorithm Used in Computer Program DPAX. Point on curve are steps of algorithm. AUC indicates area under curve.

serve as a model for an approach that might improve the performance of a more contemporary screener.

In conclusion, it can be noted that the "state of the art" in regard to screening for depression in primary care is an intersection between demonstrated accomplishments and a few points that need further attention.

The existing screeners provide a strong foundation for further development.

The questions in these screeners have now been asked of thousands and thousands of persons. There is considerable evidence that people understand the questions and are willing to answer them. While safeguards against response bias are needed, most people seem to respond in truthful and meaningful ways. Furthermore, most of these existing screeners have adequate to excellent psychometric properties. The areas for which further research is needed can be summarized as five points:

1. The importance of identifying both chronic conditions and current episodes;
2. The need for attention to the role played by comorbidity, especially the coexistence of depression and anxiety syndrome;
3. The need for well-designed validity studies and their replication;
4. The value of ROC analysis as an aid in evaluating screeners;
5. The possibility of overcoming problems about cutpoints by using diagnostic scoring rules.

References

American Psychiatric Association (1952). *Diagnostic and statistical manual* (1st ed.). Washington, D.C.: Author.

American Psychiatric Association (1980). *Diagnostic and statistical manual of mental disorders* (3rd ed.). Washington, D.C.: Author.

Beck, A. T., Ward, C. H., Mendelson, M., Mock, J., & Erbaugh, J. (1961). An inventory for measuring depression. *Archives of General Psychiatry, 4*, 561–571.

Brodman, K., Erdmann, A. J., Lorge, I., Deutschberger, J., & Wolff, H. G. (1954). The Cornell Medical Index Health Questionnaire. VI. The prediction of psychosomatic and psychiatric disabilities in army training. *American Journal of Psychiatry, 3*, 37–40.

Brodman, K., Erdmann, A. J., & Wolff, H. G. (1949). *Cornell Medical Index Health Questionnaire (manual)*. New York: Cornell University Medical College.

Dahlstrom, W. G., Welsh, G. S., & Dahlstrom, L. E. (1972). *An MMPI handbook. Vol. I, Clinical interpretation*. Minneapolis: University of Minnesota Press.

Derogatis, L. R., & Cleary, P. A. (1977). Factorial invariance across gender for the primary symptom dimensions of the SCL–90. *British Journal of Social and Clinical Psychology, 16*, 347–356.

Derogatis, L. R., Klerman, G. L., & Lipman, R. S. (1972). Anxiety states and depressive neuroses. *Journal of Nervous and Mental Disorders, 155*, 392–403.

Derogatis, L. R., Lipman, R. S., Covi, L., & Rickels, K. (1972). Factorial invariance of neurotic symptom dimensions in anxious and depressive neuroses. *Archives of General Psychiatry, 27*, 659–665.

Derogatis, L. R., Lipman, R. S., Rickels, K., Uhlenhuth, E. H., & Covi, L. (1974). The Hopkins Symptom Checklist (HSCL): A self-report symptom inventory. *Behavioral Sciences, 19*, 1–15.

Dinning, W. D., & Evans, R. G. (1977). Discriminant and convergent validity of the SCL–90 in psychiatric inpatients. *Journal of Personality Assessment, 41*, 304–310.

Dohrenwend, B. P., & Dohrenwend, B. S. (1982). Perspectives on the past and future of psychiatric epidemiology: The 1981 Rema Lapouse Lecture. *American Journal of Public Health, 72*, 1271–1279.

Dohrenwend B. P., Shrout P. E., Egri G., & Mendelsohn, F. S. (1980). Nonspecific psychological distress and other dimensions of psychopathology. *Archives of General Psychiatry, 37*, 1229–1236.

Duncan-Jones, P., & Henderson, S. (1978). The use of a two-phase design in a prevalence survey. *Social Psychiatry, 13*, 231–237.

Endicott, J., & Spitzer, R. L. (1978). A diagnostic interview: The Schedule for Affective Disorders and Schizophrenia. *Archives of General Psychiatry, 35*, 837–844.

Eysenck, H. J. (1947). *Dimensions of personality*. London: Routledge and Kegan Paul.

Finlay-Jones, R. A., & Murphy, E. (1979). Severity of psychiatric disorder and the 30-item General Health Questionnaire. *British Journal of Psychiatry, 134,* 609–616.

Frank, J. D. (1974). Psychotherapy: The restoration of morale. *American Journal of Psychiatry, 131,* 271–274.

Goldberg, D. P. (1972). *The detection of psychiatric illness by questionnaire*. London: Oxford University Press.

Goldberg, D. P. (1979). *Manual of the General Health Questionnaire*. Windsor, Berkshire: NFER Publishing.

Goldberg, D. P., & Blackwell, B. (1970). Psychiatric illness in general practice: A detailed study using a new method of case identification. *British Medical Journal, 2,* 439–443.

Goldberg, D. P., Cooper, B., Eastwood, M. R., Kedward, H. B., & Shepherd, M. (1970). A standardized psychiatric interview for use in community surveys. *British Journal of Preventative and Social Medicine, 24,* 18–23.

Goldberg, D. P., & Hillier, V. F. (1979). A scaled version of the General Health Questionnaire. *Psychological Medicine, 9,* 139–145.

Hankin, J. R., & Locke, B. Z. (1979). *Extent of depressed mood among patients seeking care in prepaid group practices*. Paper presented at the Annual Meeting of the American Public Health Association, New York, NY.

Hanley, J. A., & McNeil, B. J. (1982). The meaning and use of the area under a receiver operating characteristic (ROC) curve. *Radiology, 143,* 29–36.

Hanley, J. A., & McNeil, B. J. (1983). A method of comparing the areas under receiver operating characteristic curves derived from the same cases. *Radiology, 148,* 839–843.

Hoeper, E. W., Nycz, G. R., Cleary, P. D., Regier, D. A., & Goldberg, I. D. (1979). Estimated prevalence of RDC mental disorder in primary mental care. *International Journal of Mental Health, 8,* 6–15.

Hornstra, R. K., & Klassen, D. (1977). The course of depression. *Comprehensive Psychiatry, 18,* 119–125.

Keller, M. B., & Shapiro, R. W. (1982). Double depression: Superimposition of acute depressive episodes on chronic depressive disorders. *American Journal of Psychiatry, 139,* 438–442.

Kelman, H. C., & Parloff, M. B. (1957). Interrelations among three criteria of improvement in group therapy: Comfort, effectiveness, and self-awareness. *Journal of Abnormal and Social Psychology, 54,* 281–288.

Kessler, L. G., Burns, B. J., Shapiro, S., Tischler, G. L., George, L. K., Hough, R. L., Bodison, D., & Miller, R. H. (1987). Psychiatric diagnoses of medical service users: Evidence from the Epidemiologic Catchment Area Program. *American Journal of Public Health, 77,* 18–24.

Langner, T. S. (1962). A twenty-two item screening score of psychiatric symptoms indicating impairment. *Journal of Health and Human Behavior, 3,* 269–276.

Leighton, D. C., Harding, J. S., Macklin, D. B., Macmillan, A. M., & Leighton, A. H. (1963). *The character of danger: The Stirling County study* (vol. 3). New York: Basic Books.

Likert, R. A. (1932). A technique for the measurement of attitudes. *Archives of Psychology, 140,* 1–55.

Link, B., & Dohrenwend, B. P. (1980). Formulation of hypotheses about the true prevalence of demoralization in the United States. In B. P. Dohrenwend, B. S. Dohrenwend, M. S. Gould,

B. Link, R. Neugebauer, & R. Wunsch-Hitzig (eds.), *Mental illness in the United States: Epidemiological estimates* (pp 114–132). New York: Praeger.

Lipman R. S., Rickels, K., Covi, L., Derogatis, L. R., & Uhlenhuth, E. H. (1969). Factors of symptom distress: Doctor ratings of anxious neurotic outpatients. *Archives of General Psychiatry, 21,* 328–338.

Little, J. C., & McPhail, N. I. (1973). Measures of depressive mood at monthly intervals. *British Journal of Psychiatry,* `122, 447–452.

Macmillan, A. M. (1954). Explorations in rural community health with particular reference to psychophysiological symptoms. Unpublished doctoral dissertation, Cornell University, Ithaca, NY.

Macmillan, A. M. (1957). The Health Opinion Survey: Technique for estimating prevalence of psychoneurotic and related types of disorders in communities. *Psychological Reports, 3,* 325–339.

Mattsson, N. B., Williams, H. V., Rickels, K., Lipman, R. S., & Uhlenhuth, E. H. (1969). Dimensions of symptom distress in anxious neurotic outpatients. *Psychopharmacological Bulletin, 5,* 19–32.

Menninger, K. (1959). *A psychiatrist's world* (pp. 516–528). New York: The Viking Press.

Metz, C. E. (1978). Basic principles of ROC analysis. *Seminars in Nuclear Medicine, 8,* 283–298.

Murphy, J. M. (1980). Continuities in community-based psychiatric epidemiology. *Archives of General Psychiatry, 37,* 1215–1223.

Murphy, J. M. (1981). *Psychiatric instrument development for primary care.* (NIMH Contract No. 80M014280101D). Rockville, MD: Division of Biometry and Epidemiology.

Murphy, J. M. (1986). Diagnosis, screening, and demoralization: Epidemiologic implications. *Psychiatric Developments, 2,* 101–133.

Murphy, J. M., Berwick, D. M., Weinstein, M. C., Borus, J. F., Budman, S. H., & Klerman, G. L. (1987). Performance of screening and diagnostic tests: Application of receiver operating characteristic (ROC) analysis. *Archives of General Psychiatry, 44,* 550–555.

Murphy, J. M., Neff, R. K., Sobol, A. M., Rice, J. X., & Oliver, D. C. (1985). Computer diagnosis of depression and anxiety: The Stirling County study. *Psychological Medicine, 15,* 99–112.

Parloff, M. B., Kelman, H. C., & Frank, J. D. (1954). Comfort, effectiveness, and self-awareness as criteria of improvement in psychotherapy. *American Journal of Psychiatry, 3,* 343–351.

Radloff, L. S. (1977). The CES-D scale: A self report depression scale for research in the general population. *Applied Psychological Measurement, 1,* 385–401.

Robins, L. E., Helzer, J. E., Croughan, J. L., & Ratcliff, K. S. (1981). National Institute of Mental Health Diagnostic Interview Schedule: Its history, characteristics, and validity. *Archives of General Psychiatry, 38,* 381–389.

Schwartz, C. C., Myers, J. K., & Astrachan, B. M. (1973). Comparing three measures of mental status: A note on the validity of estimates of psychological disorder in the community. *Journal of Health and Social Behavior, 14,* 265–273.

Spitzer, R. L., Endicott, J., Fleiss, J. L., & Cohen, J. (1970). The Psychiatric Status Schedule: A technique for evaluating psychopathology and impairment in role functioning. *Archives of General Psychiatry, 23,* 41–55.

Spitzer, R. L., Fleiss, J. L., Endicott, J., & Cohen, J. (1967). Mental Status Schedule: Properties of factor-analytically derived scales. *Archives of General Psychiatry, 16,* 479–493.

Srole, L., Langner, T. S., Michael, S. T., Opler, M. K., & Rennie, T. A. C. (1962). *Mental health in the metropolis: The Midtown Manhattan study*. New York: McGraw-Hill.

Star, S. A. (1950). The screening of psychoneurotics: Comparison of psychiatric diagnoses and test scores at all induction stations. In S. A. Stouffer, L. Guttman, & E. A. Suchman (Eds.), *Measurement and prediction* (pp. 548–567). Princeton: Princeton University Press.

Swets, J. A., & Pickett, R. M. (1982). *Evaluation of diagnostic systems*. Orlando: Academic Press.

Weider, A., Mittelmann, B., Wechsler, D., & Wolff, H. G. (1944). The Cornell Selectee Index. *JAMA, 124*, 224–228.

Weinstein, M. C., Feinberg, H. V., Elstein, A. S., Frazier, H. S., Neuhauser, D., Neutra, R. R., & McNeil, B. J. (1980). *Clinical decision analysis*. Philadelphia: W. B. Saunders.

Weissman, M. M., Sholomskas, D., Pottenger, M., Prusoff, B. A., & Locke, B. Z. (1977). Assessing depressive symptoms in five psychiatric populations: A validation study. *American Journal of Epidemiology, 106*, 203–214.

Williams, H. V., Lipman R. S., Rickels, K., Covi, L., Uhlenhuth, E. H., & Mattsson, N. B. (1968). Replication of symptom distress factors in anxious neurotic outpatients. *Multivariate Behavioral Research, 3*, 199–211.

Wing, J. K., Cooper, J. E., & Sartorius, N. (1974). *The measurement and classification of psychiatric symptoms*. London: Cambridge University Press.

Worsley, A., Walters, W. A. W., & Wood, E. C. (1978). Responses of Australian patients with gynecological disorders to the General Health Questionnaire: A factor analytic study. *Psychological Medicine, 8*, 131–138.

7

Statistical Design of Screening Procedures

Patrick E. Shrout

The design of a screening procedure involves many decisions, including the choice of a screening instrument, the definition of who is designated "positive" on the screen, and the determination of a protocol for deciding who gets additional assessment beyond the screen.[1] Often these decisions are made on the basis of conventional wisdom or previous experience rather than a formal analysis of the costs and benefits of the screening procedure. When feasible, a mathematical analysis of the effects of design decisions on the efficiency of the screening procedure can lead to a design that is said to be "optimal." In order for such an analysis to be feasible, the administrator of the screening program must be able to translate service goals into statements that can be modeled mathematically. This translation process, usually done jointly by the health professional and a statistician, may be difficult if the goals are abstract or if there are multiple goals that are not consistent.

When successful, the translation process yields a quantitative index of the benefit of the screening procedure as a function of design parameters of the screening procedure. This equation, often referred to as a *utility function*, allows the effect of choices of design parameters to be studied systematically. For example, if a screening instrument that has mediocre validity is replaced with one that has excellent validity, an increase should be observed in the index of the utility of the screening procedure. When the mathematical analysis reveals design specifications that make the utility function as large as it can get, the specifications are called the *optimal design*. Note that what is optimal depends on the formulation of the utility function, which itself depends on the purpose of the screening program. Unlike the usual meaning of "optimal," a statistically optimal design is not necessarily the best across all primary care settings.

In this chapter, I review several types of screening goals and their mathematically optimal designs and show that a design that is optimal in one context may be far from optimal in another. For three specific applications, I review statistical

[1] This work was supported in part by grants MH30710 and MH30906 from the National Institute of Mental Health.

results that may be helpful in making decisions about the design of a screening program in primary care settings. Two decisions are highlighted in the chapter: (a) whether the administration of an initial screen for depression is cost-effective in the primary care setting; and (b) how the screening rule should be defined.

An initial screen for depression is usually employed in a two-phase (or two-stage) design for case identification: the screen (the first phase of assessment) is used to determine which patients should get further psychiatric evaluation (the second phase of assessment). We assume throughout this discussion that the screen is too crude an assessment to establish either the psychiatric diagnosis or the treatment protocol. The further evaluation is usually quite expensive relative to the screen; it typically involves a mental health professional and a detailed, structured assessment leading to a psychiatric diagnosis. An alternative to a two-phase design for identifying persons with depression in primary care settings should sometimes be considered. This alternative is the systematic psychiatric evaluation of all primary care patients, not simply those screened by an initial assessment. While such a procedure appears intuitively to be much more expensive than a screening procedure, it may be the most efficient method of collecting information if adequate screening instruments are unavailable or the cost of the formal psychiatric assessment is modest. We will refer to the alternative design as a single-phase design, in contrast to the two-phase screening design.

Given that a two-phase design is cost-efficient compared to a single-phase design, a second set of decisions has to do with the formulation of a screening rule. By *screening rule,* I mean the rule that defines how information from the screening interview is used to determine whether a patient is screened as positive or negative. For example, if a screening measure yields a quantitative score, one defines the screening rule by specifying the cutpoint on the continuum of the scale above which patients are considered possible cases of depression. Murphy, in chapter 6 of this volume, discusses other types of screening rules besides cutpoints on symptom scales. Corresponding to each rule is a pair of validity values, the *sensitivity* (the proportion of those who are clinically depressed who are screened as positive) and *specificity* (the proportion of those free of clinical depression who are screened as negative). When two competing rules are being considered jointly, one must determine whether sensitivity or specificity should be weighted more and whether the best pair of values is good enough to meet the needs of the screening program.

Much is written in this volume about the selection of instruments for screening for depression in primary care settings. At least two authors (Murphy, ch. 6; Cleary, ch. 12) recommend that ROC analysis be used to evaluate potential screening tools, since these analyses reveal the instrument's accuracy over a whole range of potential screening decision rules (usually cutpoints). The ROC curves show clearly the trade-off between the sensitivity and specificity for a series of decision rules based on a set of items. In general, as rules are considered that define more persons as screened as positive, sensitivity improves while specificity worsens. While the many points on an ROC curve are of academic interest, a screening program administrator must choose a single point representing the combination of sensitivity and specificity values that best serves the most important clinical goals. This choice of a specific screening rule may be informed by a mathematical analysis.

Optimal For What?
Goals of Screening In
Primary Care Settings

Screening programs for depression in primary care settings are implemented for different purposes, including clinical, referral, epidemiologic, and research reasons. Depending on the purpose of the screening program, the mathematical description of the usefulness of the program—i.e. the utility function—will take different forms. For each purpose, the costs and benefits of the program need to be quantified. In general, if two projects have different goals, they are likely to have different utility functions and different statistically optimal designs. To illustrate this principle, let us consider how a utility function could be defined for each of four generic screening goals.

Referral for Outside Treatment

Suppose that clinicians in a primary care facility believe that patients who show signs of depression should be informed about the options of mental health treatment, including names of mental health service providers. One could argue that a screening program designed to fulfill this goal should attempt to refer all those who are clinically depressed, since these persons will likely profit from treatment. That is, a screening rule should be adopted that maximizes sensitivity. Our didactic purposes will be well served for this first example if we assume that there is no easy way to quantify the cost associated with false positives and thus that the specificity of the screen is not of paramount importance.

In this simplified case, the utility function might be set equal to sensitivity itself. It is maximized by choosing a decision rule that screens positive all persons who truly have depression. This conclusion is unsatisfying, since any screening instrument can exhibit perfect sensitivity by setting a cutpoint such that 100% of the population is screened as positive. In this case it is clear that no initial screen is needed, since the information from the assessment would not be used in the screening rule. If a primary care practice simply refers patients with depression to outside providers, without explicitly planning treatment of medical disorders and taking depression into account, then any psychiatric assessment would not be cost-efficient.

Screening for Comprehensive Clinical Management

If the primary care facility provides comprehensive medical and psychiatric treatment, it will want to identify patients with affective disorders both to provide treatment for the mental disorder and to take the psychiatric condition into account in planning treatment for medical disorders. As before, it is of interest to identify all persons who are clinically depressed, but now it is also of interest to avoid *false positives* (persons without depression who are erroneously screened as positive). Patients who are false positives add cost without benefit to the screening endeavor: they require expensive further assessments and may receive improper medical and psychiatric treatment if they are presumed to be depressed when, in fact, they are not. Now both sensitivity and specificity are of concern, especially insofar as they have an impact on the screen's *positive predictive value* (PPV; or the proportion of those screened as positive who are clinically depressed). The closer PPV is to unity, the fewer false positives are included among those screened as positive.

A complementary quantity to PPV is *negative predictive value* (NPV; the proportion of those screened as negative who do not have clinical depression). For a rare disorder such as depression, this quantity will tend to be close to unity for most screening applications; it will be below 0.90 only when the rate of persons with depression exceeds 10% in the group screened as negative. While values of NPV less than unity reveal that some persons with clinical depression are missed by the screen, small variations in NPV do not have cost-benefit implications that variations in PPV have. For this reason, it can be argued that a screening program designed for clinical management of primary care patients is best served by a design that maximizes PPV, especially if the design yields a manageable number of patients who are screened as positive.[2]

Identification of Confirmed Cases for Research

As Burnam and Wells note in Chapter 8 of this volume, another goal of a depression screening program in a primary care setting may be to identify persons with depression to serve as subjects in psychiatric research. It is well known that only a portion of those experiencing depression seek treatment (e.g., Shapiro et al., 1984), and thus the recruitment of depressed cases from mental health facilities may result in nonrepresentative samples of depressed persons. Treated

---

[2] Sometimes it is possible to define explicit weighing functions that allow both PPV and NPV (or both sensitivity and specificity) to enter into a single utility function. For example, a change of .1 in specificity may be hypothesized to have the same implications as a change of .01 in sensitivity. These weights might be established by studying the actual costs associated with false negatives and false positives. Examples of the analysis of such complex utility functions have been discussed by Hand (1987).

cases are more likely to be chronic and to have special resources for payment of mental health care. A much more representative sample of depressed persons is likely to be found from screening a primary care population. The best design of the screening program in this instance is one that produces the desired number of confirmed cases while minimizing the expense of assessment.

Assessment of Prevalence in Primary Care Population

Epidemiology and services researchers may implement a screening program in a primary care setting to determine the proportion of the population served by the setting that is suffering from depression at a point in time. Unlike the three examples just discussed, which have case identification as a goal, the estimation of prevalence requires the examination of samples of both those screened as positive and those screened as negative, since both true positives and false negatives enter into the prevalence formula (see for example, Cochran, 1977; Deming, 1977; Shrout & Newman, 1989). The best design of the screening program is one that produces an unbiased estimate of the prevalence with the minimum standard error. (The *standard error* is the statistical measure of the precision of the prevalence estimate.)

Information from a prevalence study is usually needed to design a case identification screening study. Not only do the results from the prevalence study inform the administrator about the numbers of persons in the population who might profit from referral or who are available for scientific study, the results also allow estimates of sensitivity and specificity of the screening rule to be obtained for the primary care population. These estimates rely on information about the false negative rates that is obtained from the diagnostic assessment of a sample of those screened as negative.

Some Optimal Decision Rules for Screening Design

The first decision that must be faced when considering implementing a screening operation is whether a two-phase screening design is actually worthwhile. We have assumed that ultimately the clinical practitioner, the clinical researcher, and the epidemiologist would like to know which (or how many) primary care patients are clinically depressed. The initial screen of a two-phase design does not provide that information—only the detailed clinical assessment can establish the diagnosis. Instead, the initial screen attempts to identify a subset of patients who appear to have some of the symptoms of depression. When everything works well, this subset is relatively small compared to the total patient population, and the number of expensive clinical assessments is minimized. However, if the cost of administering the screen is not substantially less than the cost of the clinical assessments, or if the screening instrument does not adequately identify those with the disorder, then the two-phase design may actually be more expensive than simply providing a careful clinical assessment for all patients (i.e., assessment of all persons in a single phase). In describing two-phase designs that are optimally efficient, we will use the single-phase alternative as a benchmark.

Screening for Comprehensive Clinical Management

As discussed above, when the cost of false positives is borne by the health care organization, it will be necessary to devise a screening program with excellent positive predictive value. This quantity can be expressed as a function of sensitivity, specificity, and prevalence using Bayes' formula (see Fleiss, 1981, pp. 10–13). Let S_e and S_p represent sensitivity and specificity, respectively, of the screen, and let p represent the prevalence of depression in the primary care population. Then, positive predictive value can be expressed as

$$PPV = pS_e/[pS_e + (1 - p)(1 - S_p)]. \qquad (7.1)$$

When one has an idea of the prevalence of depression in the population to be screened, one can choose the screening decision rule that yields sensitivity and specificity values that produce the best positive predictive values. Table 7.1 shows for a range of values of S_e, S_p, and p the expected positive predictive value of the screen. This table reminds us that good values of positive predictive values are hard to attain when the prevalence is small. We also can see that for rare disorders, very good specificity is more important than good sensitivity. Consider the column corresponding to a prevalence of 5%: When both sensitivity and specificity are .95, only half of those screened as positive will truly have depression. If sensitivity remains at .95, but specificity slips to .90, then only one-third of those screened as positive will be cases. On the other hand, if specificity remains at .95, but sensitivity is reduced to .90, the positive predictive value is hardly affected at all: 49% of the screened positives are expected to be cases. If the screening decision rule is defined by selecting a cutpoint on a continuous screening scale such as the CES-D (Radloff, 1977), one would be inclined to use a rather high cutpoint in order to screen only the most symptomatic persons and to maintain high levels of specificity.

Identification of Confirmed Cases for Research

Let us now turn our attention to the problem of identifying persons with clinical depression for scientific studies. To obtain unbiased scientific results, it will be necessary to be sure that those persons assigned to the depression case group are truly depressed, while those in the comparison group are truly not depressed. While there is no universally acclaimed "gold standard" for making these true diagnostic distinctions, let us assume that there is a diagnostic procedure available that is relatively well accepted and can be used operationally to define the case group. This procedure may be extremely expensive, such as the Longitudinal,

Table 7.1. Positive Predictive Value for Combinations of Values of Sensitivity (S_e),
Specificity (S_p), and Prevalence (p)

S_e	S_p	p = .01	p = .05	p = .1	p = .2	p = .3
.95	.99	0.49	0.83	0.91	0.96	0.98
.95	.95	0.16	0.50	0.68	0.83	0.89
.95	.90	0.09	0.33	0.51	0.70	0.80
.95	.85	0.06	0.25	0.41	0.61	0.73
.95	.75	0.04	0.17	0.30	0.49	0.62
.95	.65	0.03	0.13	0.23	0.40	0.54
.90	.99	0.48	0.83	0.91	0.96	0.97
.90	.95	0.15	0.49	0.67	0.82	0.89
.90	.90	0.08	0.32	0.50	0.69	0.79
.90	.85	0.06	0.24	0.40	0.60	0.72
.90	.75	0.04	0.16	0.29	0.47	0.61
.90	.65	0.03	0.12	0.22	0.39	0.52
.85	.99	0.46	0.82	0.90	0.96	0.97
.85	.95	0.15	0.47	0.65	0.81	0.88
.85	.90	0.08	0.31	0.49	0.68	0.78
.85	.85	0.05	0.23	0.39	0.59	0.71
.85	.75	0.03	0.15	0.27	0.46	0.59
.85	.65	0.02	0.11	0.21	0.38	0.51
.75	.99	0.43	0.80	0.89	0.95	0.97
.75	.95	0.13	0.44	0.62	0.79	0.87
.75	.90	0.07	0.28	0.45	0.65	0.76
.75	.85	0.05	0.21	0.36	0.56	0.68
.75	.75	0.03	0.14	0.25	0.43	0.56
.75	.65	0.02	0.10	0.19	0.35	0.48
.65	.99	0.40	0.77	0.88	0.94	0.97
.65	.95	0.12	0.41	0.59	0.76	0.85
.65	.90	0.06	0.25	0.42	0.62	0.74
.65	.85	0.04	0.19	0.32	0.52	0.65
.65	.75	0.03	0.12	0.22	0.39	0.53
.65	.65	0.02	0.09	0.17	0.32	0.44
.55	.99	0.36	0.74	0.86	0.93	0.96
.55	.95	0.10	0.37	0.55	0.73	0.83
.55	.90	0.05	0.22	0.38	0.58	0.70
.55	.85	0.04	0.16	0.29	0.48	0.61
.55	.75	0.02	0.10	0.20	0.35	0.49
.55	.65	0.02	0.08	0.15	0.28	0.40

Expert, and All Data (LEAD) procedure (Spitzer, 1983), which involves teams of diagnosticians reviewing voluminous information, or it may be only somewhat expensive, such as a structured interview administered by a trained nonclinician. In either case, it may be thought that expense can be minimized by administering the diagnostic procedure only to primary care patients who have been identified as possibly depressed by a very inexpensive screen.

Let c_D be the cost associated with administering the diagnostic procedure to a patient and let c_S be the cost of the screen. Suppose that the screening rule identifies a proportion π of the population as positive and that in that screened positive group the rate of depression according to the diagnostic procedure is p_1, which is identical to the positive predictive value. (Later we will also need the rate among the screened negatives, p_2.) If all those screened as positive are given the diagnostic assessment, while none of those screened as negative are thus assessed, the expected number of confirmed cases out of N persons screened is $N\pi p_1$. The expected cost of this two-phase assessment is $Nc_S + N\pi c_D$. The utility function may be explicitly defined as the number of confirmed cases per cost; it can be written $U = \pi p_1/[c_D(C+\pi)]$, where C is the ratio of the screening to diagnostic costs, c_S/c_D. This function is easier to evaluate if we compare it to the ratio of confirmed cases to cost that is expected if all persons in the primary care facility were given the diagnostic assessment (possibly feasible if the diagnostic assessment is simply a structured interview). Such a one-phase case identification procedure would be expected to find N_p cases with expense Nc_D, and its benefit to cost ratio is p/c_D. If we define the efficiency of the two-phase design to be the ratio of the benefit to cost ratios in two and one-phase designs, we get the result Efficiency $= S_e/(C+\pi)$. From this expression we see that the two-phase design will be more efficient than the single phase design if the sensitivity of the screen exceeds the sum of the cost ratio and the proportion screened as positive in the first phase.

If the two-phase design were no more efficient than a one-phase assessment, most administrators would rather not oversee the complexities of a screening program. For this reason, it is of interest to see when the formula given above is equal to one. This will occur when $C = (1 - p)(S_e + S_p - 1)$. For convenience, these values of C are shown in Table 7.2 as a function of sensitivity, specificity, and prevalence. For a screening program to be more efficient in case identification than a one-phase program, the expected cost ratio of the screen to the diagnostic assessment should be less than the values shown in Table 7.2. As shown by both the equation for C and the tabled values, the two-phase design is likely to be more efficient than a single-phase design when the prevalence of the disorder is low, especially when the sensitivity and specificity of the screen are good. One can also see that for this application there is a perfect trade-off between sensitivity and specificity: Neither is more influential in determining that the screening program will be efficient.

Assessment of Prevalence in Primary Care Population

If the prevalence of depression is not known in a primary care population, or if the sensitivity and specificity of the screen is unknown, then one must design a two-phase assessment that differs in an important way from those just discussed. Instead of following all of the screened positives and none of the screened

Table 7.2. Cost Ratio of Screen to Diagnosis for Which One and Two Phase Designs Are Equally Efficient for Case Identification

S_e	S_p	p = .01	p = .05	p = .1	p = .2	p = .3
.95	.99	0.93	0.89	0.85	0.75	0.66
.95	.95	0.89	0.85	0.81	0.72	0.63
.95	.90	0.84	0.81	0.77	0.68	0.60
.95	.85	0.79	0.76	0.72	0.64	0.56
.95	.75	0.69	0.67	0.63	0.56	0.49
.95	.65	0.59	0.57	0.54	0.48	0.42
.90	.99	0.88	0.85	0.80	0.71	0.62
.90	.95	0.84	0.81	0.77	0.68	0.60
.90	.90	0.79	0.76	0.72	0.64	0.56
.90	.85	0.74	0.71	0.68	0.60	0.53
.90	.75	0.64	0.62	0.59	0.52	0.46
.90	.65	0.54	0.52	0.50	0.44	0.39
.85	.99	0.83	0.80	0.76	0.67	0.59
.85	.95	0.79	0.76	0.72	0.64	0.56
.85	.90	0.74	0.71	0.68	0.60	0.53
.85	.85	0.69	0.66	0.63	0.56	0.49
.85	.75	0.59	0.57	0.54	0.48	0.42
.85	.65	0.49	0.47	0.45	0.40	0.35
.75	.99	0.73	0.70	0.67	0.59	0.52
.75	.95	0.69	0.66	0.63	0.56	0.49
.75	.90	0.64	0.62	0.59	0.52	0.46
.75	.85	0.59	0.57	0.54	0.48	0.42
.75	.75	0.49	0.47	0.45	0.40	0.35
.75	.65	0.40	0.38	0.36	0.32	0.28
.65	.99	0.63	0.61	0.58	0.51	0.45
.65	.95	0.59	0.57	0.54	0.48	0.42
.65	.90	0.54	0.52	0.49	0.44	0.39
.65	.85	0.49	0.47	0.45	0.40	0.35
.65	.75	0.40	0.38	0.36	0.32	0.28
.65	.65	0.30	0.28	0.27	0.24	0.21
.55	.99	0.53	0.51	0.49	0.43	0.38
.55	.95	0.49	0.47	0.45	0.40	0.35
.55	.90	0.45	0.43	0.40	0.36	0.32
.55	.85	0.40	0.38	0.36	0.32	0.28
.55	.75	0.30	0.28	0.27	0.24	0.21
.55	.65	0.20	0.19	0.18	0.16	0.14

negatives, one must follow samples of both screened groups. Let f_1 be the fraction of the screened positives who are followed and f_2 be the fraction of the screened negatives. These fractions must be determined in advance, and the sample of each group to be followed must be determined randomly. We will review the choices of f_1 and f_2 that produce the smallest standard error for the estimate of p for a given budget.

As before, the rate of depression among those screened as positive is p_1, the rate among those screened as negative is p_2 and the proportion of the population screened as positive is π. These parameters can be estimated from the results of two-phase study, and the estimates (technically the "statistics") can be used to estimate the prevalence using, $p = p_1\pi + p_2(1 - \pi)$. As has been discussed in Cochran (1977) and Shrout and Newman (1989), the standard error of the estimate of p is

$$V(\hat{p}) = \frac{1}{N}\left[\frac{\pi p_1(1 - p_1)}{f_1} + \frac{(1 - \pi)p_2(1 - p_2)}{f_2} + \pi(1 - \pi)(p_1 - p_2)^2\right].$$

The values of f_1 and f_2 that minimize this expression are

$$f_1^* = \sqrt{\frac{p_1(1 - p_1)}{(p_1 - p_2)^2\pi(1 - \pi)}\frac{c_S}{c_D}}$$

and

$$f_2^* = \sqrt{\frac{p_2(1 - p_2)}{(p_1 - p_2)^2\pi(1 - \pi)}\frac{c_S}{c_D}}.$$

These values are assumed to be between 0 and 1, but Shrout and Newman (1989) have pointed out that when p is small, the obtained values may go beyond that range, especially for f_1^*. When f_1^* is larger than 1, they recommend setting f_1 to 1.0 exactly and using the following to find f_2:

$$f_2^{**} = \sqrt{\frac{p_2(1 - p_2)(\pi + c_S/c_D)}{\pi p_1(1 - p_1) + \pi(1 - \pi)(p_1 - p_2)^2}}.$$

When f_2^{**} is also greater than 1.0, one can conclude that a one-phase design must be more efficient than a two-phase screen.

When the investigators have ideas about the values of S_e and S_p, but not of p_1 or p_2, they can use Equation 7.1 to calculate p_1, the positive predictive value. A value for p_2, which is equal to the negative predictive value subtracted from one, can be obtained using, $p_2 = p(1 - S_e)/[(1 - p)S_p + p(1 - S_e)]$. Since these formulas depend on p, the value to be estimated in the two-phase design, one should try a range of plausible values to determine the stability of the planned values for f_1 and f_2.

Given rough ideas about p, S_e, and S_p, Table 7.3 can be used to evaluate the efficiency of a two-phase design for prevalence estimation relative to a single phase design. This table is constructed using the results of Shrout and Newman (1989) and is similar to a table presented in their article. The efficiency of the two-phase design depends not only on the underlying rate of the disorder (p) and the validity of the screen (S_e and S_p), but also on the ratio of the costs of the screen to the diagnostic assessment ($C = c_S/c_D$). For a given set of prevalence,

Table 7.3. Cost Ratio of Screen to Diagnosis for Which One and Two Phase Designs Are Equally Efficient for Prevalence Estimation

S_e	S_p	p = .01	p = .05	p = .1	p = .2	p = .3
.95	.99	0.62	0.58	0.54	0.45	0.36
.95	.95	0.59	0.55	0.51	0.42	0.34
.95	.90	0.55	0.51	0.47	0.39	0.31
.95	.85	0.51	0.48	0.44	0.36	0.29
.95	.75	0.43	0.40	0.37	0.30	0.24
.95	.65	0.35	0.33	0.30	0.25	0.19
.90	.99	0.50	0.47	0.43	0.35	0.27
.90	.95	0.47	0.44	0.40	0.32	0.25
.90	.90	0.44	0.41	0.37	0.30	0.23
.90	.85	0.40	0.37	0.34	0.27	0.21
.90	.75	0.33	0.31	0.28	0.22	0.16
.90	.65	0.26	0.24	0.22	0.17	0.13
.85	.99	0.43	0.40	0.36	0.28	0.21
.85	.95	0.40	0.37	0.33	0.26	0.19
.85	.90	0.36	0.34	0.30	0.24	0.18
.85	.85	0.33	0.31	0.27	0.21	0.16
.85	.75	0.26	0.24	0.22	0.17	0.12
.85	.65	0.20	0.19	0.16	0.12	0.09
.75	.99	0.32	0.29	0.26	0.20	0.14
.75	.95	0.29	0.27	0.24	0.18	0.13
.75	.90	0.26	0.24	0.21	0.16	0.11
.75	.85	0.23	0.21	0.19	0.14	0.10
.75	.75	0.17	0.16	0.14	0.10	0.07
.75	.65	0.12	0.11	0.10	0.07	0.04
.65	.99	0.24	0.22	0.20	0.14	0.10
.65	.95	0.22	0.20	0.18	0.13	0.09
.65	.90	0.19	0.17	0.15	0.11	0.07
.65	.85	0.16	0.15	0.13	0.09	0.06
.65	.75	0.11	0.10	0.09	0.06	0.04
.65	.65	0.07	0.06	0.05	0.04	0.02
.55	.99	0.19	0.17	0.15	0.11	0.07
.55	.95	0.16	0.15	0.13	0.09	0.06
.55	.90	0.14	0.12	0.11	0.07	0.05
.55	.85	0.11	0.10	0.09	0.06	0.04
.55	.75	0.07	0.06	0.05	0.03	0.02
.55	.65	0.03	0.03	0.02	0.02	0.01

sensitivity, and specificity values, if the anticipated cost ratio is less than the values shown in Table 7.3, then a two-phase design is likely to be more efficient than a one-phase design.

Like the results for case identification shown in Table 7.2, the values in Table 7.3 reveal that two-phase designs have greater relative efficiency when the prevalence of the disorder under study is very low. Unlike the case identification application, however, there is not a complete trade-off between sensitivity and specificity; losses in specificity appear to have a greater impact than losses of sensitivity. Also, compared to the case identification application, for the two-phase design to be efficient for prevalence estimation, the relative cost of the screen to the diagnostic assessment must be much lower. If the screen is not less than half as expensive as the diagnostic evaluation, then the two-phase design is likely to be less efficient than the single phase design. Moreover, for many plausible values of S_e, S_p and p, the pay-off for a two-phase design is realized only when the screen is five to ten times less expensive than the diagnostic assessment.

Discussion

To illustrate how different screening goals lead to different screening program designs, let us imagine that there exists a primary care population in which it is thought that about 5% of the patients have a depressive disorder and for which a screen has been shown to have moderate validity. Suppose that when a relatively high cutpoint is employed on the screen, the sensitivity is .75 and the specificity is .85. When the cutpoint is lowered to include less symptomatic persons, the sensitivity rises to .85, while the specificity drops to .75.

If we are interested in simply referring the depressed persons to a mental health specialist within the same health care organization on the basis of the screening results, we see from Table 7.1 that we can expect either 21% or 15% of the referred cases to truly have the disorder, depending on the cutpoint used. Clearly, if the mental health facility were overburdened, we would tend to recommend that the screening rule employ the higher cutpoint. Put another way, we would choose the cutpoint that improves specificity at the expense of sensitivity. In any case, we might not be too impressed with the efficiency produced by the screen; while the prevalence in the screened positive group is three to four times that in the total population, more than 75% of those screened as positive will not have clinical depression.

If we were interested in identifying persons with depression for a case-control study, and if the diagnosis were to be made on the basis of a structured diagnostic procedure that is approximately four times more expensive to administer than the screen, we can see from Table 7.2 that a two-phase screening design is likely to be more efficient than the alternative of subjecting a whole series of persons to the diagnostic assessment. Regardless of the choice of cutpoints on the screen in this case, the two-phase design is expected to be more efficient as long as the screen is 57% or less expensive than the diagnostic assessment.

For prevalence estimation, however, the two-phase design might not be preferable to a single-phase diagnostic study. From Table 7.3 we see that the two-phase design will not be more efficient when using this screen, unless the cost of the screen is less than 24% the cost of the diagnosis. This conclusion is based on the use of the more inclusive cutpoint, which improves sensitivity at the expense of specificity.

This illustration shows that the utility of employing a two-phase screening design depends on the goals of the screening program. It also shows that the relative importance of sensitivity versus specificity varies with the application. A cutpoint on a screening scale that works well for one application may be far from optimal for another purpose. In practice, it may not be possible to decide which screening goal should be given priority in the design of the procedure, because administrators and scientists may each have their own interest in the results. When a screening program is designed both to collect cases and to estimate prevalence, for example, there is no single design that can jointly optimize the procedure. For more discussion of this point from a statistical perspective, see Hand (1987).

In this illustration, we assumed that we knew about the sensitivity and specificity of the screen and had some idea about the prevalence of the disorder. We can note from the tables that the calculation of positive predictive value is very much affected by the assumption of the underlying prevalence (Table 7.1), but the efficiency of the two-phase design for confirmed case identification and prevalence estimation is not much affected, unless the prevalence gets quite large (Tables 7.2 & 7.3). All sets of values, however, are affected by the assumed values of sensitivity and specificity, and thus it is especially important to make use of realistic values of these quantities.

Unfortunately, there is limited information about the sensitivity and specificity of screening scales for depression that is based on representative samples from primary care facilities. Many of the reports of sensitivity and specificity come from studies of clinical samples from psychiatric facilities. One should anticipate that episodes of depression among persons who have not sought psychiatric treatment will be diagnostically less clear cut than episodes reported by cases recruited from a mental health facility and thus that the sensitivity of any measure will be worse in nonpsychiatric populations than in psychiatric populations. On the other hand, the specificity of measures tested in populations other than psychiatric populations is often improved, since the proportion of population with symptoms that are similar to symptoms of depression is low.

If the sensitivity and specificity of a screen are not known when applied to a primary care population, it is strongly recommended that appropriate data be collected to evaluate these validity statistics. Keep in mind that it is not possible to estimate these values from a simple case-finding design, unless provisions are made to also estimate false negative rates by evaluating samples of persons screened as negative. Such samples must be quite large if one is to have confidence that false negatives are truly rare.

While the case identification exercise we described is most efficient when only persons who are screened as positive are followed with the diagnostic evaluation, there are important scientific reasons for following samples of negatives even in this application. The statistical model assumes that all cases are interchangeable, but in fact a sample of cases obtained on the basis of a few simple screening questions may not be representative of all cases in the primary care population. False negatives may have disproportionately less education, be cognitively impaired, or may have comorbidity that accounts for the failure of the screen. Risk factor studies or treatment efficacy studies may be biased by including only persons who were positive on the simple screen.

To conclude, there do exist statistical rules for designing optimal screening studies when the goals of the study are simple and can be translated into a mathematical utility function. In this chapter, several such rules have been reviewed. In practice, there may be multiple goals that cannot be given quantitative priority in a single utility function. Designers of screening procedures in these cases may use the results we have reviewed to determine whether the procedures are at all efficient and informative, even if not optimal. Some deviations from optimal designs, such as obtaining complete diagnostic assessments of a sample of screened negatives, are particularly important in order to monitor the overall quality of the screening procedure.

References

Cochran, W. G. (1977). *Sampling techniques* (3rd ed.). New York: Wiley.

Deming, W. E. (1977). An essay on screening, or on two-phase sampling, applied to surveys of a community. *International Statistical Review, 45,* 29–37.

Fleiss, J. L. (1981). *Statistical methods for rates and proportions* (2nd ed.). New York: Wiley.

Hand, D. J. (1987). Screening vs. prevalence estimation. *Applied Statistics, 36,* 1–7.

Radloff, L. S. (1977). The CES-D scale: A self-report depression scale for research in the general population. *Applied Psychological Measurement, 1,* 385–401.

Shapiro, S., Skinner, E. A., Kessler, L. G., Von Korff, M., German, P. S., Tischler, G. L., Leaf, P. J., Benham, L., Cottler, L. (1984). Utilization of health and mental health services: Three epidemiologic catchment area sites. *Archives of General Psychiatry, 41,* 971–978.

Shrout, P. E. & Newman, S. (1989). Design of two-phase prevalence surveys of rare disorders. *Biometrics, 45,* 549–555.

Spitzer, R. L. (1983). Psychiatric diagnosis: Are clinicians still necessary? *Comprehensive Psychiatry, 24,* 399—411.

8

Use of a Two-Stage Procedure to Identify Depression: The Medical Outcomes Study

M. Audrey Burnam and Kenneth B. Wells

This chapter describes the method used to identify persons with depressive disorder in a large-scale health policy study, the National Study of Medical Care Outcomes (MOS)[1]. The MOS, currently being fielded, was designed to compare the processes and outcomes of health care for adults with selected chronic disorder conditions across three types of health care systems: single specialty fee-for-service practices, multispecialty group practices, and health maintenance organizations (HMOs). The study will also compare processes and outcomes of medical care across provider specialty types (primary care physicians and mental health specialists). The conditions being studied are unipolar depressive disorder, hypertension, diabetes, and advanced coronary artery disease. The MOS uses a nonexperimental design to study effects of the health care systems as they naturally occur; patient selection factors are being comprehensively assessed and statistically controlled.

The MOS is being conducted at three U.S. sites (Los Angeles, Boston, and Chicago). At each site, providers were randomly selected from the total eligible population of providers in fee-for-service practices, and from selected large multispecialty group practices and HMOs. All patients seen in the practices of participating providers over a period of one to two weeks were screened for eligibility for the MOS. Across all sites and systems of care, over 25,000 patients were screened. From among the screened patients who had one of the conditions upon which the study focused (depression, hypertension, diabetes, and coronary artery disease) and who met other study eligibility criteria, a sample of over 2,500

[1] This research was supported by grants from the Robert Wood Johnson Foundation, The Henry J. Kaiser Family Foundation, the Pew Memorial Trust, and the National Institute of Mental Health. Portions of tables and text of this Chapter appeared originally in: (a) Burnam, M.A., Wells, K.B., Leake, B., & Landsverk, J. (1988). Development of a brief screening instrument for detecting depressive disorders. *Medical Care, 26,* 775–789; and (b) Wells, K.B., Burnam, M.A., Leake, B., Robins, L.N. (1988). Agreement between face to face and telephone administered versions of the depression section of the NIMH Diagnostic Interview Schedule. *Journal of Psychiatric Research, 22,* 207–220. Permission to reproduce these materials has been granted by Pergamon Press and Lippincott, Harper & Row, respectively.

was recruited into a two-year longitudinal panel study, designed to describe changes in health status over time and to explain these changes in terms of system of care, provider specialty, style of practice, and the intensity of utilization of health care resources.

The MOS focuses on unipolar depressive disorders, rather than on the broader phenomenon of depressive symptoms, in order to have a relatively homogeneous "tracer" group for whom treatments of known efficacy are clearly indicated. The ambitious design of the MOS presented us with the methodologic challenge of developing a depression case-identification procedure that would have clinical validity and that would be feasible given the scope and budget constraints of the study.

We considered a variety of strategies that might be used to identify persons with clinically significant depression, including the clinical diagnosis of a treating physician or clinician, self-reported symptoms comprising a depression scale, structured diagnostic interviews, or a variety of laboratory tests (e.g., the dexamethasone suppression test). For the MOS, the assessment of depression had to be independent of the diagnosis of the treating physician/clinician because the detection of depression by the clinician is one of the treatment components being studied. While self-report scales of depression provide an independent assessment of depressive symptoms, they do not provide a specific diagnosis of depressive disorders. Laboratory tests may increase the suspicion of affective disorder, but do not provide a definitive diagnosis. Structured diagnostic interviews are appropriate for this purpose, but they are prohibitively expensive to administer to every patient needing to be screened for such a large study.

Our resolution to this problem was to design a two-stage case identification approach. At the first stage, a simple self-report screening scale would be used, while at the second stage, only those having a high probability of being depressed would be given a structured diagnostic interview. There are two reasons why this approach seemed particularly appropriate for the MOS. First, a two-stage procedure could potentially reduce the cost of case-finding to feasible levels if, using a simple screen, the number of persons requiring a diagnostic interview could be greatly reduced from 25,000. Secondly, current methods for assessing psychiatric disorder readily lend themselves to a two-stage procedure. Self-report symptom scales tend to have good reliability and high sensitivity for psychiatric disorders in general populations and are simple and inexpensive to administer, making them appropriate for a first-stage screen. Structured psychiatric interviews, on the other hand, are designed to have a high degree of specificity, are time-consuming and expensive to administer, and may be more valid indicators of disorder among persons who are highly symptomatic, making them most useful as second-stage assessment instruments (see Dohrenwend & Shrout, 1982). Recently, several other researchers have studied depression in primary care populations using a two-stage case identification procedure (e.g., Hoeper, Ncyz, Cleary, Regier, & Goldberg, 1979; Schulberg et al., 1985), giving us further confidence that this was a strategy that could be successfully employed in the MOS.

The next sections present the MOS two-stage depression case-identification strategy in greater detail. First, the specific definition of depression chosen for the study is explained. Next, the selection of the second-stage diagnostic instrument and modifications made for its use in the MOS are described. Finally, results of the development and testing of a first-stage screener are presented.

Definition of Depression

The MOS definition of depressive disorders is based on DSM-III criteria because this diagnostic nomenclature reflects the current state of understanding of depressive disorders, and because it is widely accepted by both clinicians and researchers in the U.S. Two DSM-III disorders falling into the larger classification of unipolar affective disorders were selected to be the focus of the MOS study: *major depression* and *dysthymia*. These disorders were selected because of: (a) their high prevalence, relative to other affective disorders in the general population and in the practices of general medical physicians and mental health specialists; (b) their association with significant impairment in functioning; and (c) the availability of research instruments for diagnosing these disorders. Although most previous clinical and epidemiological research has focused on major depression alone, we included dysthymia because many patients with major depression also have preexisting dysthymia, and this tends to result in a more pernicious course of disorder (Keller et al., 1982; Keller, Lavori, Endicott, Coryell, & Klerman, 1983; Keller, Lavori, Lewis, & Klerman, 1983; Keller, Shapiro, Lavori, & Wolfe, 1982a; Keller, Shapiro, Lavori, & Wolfe, 1982b). Additionally, although dysthymia is almost as prevalent in the general population (2 to 4% lifetime) as major depression (around 5% lifetime) (Robins et al., 1984), it is a recently defined disorder and therefore relatively little research is available on it. Finally, dysthymia may be especially prevalent among patients with chronic medical conditions as a response to loss of functioning.

According to DSM-III, major depressive disorder is characterized by one or more major depressive episodes and the absence of manic episodes (e.g., elated mood). A *major depressive episode* is characterized by persistent depressive mood or loss of interest or pleasure in nearly all usual activities for a period of at least two weeks, accompanied by symptoms in four of eight symptom groups. The symptom groups are disturbances in appetite or weight; sleep disturbances; psychomotor agitation or retardation; decreased interest or pleasure in things usually enjoyed; decreased energy; feelings of worthlessness or guilt; difficulty concentrating or thinking; and thoughts of death or suicide, or suicidal attempts. According to DSM-III, the diagnosis does not apply when the syndrome is superimposed on certain psychiatric conditions (i.e., schizophrenia, schizophreniform disorder, paranoid disorder) or when due to an organic mental disorder or uncomplicated bereavement.

A *dysthymic disorder* is characterized by depressed mood or loss of interest in nearly all usual activities. However, the depression is not of sufficient severity or persistence to meet the criteria for major depression. According to DSM-III, the disorder must be present at least two years, and there may be periods of normal mood lasting a few days to weeks, but not exceeding a few months at a time. The diagnosis requires three associated symptoms from thirteen symptom groups, many of which are similar to, or represent less severe expressions of, the major depression symptom groups.

DSM-III does not propose a specific time frame for defining current as opposed to past disorder. We decided to consider the depressive disorder current if the patient met criteria for the disorder within the preceding twelve months and had not experienced a remission since meeting criteria. After Keller and colleagues (Keller et al., 1982b), we defined a remission as eight or more weeks during which no more than two symptoms of depression were experienced.

Second-Stage Diagnostic Assessment

The Diagnostic Interview Schedule (DIS) (Robins, Helzer, Croughan, & Ratcliff, 1981) was selected as the second-stage instrument for identifying DSM-III depressive disorders in the MOS. The DIS is relatively unique among structured diagnostic interview degree of specification of its questions, probes, and scoring system, and because of this specificity, it can be administered by lay interviewers. This was an advantage over alternative diagnostic interviews, such as the Schedule for Affective Disorders and Schizophrenia (SADS) (Endicott & Spitzer, 1978), which require clinician interviewers, because it considerably reduces the cost of the second-stage identification. Unlike the SADS, the DIS does not assess level of functioning. However, the MOS is collecting very extensive data on functioning of patients enrolled into the longitudinal panel, making it unnecessary to do so as part of the case-finding procedures.

The DIS has been used in a number of large-scale epidemiologic studies in the United States, most notably in the NIMH Epidemiologic Catchment Area program (Eaton & Kessler, 1985; Regier et al., 1984). A number of studies have been conducted to evaluate the validity of diagnoses as classified by the DIS (see review by Burke, 1986). Because there is no widely accepted gold standard for specifying diagnoses in psychiatry, and because inherent methodologic and statistical problems have made it difficult to clearly interpret the results of validity studies (see Robins, 1985), there is controversy over the validity of the DIS. Although similar controversy surrounds other diagnostic measures, it is probably heightened for the DIS because of its nontraditional methods—use of lay interviewers and assignment of diagnoses through computer algorithm rather than clinical judgement. Nevertheless, the DIS compares favorably to other diagnostic interviews in terms of its reliability and validity results, and it is superior to other instruments with respect to availability of national comparative data and feasibility of administration to large samples.

For the purposes of determining current depressive disorder for the MOS, the depression section of the DIS was modified. The modifications included expanding the information collected on depressive symptoms and episodes, using a telephone interview rather than a face to face administration, and using a computer-assisted interview. Each modification is described below.

Additional Information on Depression

First, information collected on current episodes of depression was expanded. The original DIS was structured to make lifetime diagnoses, with little information collected on current episodes. We added questions to determine the most recent occurrence of each depressive symptom and to determine whether the worst episode of depression occurring in the past year met full DSM-III criteria. Second, the instrument was modified to collect more extensive information regarding dysthymia. In the original DIS, not all dysthymia symptom groups (as specified in DSM-III) were included, nor was recency or onset of dysthymia determined. Our modifications included questions to assess all dysthymia symptom criteria, to determine whether dysthymia was ongoing in the previous year, and to determine first age of onset of dysthymia. Third, we added several questions to identify the melancholia subtype of major depression, because this distinction may be prognostically significant. Finally, we added questions regarding periods of remission in the past year, since the MOS definition of current depressive disorder requires that no eight-week remission has occurred since meeting full criteria for disorder in the past year. If such a remission occurred, questions then determined whether a new full-criterion episode of depression followed the remission.

Telephone Administration

The original DIS was designed be to given as part of a face to face interview. A telephone interview method was preferable for the MOS because of the large number of persons to be interviewed, their dispersion both within cities and across sites, and the necessity of recontacting them at home following the first-stage screening conducted in doctors' offices. We decided, therefore, to undertake a pilot study that would test the equivalence of the DIS depression instrument when given by telephone compared to a face to face interview (Wells, Burnam, Leake, & Robins, 1988).

This study was designed as a follow-up of the Los Angeles Epidemiologic Catchment Area (ECA) project, in which household adults received two face to face DIS interviews over a one-year interval. A subsample of persons completing the second (Wave II) face to face interview was selected to subsequently receive the DIS depression telephone interview. The sample was randomly selected among persons completing a Wave II interview in English between August 1984 and September 1985. The sample was stratified by presence or absence of two indicators of lifetime depression, with persons having neither depression indicator undersampled so that they formed only half of the study sample.

A total of 230 persons completed the telephone interview, representing a completion rate of 68% among eligible selected individuals. An average interval of 3 months separated the Wave II and the telephone interviews.

Table 8.1 shows the results of the study for lifetime major depression and dysthymia diagnoses. Sensitivity and specificity of the telephone interview diagnosis (using the Wave II diagnosis as the criterion) is given, as is overall agreement between Wave II and telephone diagnoses, and the kappa statistic (a measure of overall agreement corrected for chance agreement). Sensitivity and specificity are reasonably high for the combined diagnosis of major depression or dysthymia, and overall agreement is acceptable as indicated by percentage of agreement and kappa. There was no significantly detectable bias in the tendency for the telephone interview either to underdiagnose or to overdiagnose depressive disorders relative to the Wave II interview. In this subsample, the Wave II interview resulted in a lifetime prevalence rate of 21% for major depression or dysthymia, while the telephone interview resulted in a prevalence rate of 23%.

Although concordance between the Wave II and telephone interviews was reasonably high, it was far from perfect. When the Wave II and telephone interview diagnoses were discordant, this could be attributable to differences between face to face and telephone protocols, or it could have been due to one of two other factors. First, it is possible that the interval between interviews was long enough to result in new incidence of disorder, which would result in a valid Wave II negative diagnosis and a valid telephone positive diagnosis. When results were corrected for this possibility by rescoring telephone diagnoses as negative if their onset was within the interval between interviews, this resulted in trivial

Table 8.1 Test-Retest Agreement between DIS Diagnosis

	% Agreement	Sensitivity	Specificity	Kappa	Bias
Major Depression					
Wave II vs. Telephone	83	56	89	.45	No
Wave I vs. Wave II	83	52	90	.45	No
Dysthymia					
Wave II vs. Telephone	91	55	95	.48	No
Wave I vs. Wave II	90	52	95	.46	No
Either Diagnosis					
Wave II vs. Telephone	85	71	89	.57	No
Wave I vs. Wave II	81	54	89	.45	No

Note: Data are reprinted with permission from Pergamon Press (K. B. Wells et al. [1988]).

differences in concordance across interviews. A second and more plausible reason for differences between the Wave II and telephone diagnosis is the unreliability of DIS depression diagnoses generally, which would exist even when test and retest interviews are both administered face to face. To examine this possibility, we compared concordance of lifetime depression diagnoses across Wave I and Wave II interviews, both of which were given face to face. Results are shown in Table 8.1, which shows that concordance between these two interviews was very similar to that obtained when we compared the Wave II to the telephone interview. When the statistics were corrected for the one-year interval between the Wave I and Wave II interviews for major depression, the results did not substantially change (results not shown). We therefore concluded that the telephone administration of the DIS depression instrument was equivalent to a face to face administration, and that unreliability of the telephone interview was attributable largely, if not entirely, to the unreliability of the instrument generally.

Computer-Assisted Administration

For the MOS, the DIS depression instrument was administered using computer-assisted telephone interview (CATI) methods. In this technique, survey questions are presented to the telephone interviewer on a computer video screen. The interviewer reads the question to the survey participant and enters the response using the computer keyboard. The computer is programmed to make the appropriate decisions regarding the next question to be presented. Although the CATI method requires the availability of special equipment and the initial effort required to program the instrument, it offers a number of advantages: (a) interviewer errors in skip patterns are eliminated, which is a great advantage when the skip patterns are complicated as is the case with the DIS; (b) interviewer training time is decreased since the complicated skip patterns (e.g., the probe flow chart) do not require extensive explanation or practice; (c) data are entered as part of the interview process and therefore no separate data entry step is required; (d) little editing of completed interviews is required since a large source of interview error (incorrectly following skip patterns) is prevented; and (e) interviews can be conveniently monitored at a central location. A final advantage of the CATI for our purposes was that the computer could be programmed to give a diagnosis as soon as the respondent completed the interview. As a result, those meeting study criteria could be immediately invited to participate in the longitudinal study as part of the same call. This facilitated recruitment into the study and saved time and effort that would otherwise have been required if it had been necessary to recontact individuals to invite them to participate.

First-Stage Screener

The MOS design required a self-report instrument to be given to patients while visiting health providers' offices that screened for three chronic medical diseases as well as depression and also obtained data on use of services, demographic characteristics, general health, and functional status. Pretesting suggested that the total questionnaire could take no more than ten minutes to complete to achieve an acceptable response rate. Thus, the depression screener included in this short questionnaire had to be extremely brief, limited to only five to ten items. There were two additional requirements for this first-stage depression screener. First, it had to have high sensitivity to current major depression and/or dysthymia so that the MOS would obtain a sample representative of all patients with one of these depressive disorders. That is, we wished to minimize the number of false negative errors made by the screener. A sensitivity of 85% or greater was considered satisfactory. Secondly, the screener should have a relatively good positive predictive value. That is, among those screened positive, the proportion subsequently determined to have depressive disorder should be high. To keep the cost of the second-stage assessment within budget, we wanted the screener to result in at least one-third of those positive at the first-stage screening to be identified as positively diagnosed cases at the second stage.

Sensitivity and positive predictive value, however, are inversely related. Raising the threshold or cutpoint on a screener, for example, will increase sensitivity and will also increase the proportion of false positive errors. Therefore, the positive predictive value of the screener will decrease. In order to have both high sensitivity and good positive predictive value, then, the MOS screener as a continuous scale had to be highly related to the probability of having a depressive disorder.

To select items for a first-stage screener, Wells (1985) reviewed existing self-report measures of depressive symptoms and general psychological distress, including the Beck Depression Inventory (Beck, Ward, Mendelson, Mock, & Erbaugh, 1961), the General Health Questionnaire (Goldberg, 1972), the Zung Self-Assessment Scale (Zung, 1965), the Hopkins Symptoms Checklist (Kelman & Parloff, 1957), the Mental Health Inventory (Ware, Johnson, Davies-Avery, & Brook, 1979), and the Center for Epidemiologic Studies Depression Scale (Radloff, 1977). The Center for Epidemiologic Studies Depression Scale (CES-D) was selected as the basis for the screener because its test-retest reliability is acceptable (Radloff, 1977), and it is short and easy to administer. Furthermore, the CES-D has been consistently predictive of depression and other psychiatric disorders (Hough et al., 1983; Myers & Weissman, 1980; Roberts & Vernon, 1983; Weissman, Shalomskas, Pottenger, Prusoff, & Locke, 1977). Other screener scale candidates were not consistently correlated with measures of depression (the Zung Self-Assessment Scale and the Hopkins Symptoms Checklist), were developed to assess severity of depression rather than to ascertain caseness (the Beck Depression Inventory), had not been evaluated against the presence or absence of depressive disorders (the Mental Health Inventory), or were much too long (the General Health Questionnaire). Finally, the high internal reliability of the CES-D scale suggested that it could be shortened from its original twenty items to a length that was feasible for the MOS screener. Although previous studies of the CES-D suggest that it is a sensitive indicator of psychiatric disorders, they also show that it does not adequately differentiate depression from other psychiatric disorders (Myers & Weissman, 1980). We hypothesized that the overall predictive power, and therefore the positive predictive value, of the CES-D might be increased in two ways: by using an alternative scoring method and by adding items that asked about persistent periods of depressed mood. The CES-D is scored by summing values for the 20 items, each of which has values ranging from 0 to 3. This scoring strategy does not take into account the possibility that some items may be better predictors of depressive disorders than others. Differentially weighing items might therefore increase the ability of the items to predict depressive disorder, especially when the number of items is restricted to only 5 or 10. Adding items to the screener that ask about persistent periods of depressed mood may also add predictive power to the screener. DSM-III criteria require that the duration of depressed affect for major depression is at least 2 weeks and for dysthymia is at least 2 years. The CES-D, however, asks about symptoms of depression over the past week. The DIS contains 2 items that determine whether persistent periods (for 2 weeks and 2 years) of depressed affect have occurred. We hypothesized that adding these items to a CES-D based screener would increase specificity without reducing sensitivity because all persons with major depression or dysthymia must have one of these two indications to meet DSM-III criteria for depressive disorders (i.e., they represent Criteria A for major depression and dysthymia).

In order to select the final items, weights, and cutpoint of the screener to be used in the MOS, it was necessary to empirically test the relationship between the potential 20 CES-D and 2 DIS screener items and current depressive disorder as defined in the MOS and operationalized by the DIS. The empirical development and testing of the screener is described in detail by Burnam, Wells, Leake, and Landsverk (1988). Fortunately, we were able to obtain access to data from two prior studies for this purpose, each of which had survey data on both the CES-D and the DIS. These studies were the ECA survey mentioned earlier, and a study of Psychiatric Screening Scales in Primary Care (PSP) survey conducted by Hough and colleagues (1983).

Development of Screener

The total household sample from Wave I of the ECA survey ($N = 3132$) was used to develop the screener model. The specific DIS depressive disorder definitions used to develop the screener required, for major depression, a lifetime diagnosis meeting full DSM-III criteria and an episode reported in the previous year. For dysthymia, a lifetime diagnosis was required, along with 2 or more years of depressed mood that was current or persisted into the past year. For both major depression and dysthymia, evidence of continuing depressive symptoms was required, as indicated by the presence of a symptom in at least three DSM-III-defined symptom groups or the presence of a symptom in two symptom groups plus a period of depressed mood within the past month. Presence of either major depression or dysthymia according to these definitions was used as the criterion for "true" current disorder in the development of the screener.

To select the best subset of items for the screener, multiple logistic regression analysis was employed, with the 20 CES-D and 2 DIS items tested as predictors of the probability of having current depression or dysthymia. Because there were so many correlated predictors to be tested, a two-step analytic strategy was used. At the first step, an all possible subsets regression procedure was used to uncover underlying dimensions in the data and identify good sets of predictors. The best set of predictive items at step one was then submitted to a logistic regression program with stepwise backward elimination being used to produce a final reduced model. The final set of items included in this model were 6 CES-D items and the 2 DIS items. The prediction equation is given in Table 8.2. Using this equation, the screener was scored by solving for the probability of being depressed and assigning this value as a scale score for each individual.

Table 8.2. Screener Items and Unstandardized Coefficients Derived From Logistic Regression

Screener Item	Possible values	Coefficient
1. I felt depressed	0—3	1.078
2. My sleep was restless	0—3	0.185
3. I enjoyed life (reverse scored).	0—3	−0.269
4. I had crying spells.	0—3	0.329
5. I felt sad.	0—3	−0.280
6. I felt that people disliked me.	0—3	0.288
7. In the past year, have you had 2 weeks or more during which you felt sad, blue, or depressed, or lost pleasure in things that you usually cared about or enjoyed?	0—1	2.712
8. Have you had 2 years or more in your life when you felt depressed or sad most days, even if you felt okay sometimes? (If yes) Have you felt depressed or sad much of the time in the past year?	0—1	2.182

$$p = \frac{e^{A + Bx}}{1 + e^{a + Bx}}, \text{ where}$$

e = natural logarithm

$a = -6.543$

$Bx = (1.078 \times \text{Item 1}) + (0.185 \times \text{Item 2}) - (0.269 \times \text{Item 3})$
$+ (0.329 \times \text{Item 4}) - (0.280 \times \text{Item 5}) + (0.288 \times \text{Item 6})$
$+ (2.712 \times \text{Item 7}) + (2.182 \times \text{Item 8})$

Evaluation of Screener

The effectiveness of this screener score for detecting depressive disorder was evaluated in four samples. Two were subsamples of ECA survey of particular interest to the MOS: (a) those who used outpatient health care services for a physical problem in the past six months, which we call the *primary care sample;* and (b) those who used health services for a mental health problem in the past six months, or the *mental health sample.* The two other samples in which the screener was tested were from the PSP study and were therefore completely independent from the ECA sample in which the screener was developed. The PSP study interviewed a sample of patients randomly selected from those scheduled for primary care visits in an HMO in Southern California ($n = 525$). The second PSP study sample was selected from adult outpatients of a community mental health center in Los Angeles ($n = 101$). The PSP study samples are therefore also distinguished as primary care and mental health samples.

First, we examined the sensitivity, specificity, and positive predictive value of the screener for current depressive disorder as defined in the MOS study using a range of different screener cutpoints. Table 8.3 shows these results for several

Table 8.3. Screener Detection of Current Depressive Disorder as Defined in MOS Using Varying Cutpoints

	ECA		PSP	
	Primary Care (N = 1416)	Mental Health (N = 206)	Primary Care (N = 497)	Mental Health (N = 97)
Sensitivity for cutpoint				
.009	100	100	86	100
.026	93	96	86	92
.043	91	92	86	92
.060	86	89	86	92
.080	86	88	79	81
Specificity for cutpoint				
.009	83	63	75	38
.026	92	83	85	56
.043	94	86	88	62
.060	95	87	90	63
.080	96	89	91	69
Positive predictive value for cutpoint				
.009	16	28	9	37
.026	26	46	14	44
.043	33	48	17	47
.060	37	50	20	48
.080	39	55	20	49
% criterion pos.	3.0	12.5	3.0	26.5

Note: Data are reprinted with permission from Pergamon Press (K. B. Wells et al. [1988]).

cutpoints that were in a good range for maintaining high sensitivity of the screener. We decided that the cutpoint of .060 would give the best results for the MOS, given our requirements for sensitivity of at least 85% and high positive predictive values. Base rates of depressive disorder are higher in the mental health than the primary care samples, as we would expect, and the screener tends to have higher sensitivity and lower specificity in the mental health samples. In spite of reduced specificity, positive predictive power in the mental health samples is very good because of the relatively higher prevalence of disorder in this population.

We tested the screener using the standard DIS definition of current major depression and dysthymia (within the past month) and a more stringent DIS definition of current disorder suggested by Von Korff and Anthony (1982), in which individuals must have experienced the complete DSM-III symptom criteria within the past month. Table 8.4 shows these results using a screener cutpoint of .060. Of those with current depressive disorder using the standard DIS definition, only half meet the stringent definition, similar to Von Korff and Anthony's prior findings. Screener sensitivity is higher and specificity only slightly lower for the stringent compared to the standard DIS definition, suggesting that the screener is better for detecting depressive disorder during more severe or acute stages of the disorder than during periods of diminished or residual symptomatology. We tested the ability of the screener to detect depressive disorders across different prevalence periods that can be defined using the DIS: lifetime, within the past year, within the past six months, and within the past month. Table 8.5 shows the results of this analysis when current prevalence periods were defined according

Table 8.4. Screener Detection of Depressive Disorder Within the Past Month Using Standard and Stringent DIS Definition*

	ECA			PSP	
	Total (N = 3015)	Primary Care (N = 1416)	Mental Health (N = 206)	Primary Care (N = 501)	Mental Health (N = 97)
Sensitivity					
Stringent	89	96	94	86	94
Standard	72	70	75	71	87
Specificity					
Stringent	95	95	85	90	58
Standard	96	96	87	91	65
Positive Predictive Value					
Stringent	23	24	37	20	32
Standard	41	40	52	33	54
% Criterion Positive					
Stringent	1.5	1.8	8.7	2.8	17.5
Standard	3.4	4.0	15.5	5.6	32.0

* Screener Cutpoint = .060

Note: Data are reprinted with permission from Pergamon Press (K. B. Wells et al. [1988]).

Table 8.5. Screener Detection of Depressive Disorder Defined for Lifetime and Three Current Prevalence Periods Using Stringent DIS Definition

	ECA						PSP			
	Total (N = 3015)		Primary Care (N = 1416)		Mental Health (N = 206)		Primary Care (N = 501)		Mental Health (N = 97)	
	.060	.009	.060	.009	.060	.009	.060	.009	.060	.009
Sensitivity										
Lifetime	37	71	34	72	47	80	41	72	75	91
Past year	67	95	61	95	74	96	68	88	87	100
Past 6 mos.	74	9	70	93	83	96	76	91	90	100
Past month	89	98	96	100	94	100	86	93	94	100
Specificity										
Lifetime	97	89	97	88	88	70	93	81	79	52
Past year	96	86	95	84	85	63	91	76	67	46
Past 6 mos.	96	85	95	83	86	62	91	76	69	41
Past month	95	84	95	82	85	61	90	75	58	34
Positive predictive value										
Lifetime	36	40	33	45	47	52	48	38	82	71
Past year	36	18	35	20	43	28	28	16	66	54
Past 6 mos.	31	14	31	15	43	25	26	14	56	44
Past month	23	9	24	9	37	20	20	10	32	24
% criterion positive										
Lifetime	9.6		12.2		29.1		14.2		56.7	
Past year	3.2		4.0		13.1		5.0		39.2	
Past 6 mos.	2.5		3.1		11.7		4.2		32.0	
Past month	1.5		1.8		8.7		2.8		17.5	

Note: Data are reprinted with permission from Pergamon Press (K. B. Wells et al. [1988]).

to the stringent DIS definition, but similar variations by time periods were found when using the standard DIS definition. Using the cutpoint of .060, selected for the MOS study, sensitivity of the screener is best for more recent diagnoses, and specificity drops only slightly from lifetime to more recent diagnoses. Thus, it appears that the screener is best for detecting very recent disorder. We lowered the cutpoint of the screener to determine if a reduced threshold would better screen for longer prevalence periods. The table shows the screener's ability to detect depressive disorder using a .009 cutpoint. With this lower cutpoint, sensitivity reached more acceptable levels even for lifetime prevalence. However specificity dropped, especially for current prevalence periods. Overall, a cutpoint of .009 resulted in quite good performance of the screener for detection of lifetime, but not current, depressive disorder. Up to this point, we have shown the ability of the screener to detect the diagnosis of either major depression or dysthymia. One remaining question is whether the screener is relatively better at detecting one versus the other of these depressive disorders. Dysthymic disorder, for example, might be less effectively detected, since it tends to be less severe.

Table 8.6 shows the ability of the screener to detect the specific disorders of lifetime major depression and lifetime dysthymia, using the cutpoint of .009. The screener tended to have somewhat higher sensitivity for dysthymia than for major depression, while specificities and positive predictive values were similar for the two types of depressive disorder. The results were similar when we examined recent diagnoses of major depression and dysthymia.

Finally, we examined the ability of the screener to detect other noneffective psychiatric disorders relative to its ability to detect depressive disorder. Table 8.7 presents the results when persons with lifetime major depression or dysthymia (with or without manic episodes) were compared to persons with any other lifetime nonaffective DIS/DSM-III psychiatric disorder. Those with both a depressive disorder and a nonaffective disorder were excluded from this analysis.

Each disorder category was compared to those with no disorder, resulting in identical screener specificities for depressive and nonaffective disorders. The screener had much lower sensitivity for nonaffective relative to depressive disorder. This resulted in a much greater proportion of those with nonaffective disorder being incorrectly classified than those with depressive disorder, as can be seen by examining the false-negative rates. Although the positive predictive value of the screener for nonaffective disorder exceeds to a moderate extent that of affective disorders, the high positive predictive value can be explained by the higher base rates of nonaffective disorders relative to the depressive disorders. These results suggest that the instrument is a much better screener for depressive disorders specifically than for psychiatric disorder generally.

Table 8.6. Screener Detection of Lifetime Major Depression and Lifetime Dysthymia*

	ECA			PSP	
	Total (N = 3051)	Primary Care (N = 1416)	Mental Health (N = 206)	Primary Care (N = 501)	Mental Health (N = 97)
Sensitivity					
Major depression	65	66	76	67	100
Dysthymia	90	90	89	85	92
Specificity					
Major depression	87	85	65	78	34
Dysthymia	87	85	62	78	35
Positive predictive value					
Major depression	29	32	41	25	24
Dysthymia	25	26	26	26	33
% criterion positive					
Major depression	7.0	9.5	24.0	10.3	48.5
Dysthymia	4.7	5.7	13.1	8.3	25.8

* Screener cutpoint = .009

Note: Data are reprinted with permission from Pergamon Press (K. B. Wells et al. [1988]).

Table 8.7. Screener Detection of Lifetime Affective Disorder Only and Lifetime Nonaffective Disorders Only Versus No Lifetime Disorders*

	Total (N = 2074) (N = 2697)	ECA		PSP	
		Primary Care (N = 934) (N = 1227)	Mental Health (N = 91) (N = 141)	Primary Care (N = 327) (N = 421)	Mental Health (N = 21) (N = 37)
Sensitivity					
Affective	69	75	84	69	100
Nonaffective	19	18	33	22	58
Specificity					
Affective	92	90	74	83	72
Nonaffective	92	90	74	83	72
Positive predictive value					
Affective	32	36	46	28	73
Nonaffective	45	42	55	34	83
False negative rate					
Affective	2	2	5	44	20
Nonaffective	25	27	46	28	58
% criterion positive					
Affective	5.3	6.9	20.9	8.9	47.7
Nonaffective	27.2	29.1	48.9	29.2	70.3

* Cutpoint = .009

Note: Data are reprinted with permission Pergamon Press (K. B. Wells et al. [1988]).

Conclusions

Using the two-stage case identification methods that we have described, we were able to identify and enroll 424 patients with current depressive disorder (who also met other study inclusion criteria) into the longitudinal panel of the MOS. These depressed patients were identified from among 25,000 patients of primary care and mental health providers across different health care systems and in different U.S. cities. This case identification method has the advantage of being relatively easy and inexpensive to implement, and yet results in the identification of most persons with clinically significant depressive disorder. A strategy such as the one described here is therefore particularly useful for detecting depressive disorder in populations in which the prevalence of the disorder is low. Not only would it be a cost-effective method of detection not only in studies of large samples from primary care or community settings, but it might also be used by primary health care providers as an efficient means of detecting depressive disorder to more appropriately treat or refer their patients. The pilot studies we conducted to develop and evaluate the components of this two-stage case identification procedure suggest that it is possible to significantly modify existing depression assessment tools to make them more usable for large scale policy studies like the MOS and for other situations in which large populations with low prevalence of depressive disorder must be screened. At the first stage, we were able to use the CES-D and two items from the DIS to develop a very brief (eight-item) screener that had high sensitivity and good positive predictive value for current depressive disorder. The coefficients derived from our logistic regression model suggested that, in fact, we might be able to reduce the screener to four items with little loss of information. The fact that we were able to use so few items and still effectively screen for depression is due in large part to the inclusion of two DIS items in the screener. Because these items ask about persistent periods of depressed mood that correspond to the mood criteria for major depression and dysthymia of DSM-III, they may more effectively discriminate between normal depressed mood and clinically significant depression than traditional screener items such as those in the CES-D.

At the second stage, we modified the DIS depression instrument so that it could be administered by telephone. The telephone administration greatly reduced the cost of administering the DIS as the second-stage diagnostic assessment in the MOS. Using the CATI technology in concert with telephone interviewing added advantages such as reduced interviewer training, reduced interviewer error, and direct data entry onto a computer file. In addition, since CATI could be programmed to give an immediate diagnosis at the termination of the interview, the interviewer could recruit positive cases into the longitudinal panel at the end of the interview, which saved subsequent recruitment calls. The DIS was further modified to collect more extensive information on symptoms of dysthymia and melancholia and on current episodes of disorder. These modifications, while relatively minor in terms of their impact on the structure and style of the DIS, were crucial for operationalizing current depressive disorder in a way that had relevance for the MOS.

The brief screener used as the first-stage of the MOS case identification procedure may not be suitable as a screening measure when using other definitions of depressive disorder. The screener was tailored to the specific definition of depressive disorder used in the MOS—DSM-III major depression or dysthymia emphasizing a recent episode and continuing symptoms. The screener detects very recent and acute depressive disorder better than past or residual disorder. It detects both dysthymia and major depression and may therefore not be appropriate for studies in which major depression must be discriminated from dysthymia. Other self-report symptom scales, however, would seem likely to share this inability to discriminate major depression from dysthymia. The overall effectiveness of our screener may in part be the result of including those with dysthymia in the definition of depression. Finally, we do not know how the screener is related to depression defined according to other diagnostic criteria. As a general recommendation, we think it is important for researchers and practitioners to consider carefully the definition of depression appropriate for their purposes (e.g., depressive disorders covered, diagnostic criteria, time frame, and current severity) and to develop or select a screener that is closely related to and predictive of that specific definition. One limitation of the analyses used to develop and test the first-stage screener is that the screener instrument and the DIS were not independently administered. This was due to practical constraints that necessitated our reliance upon existing survey data in which the CES-D and the DIS were administered as part of a single instrument. We would not expect this problem to substantially influence the findings regarding the CES-D items in the screener. However, the two DIS items that were included in the screener were also used to define the criterion measure. In a true two-stage case identification procedure, where the screener and DIS diagnostic instrument are independently administered, we would expect a high correlation between the two DIS items from a first to a repeat administration, but not a perfect correlation since some measurement error will exist. If the test-retest reliability of these two items is high, as suggested by the results of a study by Wells et al. (1988), then independent administration of the screener and the DIS diagnostic instruments would not be expected to change our conclusions regarding the effectiveness of the screener.

A final caution regarding the first-stage screener we have developed: It has been examined only in a community household population and among primary care and mental health specialty outpatients. We do not know whether it would operate similarly among inpatient populations or those with specific chronic diseases.

In sum, we have found that existing measures of depressive symptoms and disorders can be modified to develop a case finding strategy that is clinically valid and feasible for a large-scale health policy study. It appears to be particularly important to consider the particular group of depression disorders to be studied, the time frame for defining caseness, matching screening characteristics to definitional criteria, and using scoring techniques that maximize the predictive value of screening items.

References

Beck, A. T., Ward, C. H., Mendelson, M., Mock, J. & Erbaugh, J. (1961). An inventory for measuring depression. *Archives of General Psychiatry, 4,* 561–571.

Burke, J. D. (1986). Diagnostic interview categorization by the Diagnostic Interview Schedule (DIS): A comparison with other methods of assessment. In J. E. Barrett & R. M. Rose (eds.), *Mental disorder in the community: Progress and challenge* (pp. 255–285). New York: Guilford Press.

Burnam, M. A., Wells, K. B., Leake, B., & Landsverk, J. (1988). Development of a brief screening instrument for detecting depressive disorders. *Medical care, 26,* 775–789.

Dohrenwend, B. P., & Shrout, P. E. (1981). Toward the development of a two-stage procedure for case identification and classification in psychiatric epidemiology. In R. G. Simmon (ed.), *Research in community and mental health,* vol. 2 (pp. 295–323). Greenwich, CT: JAI Press.

Eaton, W. W., & Kessler, L. G. (eds.) (1985). *Epidemiologic field methods in psychiatry: The NIMH Epidemiologic Catchment Area Program.* Orlando: Academic Press.

Endicott, J., & Spitzer, R. L. (1978). A diagnostic interview–The Schedule for Affective Disorders and Schizophrenia. *Archives of General Psychiatry, 35,* 837–844.

Goldberg, D. P. (1972). *The detection of psychiatric illness by questionnaire: A technique for the identification and assessment of nonpsychotic psychiatric illness.* London: Oxford University.

Hoeper, E. W., Ncyz, P. D., Cleary, P. D., Regier, D. A., & Goldberg, I. D. (1979). Estimated prevalence of RDC mental disorder in primary medical care. *International Journal of Mental Health, 8,* 6–15.

Hough, R. L., Landsverk, J. A., Stone, J. D., Jacobson, G. F., Forsythe, A. B., & McGranahan, C. (1983). *Psychiatric screening scale project: Final report* (Contract No. DB–81–0036). Bethesda: National Institute of Mental Health.

Keller, M. B., Klerman, G. L., Lavori, P. W., Fawcett, J. A., Coryell, W., & Endicott, J. (1982). Treatment received by depressed patients. *Journal of the American Medical Association, 248,* 1848–1855.

Keller, M. B., Lavori, P. W., Endicott, J., Coryell, W., & Klerman, G. J. (1983). Double depression two-year followup. *American Journal of Psychiatry, 140,* 689–694.

Keller, M. B., Lavori, P. W., Lewis, C. E., & Klerman, G. L. (1983). Predictors of relapse in major depressive disorder. *Journal of the American Medical Association, 250,* 3299–3304.

Keller, M. B., Shapiro, R. W., Lavori, P. W., & Wolfe, N. (1982a). Relapse in major depressive disorder–Analysis with the Life Table and Regression Models. *Archives of General Psychiatry, 39,* 911–915.

Keller, M. B., Shapiro, R. W., Lavori, P. W., & Wolfe, N. (1982b). Recovery in major depressive disorder–Analysis with the Life Table and Regression models. *Archives of General Psychiatry, 39,* 905–910.

Kelman, H. C., & Parlof, M. B. (1957). Interrelations among three criteria of improvement in group therapy: Comfort, effectiveness, and self-awareness. *Journal of Abnormal & Social Psychology, 54,* 281–288.

Myers, J. L., & Weissman, M. M. (1980). Use of a self-report symptom scale to detect depression in a community sample. *American Journal of Psychiatry, 137,* 1081–1084.

Radloff, L. S. (1977). A self-report depression scale for research in the general population. *Applied Psychological Measurement, 1,* 385–401.

Regier, D. A., Myers, J. L., Kramer, M., Robins, L. N., Blazer, D. G., Hough, R. L., Eaton, W. W., & Locke, B. Z. (1984). The NIMH Epidemiologic Catchment Area Program: Historical context, major objectives, and study population characteristics. *Archives of General Psychiatry, 41,* 934–941.

Roberts, R. E., & Vernon, S. W. (1983). The Center for Epidemiological Studies Depression scale: Its use in a community sample. *American Journal of Psychiatry, 140,* 41–46.

Robins, L. N. (1985). Epidemiology: Reflections on testing the validity of psychiatric interviews. *Archives of General Psychiatry, 42,* 918.

Robins, L. N., Helzer, J. E., Croughan, J., & Ratcliff, K. S. (1981). National Institute of Mental Health Diagnostic Interview Schedule: Its history, characteristics, and validity. *Archives of General Psychiatry, 38,* 381–389.

Robins, L. N., Helzer, J. E., Weismann, M. M., Orvashel, H., Gruenberg, E., Burke, J. D., & Regier, D. A. (1984). Lifetime prevalence of specific psychiatric disorders in three sites. *Archives of General Psychiatry, 41,* 949–958.

Schulberg, H. C., Saul, M., McClelland, M., Ganguli, M., Christy, W., & Frank, R. (1985).

Assessing depression in primary medical and psychiatric practices. *Archives of General Psychiatry, 42,* 1164–1170.

Von Korff, M. R., & Anthony, J. C. (1982). The NIMH Diagnostic Interview Schedule modified to record current mental status. *Journal of Affective Disorder, 4,* 365–371.

Ware, J. C., Jr., Johnson, S. A., Davies-Avery, A., Brook, R. H. (1979). *Conceptualization and measurement of health for adults in the Health Insurance Study: Volume 3, mental health* (Report No. R–1987/3-HEW). Santa Monica: Rand Corporation.

Weissman, M. M., Shalomskas, D., Pottenger, M., Prusoff, B. A., & Locke, B. Z. (1977). Assessing depressive symptoms in five psychiatric populations: A validation study. *American Journal of Epidemiology, 106,* 203–214.

Wells, K. B. (1985). *Depression as a tracer condition for the national study of medical care outcomes* (Report No. R–3293-RWJ/HJK). Santa Monica: Rand Corporation.

Wells, K. B., Burnam, M. A., Leake, B., Robins, L. N. (1988). Agreement between face to face and telephone administered versions of the depression section of the NIMH Diagnostic Interview Schedule. *Journal of Psychiatric Research, 22,* 207–220.

Zung, W. W. K. (1965). Self-rating depression scale. *Archives of General Psychiatry, 12,* 63–70.

9

Studies in the Screening and Feedback of Depression and Anxiety in Primary Care Outpatient Populations

Joel Yager and Lawrence S. Linn

The reported prevalence of symptoms and diagnoses of depression in primary care outpatient medical settings has varied from about 4% to 30% in various studies (Hoeper, Nycz, Regier, Goldberg, & Hankin, 1980; Rodin & Voshart, 1986; Schulberg et al., 1985; Zung, Magill, Moore, & George, 1983). Differences among the estimated prevalence rates have been attributed to the nature of case-finding or screening instruments, differences in cut-off points for depression used on these screening instruments, the use in some studies of structured diagnostic interviews rather than self-report instruments, and differences in the patient populations themselves (Rodin & Voshart 1986; Schulberg et al., 1985). Many questions regarding the true prevalence of depression seen in primary care settings remain. Even more fundamental, important unanswered questions concern relationships of symptoms and syndromes of depression to medical illnesses and their treatments, the concept of *masked depression,* and the very concept of *depression* itself as a group of diagnostic entities (Katon, 1984).

Studies concerning how often the diagnosis of and interventions for depression are made in primary care settings have also focused on physician factors in awareness, their knowledge about depression, their notation of depression in medical records, and their notation of the specific interventions employed (Daniels, Linn, Ward, & Leake, 1986; Jencks, 1985; Keller et al., 1982; Magill & Zung 1982; Uhlenhuth, 1982; Zung et al., 1983).

This chapter will review several studies that we conducted with screening instruments in a primary care medical clinic population, initially to assess the prevalence of depression and subsequently of anxiety as well (Linn & Yager, 1980, 1982, 1984; Yager & Linn, 1981). We examined the immediate effect of feedback regarding these conditions on physicians' clinical behavior, and we examined effects of being diagnosed as depressed on the medical care of patients during the ensuing year.

Background

Several studies have examined the general use of data feedback, including psychological screening, as a means of modifying physician performance in the work setting (Brody, 1980; Greene & Simmons, 1976). In these studies new patients are asked to complete standard psychological tests that measure such syndromes as depression and anxiety. The results are immediately given to the physician much like information regarding weight, temperature, and blood pressure. One such effort, the report by Moore and colleagues (Moore, Silimperi, & Bobula, 1978), provided the background for our research. These researchers attempted to determine whether a depression-screening questionnaire in a family medicine practice would alter the degree to which physicians noted depression as a problem in their patients' medical records. All patients 20 to 60 years old (n = 212) seen during an eight-week period were asked to complete the Zung Self-Rating Depression Scale (SDS) (Zung, 1965) before being seen by a physician. The scale was scored immediately, and patients who scored 50 or greater (thought to represent at least mild depression) were randomly assigned to two groups (n = 96). For the experimental group (n = 50) physicians were informed by a note attached to the medical chart that the patient had been found to be either mildly or severely depressed. For the control group (n = 46) physicians received only a note indicating that the patients had been screened for depression but without specific results. The charts of all 96 patients were audited to determine whether any notations were made regarding depression. Notations were found in 56% of charts in the experimental group and 22% in the control group. These investigators concluded that use of a depression-screening instrument could significantly increase physician diagnosis of such a problem.

Although the findings of the Moore study were noteworthy, several limitations in its design indicated a need for replication, modification, and extension. First, in the Moore study, charts were audited only for patients with Zung scores of 50 or greater; the other patients (the majority for the study period) were excluded from analysis, so that the frequency of notation of depression for this group of patients was unknown. Second, because physicians seeing patients assigned to the "control group" were told that their patient visits had been screened for depression, it could be argued that these physicians comprised an additional experimental group, whereas an appropriate control group, which should have been told nothing about depression, was absent from the study. Third, all patients seen in the clinic were included in the study, regardless of whether or not the physicians had seen them previously. The relative percentages of follow-up visits versus new patients may have influenced the notations of depression during the study period. Finally, the study concerned only whether or not depression was noted as a problem. It did not examine treatment.

Study no. 1

To extend the work of Moore and coworkers (Moore et al., 1978) to a general medical population, we first undertook a study of the relative effects of sensitization and screening on the frequency of medical record notations of depression as well as on notations regarding treatment. Also, since about 30% of patient encounters in our clinic were with physicians who had participated in an intensive course in interpersonal skills training and the psychosocial aspects of patient care, it was possible for us to examine whether or not exposure to such course work results in differences in the frequency of recording depression or in treatment.

Another aspect of our study was related to the need to identify quickly administered instruments that might be used to study how well physicians and patients agree about the nature and severity of presenting problems. This need is underscored by several studies. Starfield et al. (1979) found that when physicians and patients agreed on what the problems were, physicians were more likely to investigate them, and patients were more likely to report improvement. Francis, Korsch, and Morris (1969) also found that such patient-provider agreement generally yielded a higher likelihood of patient cooperation with treatment. Thus, since high agreement may lead to better health outcomes (Lazare, Eisenthal, & Wasserman, 1975), we attempted to develop a way to assess physician-patient agreement about patient depression in connection with the Zung SDS and to study how physician-patient agreement related to diagnosis.

Patient Participants

The study was conducted during a six-week period beginning August 1979 in the UCLA Medical Ambulatory Care Center in which all house staff and faculty members in the Department of Medicine see general medical outpatients. All new English-speaking patients were asked, prior to seeing their physicians, to participate until a sample size of 150 was attained. These patients were randomly assigned to one of six groups (five treatment and one control). Only nine patients refused to participate and were replaced by the next new patients to arrive. A new patient was defined as a person who had not previously seen the physician with whom he or she had an appointment. Therefore, the patient was not required to be new to the clinic or institution, only to the physician. The median age of the patient sample was 56 years, 71% of the subjects were female, 40% were from a racial minority group (two-thirds black and one-third Latino), and 82% of visits were related to chronic disease.

Physician Participants

The physician group consisted of interns, residents, and faculty members of the Department of Internal Medicine. Of the 150 patient encounters, 40% were with interns, 22% with first-year residents, 21% with second-year residents, and 17% with faculty members or fellows. Of these encounters 30% were with house staff or faculty members in the General Internal Medicine Program, in which interpersonal skills and the psychosocial aspects of patient care were stressed. Although sampling was determined by a random assignment of patients, the physician sample that resulted very closely approximated the distribution of physicians in the two programs (i.e., General Internal Medicine, in which psychosocial aspects were emphasized, and the Traditional Internal Medicine Program) and across all levels of training: Of the 85 physicians in the clinic, 78% participated in the study. The mean number of patient encounters per physician was 2.3. Therefore, the encounters seemed representative for the physicians practicing in the clinic.

Design and Instruments

Patients who signed consent forms indicating their willingness to participate in the study were randomly assigned to one of six groups.

Group I

Patients were first asked to complete the Zung Self-Rating Depression Scale (SDS) (Hedlund & Vieweg, 1979; Zung, 1965, 1968, 1969, 1971, 1972; Zung & Wonnacott, 1970). A research assistant read items to patients who were unable to read or complete the instrument. The scale was scored immediately upon completion, photocopied, and attached to the chart with a note that provided the physician with the patient's adjusted scale score and a key of norms to interpret the findings. This information was given to each doctor before the encounter began. Immediately after each patient encounter, the physician was asked to complete the Global Depression Index (GDI), a ten-rung ladder in which the top rung represented feeling extremely sad, down-hearted, and blue, based on the physician's perception during the interview of how the patient was feeling. Therefore, for patients assigned to this group, information about depression was provided to the physician prior to seeing the patient and requested from the physician prior to charting the visit in the patient's medical records.

Group II

As in Group I, patients were asked to complete the SDS. However, SDS scores were not given to the physician until after the encounter was completed (but before the doctor wrote in the medical record). In this group, immediately after each encounter, the research associate first asked the physician to rate the patient's level of depression by use of the GDI. After this was completed, the doctor was given feedback from the SDS screening.

Group III

Patients in this group also completed the SDS, and results were given to the physician before the encounter. However, physicians were not asked to rate the patients' level of depression on the GDI.

Group IV

Patients in this group were asked to complete the SDS, but results were given to the physicians only after the patient encounter was terminated. As in Group III the physicians were not asked to rate the patients' level of depression on the GDI.

Group V

Patients in this group were not screened for depression. However, after each visit was completed, the physicians were asked to evaluate the patients' level of depression on the GDI. Thus, physicians were sensitized to depression but received no feedback from screening.

Group VI

Patients in this group were not screened, and physicians were not asked to evaluate their depression.

Chart Audit

Shortly after the patient visits, medical records of the visits were reviewed for notations regarding depression and its treatment. In addition, the patients' age, sex, race, and the stated reason for the visit were recorded. Details of the statistical analyses of this study are reported elsewhere (Linn & Yager, 1980; Yager & Linn, 1981).

Summary of Study no. 1 Results

Depressive Symptoms

Of the 100 patients screened for depression, 42% endorsed symptoms of depression with a frequency higher than the normal range. Although this figure was derived by sampling only new patients seeking care in our medical clinic, the percentage is strikingly similar to that of Moore's study at a family medicine center. In Moore's investigation, 45% of patients had depression scores outside the normal range. Clearly, such symptoms are highly prevalent among patients who seek outpatient medical care in university medical centers.

In spite of the high frequency of symptoms of depression among unscreened patients ($n = 50$), notation of depression in the medical record was found for only 8%. Therefore, for first encounters with complex medical patients, internists are not likely to recognize depression or consider it a problem worthy of notation.

Without some external cue, depression in this population is not usually recorded as a problem.

Notation of Depression and Its Treatment

Screening for depression by means of Zung's SDS, together with feedback and interpretation of the results to physicians, increased the incidence of notation of depression from 8% (Groups V and VI) to 25% (Groups I—IV). Providing the results of screening after the patient visit (Groups II and IV) resulted in essentially the same effect on notation of depression as providing the information at the beginning of the encounter (Groups I and III). Sensitization of physicians (asking for the physician's opinion about the patient's level of depression via the GDI) alone has no more influence on the notation of depression than doing nothing at all. However, when such sensitization is combined with screening and feedback, notation increases from 18% (Groups III and IV) to 32% (Groups I and II).

Although the prevalence of symptoms of depression in the patients sampled was high, notation regarding treatment for depression was not. Only 12% of the total sample received any advice or treatment for depression during the visit, and only 14% of the 100 screened patients were treated. Although patients who had the highest depression scores were those most likely to be noted in the record, screening and feedback alone did not lead to the initiation of treatment. High scores on the Zung SDS scale do not, however, automatically predict the clinical syndrome or diagnosis of depression; correlations between Zung scores and clinically diagnosed full-blown depression have been found to range from .40 to .60 (Zung, 1968). Similarly, the fact that depression was noted for 14% of patients whose SDS scores fell within the normal range suggests that the Zung self-report scale does not capture all information used by physicians to assess depression.

Nevertheless, the low frequency of medical record notations regarding treatment of depression may indicate a general lack of awareness and/or of attention to such issues by internal medicine house staff and faculty. Biases against such perceptions and related activities may occur for several reasons: physicians may lack knowledge about assessment and intervention techniques; such symptoms may be viewed as unpleasant and better avoided; patients' medical problems may be considered more important and are given higher priority; assessment and treatment of such symptoms may require more frequent visits than permitted by a half-day a week clinic rotation; counseling also may be perceived as being time consuming and as having little educational value; the treatment of such symptoms with medication may be viewed as problematic; and such symptoms may be thought to have a high probability of disappearing on their own once medical complaints are brought under control.

Overall, the findings suggest that medical clinics may wish to employ simple ways of alerting physicians and other primary care providers about commonly undocumented patient complaints and needs. Physicians are very responsive to specific patient information presented in the form of laboratory test results. The use of the Zung SDS scale, therefore, seems to be very effective in alerting physicians to consider depression as a potential patient problem that may need attention.

Physician Training

There were no significant differences between notations regarding depression and whether or not the physicians in the sample had been exposed to interpersonal skills and psychosocial medicine training. However, caution should be used in drawing conclusions from this finding. Although recognition and treatment of depression occurred at the same rate among physicians in both medicine programs, the quality of care actually rendered may have differed. Finally, physicians in the General Internal Medicine program tended to rate their patients as more depressed than did physicians in the Traditional Medicine residency program. While this may reflect a greater sensitivity in the former group toward the recognition of patient affect, the two residency groups did not differ in their medical record notations regarding depression; sensitivity to patient mood was not translated into action as measured by chart review.

Patient-Physician Agreement

Physicians and their patients were generally in close agreement on their global assessment of depression, as indexed by the GDI, with an average discrepancy of 2.2 points on a 10-point scale. GDI scores were significantly correlated with patient's SDS scores and with the notation of depression by physicians in the medical record.

The correlations between physicians' and patients' GDIs and SDS are consistent with findings of other studies (Zung, 1969). They suggest that a ladder-shaped, ten-point self-rating scale for depression may be a simple, useful screening device to enable primary care physicians to become aware of their patients' moods. The data also suggest that notation is a function of both the physician's awareness and judgment and that the latter is quite congruent with how patients perceive themselves.

The Zung SDS has been criticized as a measure of depression in that the endorsement of certain of its items may actually be due to the reporting of symptoms related to syndromes other than depression, such as medical problems (Blumenthal & Dielman, 1975). The high percentage of scores in the depressive ranges may therefore reflect both true depression and also the high prevalence of somatic symptoms common to both serious medical problems and depressive syndromes (e.g., sleep and appetite disturbances). The finding that minority group patients were less likely to report depressive symptoms on the Zung SDS but that they were no different on the GDI may suggest that the interpretation and meaning of items on the Zung scale may vary with ethnic background or its socioeconomic correlates (Blumenthal & Dielman, 1975).

To summarize, this study provided evidence suggesting that internists and their new outpatients are in reasonably close agreement on the degree to which patients feel sad or depressed. Yet notations about mood or depression in the medical record occurred for only 71% of patients rated as highly sad on the GDI. Furthermore, such notation occurred for fewer than half of those patients whose Zung scores put them in the moderately to severely depressed range, and mention of intervention was made only for about 40% of such cases. While many would agree that internal medicine house staff should perhaps not initiate medical treatment for depression on a first visit before obtaining more information and consultation, the present findings suggest that additional education and the use of screening methods to alert primary care physicians about such complaints are helpful.

Study no. 2

Several studies indicate that outpatient mental health services provided to symptomatic patients may result in a significant decrease in subsequent utilization of general medical services (Follette & Cummings, 1967; Goldberg, Krantz, & Locke, 1980). Thus, the process by which primary care physicians identify psychiatric and psychosocial problems, the decisions that they make about them, and their relationship to subsequent patient and physician behaviors warrant additional research. In this light, as a second study we conducted a further examination and a one-year follow-up of the patients who participated in study no. 1.

In study no. 2 we further examined:

1. Physician behavior during the initial visit as reflected by the number of laboratory tests and medical procedures ordered and medications prescribed;
2. Chart notation of depression in subsequent encounters;
3. Patient use of institutional facilities during the year following screening, as indicated by the number and types of visits made, and providers seen; and,
4. Physician behavior as indicated by the total number of tests and procedures ordered, and drugs prescribed.

The patient and physician sample were those described for study No. 1. Retrieval of the medical records for the 150 patients entered into the initial study resulted in 10% ($n = 15$) of the charts being unobtainable. Thus, the present report is based upon the remaining 135 patients. The 15 missing charts were randomly distributed across all six patient groups.

Chart Audit

The period of examination for this study was the twelve months following the date of patient entry in the first study. The initial visit, which had previously been audited for notations regarding depression and its treatment, was reexamined for two additional factors: the number of laboratory tests and medical procedures ordered and the number of medications prescribed. Each subsequent visit was audited for the following information: total number of outpatient visits, hospitalizations, and visits to the emergency room; total number of tests ordered and medications prescribed; and the total number of notations regarding depression. Audits were performed by a skilled medical records technician supervised by the investigators.

For a detailed description of statistical analyses see Linn and Yager (1982).

Summary of Results of Study no. 2

To begin, as with the first study, the follow-up study has several limitations. First, it examined only the relationship between the prevalence of depressive symptoms and subsequent patient and physician behavior. It was not a study of the incidence of depression per se. Although a longitudinal design was employed, there was no way of knowing the course of the depression when these symptoms were measured. That is, neither the time of onset nor the pattern of development were known, nor do we know whether or not these symptoms changed after the initial date of measurement. Therefore, statements about the effect of notification about "depression" on patient or physician behavior should be made with extreme caution.

A second limitation was that patient utilization of services before the initial visit was not studied. However, since all patients were seen by their physicians for the first time and since patients were randomly assigned into screened and unscreened groups, it was assumed that the effect of previous patterns of health service utilization also should have been randomized and, therefore, should not have affected the results. However, a more important concern is that only utilization of our own medical surgical and emergency room institutional services was investigated. Care sought outside the university hospital and clinics or in the Department of Psychiatry located in an administratively separate hospital was not studied, and this must be kept in mind when interpreting the findings.

Notation of Depression

For the patient sample as a whole, depression was infrequently mentioned in the medical record over the twelve-month study period. Only 10% of charts of the 135 patients contained such a notation, although the prevalence of depression scores beyond the normal range among screened patients was initially found in

42% of the sample. However, there was a high correlation between subsequent notations of depression and notations made at the time of screening, provided that feedback about depression to the physician was made before the encounter. This pattern also characterized notations regarding treatment or referral of depression as well. Therefore, screening and the timing of feedback seem to have an important relationship to physician behavior around the diagnosis of depression. The majority of notation behavior clearly resulted from screening and feedback. Among patients for whom depression was not noted on the original visit, subsequent depression was noted in only three patients. In spite of its prevalence, problems of depression are not frequently noted without extra prompting by physicians who work in ambulatory care settings.

Curvilinearity

One interesting finding in this study was the curvilinear rather than linear relationship between the degree of depression and utilization of health services. Patients with mild depression sought care most frequently and were seen by more providers. Patients in the moderate depression range sought care more frequently and were seen by more providers than patients whose depression scores were in the normal range. The lowest utilization rate, however, was found in the severely depressed patient group. Because of small samples in each category of depressed patients, this finding is certainly in need of further study. However, it points out that researchers should be cautioned not to make assumptions of linearity in their conceptualizations about depression or in the statistical techniques employed to analyze their data.

Timing of Feedback

For mildly or moderately depressed patients, the timing of feedback dramatically affected physician behavior on the initial visit. Significantly fewer laboratory tests or procedures were ordered when feedback was provided before the encounter with the physician (mean = 2.85 tests compared with 8.12 tests).

The timing of feedback on the initial visit for mildly and moderately depressed patients was also significantly related to subsequent physician and patient behavior. When compared with the "feedback after" group, patients in the "feedback before" group made three times more visits to the institution, saw twice as many physicians, made almost twice as many visits to their initial physician, had three times the number of tests ordered, and had twice as many medications prescribed for them.

Subsequent medical record notation of depression during the ensuing twelve months was most likely to occur among the depressed patient group where feedback was provided to the physician before the initial encounter. Notations regarding treatment of depression also were more frequent for this patient group.

The timing of feedback made only a small difference in the number of tests the physician ordered on the initial visit for patients who scored in the normal range of depression scores.

The timing of feedback for patients in the normal range of depression scores also seemed to bear little relationship to the total number of visits made, providers seen, tests ordered, or medications prescribed.

This research strongly indicates that careful attention must be paid to when and how results of screening are presented to physicians and other providers. In general, fewer tests and procedures will be ordered when the results of screening for depression are provided before the encounter begins. The dramatic difference in the number of such tests ordered for the depressed patient group has several potential implications. First, alerting a primary care physician in advance that a new patient to be seen might be significantly depressed seems to alter the physician's perception and judgment of the patient's problems, reducing the number of tests and procedures ordered. On the other hand, physicians who see depressed patients without recognizing depression or without having attention drawn to it as a possible diagnosis seem more likely to order an abundance of tests, perhaps more than necessary, but certainly more than routinely ordered on initial visits for patients who are not depressed. Therefore, assessing and labeling depression and providing feedback early in the course of care has the potential for reducing costs, since laboratory tests and procedures constitute major sources of charges for outpatient visits. However, since medical records were not audited for *quality* of care in this study, it should not be assumed that fewer tests necessarily mean better care.

Return visits to the initial provider were most frequent among those depressed patients who were so labeled before their encounters. Apparently, the internists in the present study were not only willing to provide continuing care to depressed patients but seemed willing to see them more often, consistent with an appropriate course of treatment for depression. However, labeling depression by prescreening in this study was not related to a decrease in physician visits or to a decrease in the subsequent ordering of lab tests, procedures, and medication. In fact, it is correlated with an overall increased utilization of services.

What are the cost implications of these findings? For patients who are depressed, prescreening and feedback to physicians before the initial visit begins may reduce first visit costs since fewer laboratory tests were ordered for this group. However, since during the ensuing year these patients made more visits and received more prescriptions and laboratory tests, the ultimate effect of prescreening and feedback may be to increase costs.

How can we account for the increased utilization of services among patients who rated themselves as mildly or moderately depressed? There are several possible explanations. First, such patients may solicit a higher level of service in an attempt to alleviate discomfort. Second, physicians may sense greater needs for services for such patients. In either case, it is difficult to know from this study if this increased utilization is directly related to patient depression, if these patients are being properly or improperly treated for their symptoms of depression, or if these patients are ultimately happier or healthier as a result of increased utilization.

Finally, it should be emphasized that this study did not consider the severity of medical illness or the nature of medical problems in relation to symptoms of depression. While this patient population as a whole can be characterized as significantly and chronically ill, patients in the mildly and moderately depressed groups also may have been medically sicker, having medical problems that required more visits, tests, procedures, and medications over time. The data are consistent with this formulation. However, the effect of feedback and level of depression on the number of tests ordered during the initial visit or in subsequent medical record notations cannot be accounted for by this interpretation. Although further research is needed to examine interrelationships between medical illness and depression, this study affirms that simple prescreening and feedback techniques may have significant and prolonged influences on several important dimensions of patient and physician behavior.

Study no. 3

To extend this work further, we screened a new group of general medical patients for both anxiety and depression, since both are common in primary care settings and since the interrelationship of these problems has been of interest (Derogatis, Klerman, & Lipman, 1972; Mendels, Weinstein, & Cochrane, 1972; Zung, 1971). In addition to examining the prevalence of these two problems, the study was designed to explore how primary care physicians responded to these conditions in their patients as well as how they were influenced by specific information about one or both conditions provided to them under experimentally controlled conditions. The research was designed to assess whether primary care physicians respond differently to anxiety and depression in their patients as reflected by their notations in the medical record regarding diagnosis or treatment, and the extent to which information about these conditions that physicians receive prior to seeing their patients makes a difference.

Design

The third study involved ninety-five English-speaking patients who were seeing their primary care physicians for the first time, as close to a consecutive sample of patients seen in the clinic as practical limitations permitted. The physicians involved were house staff and faculty of the Department of Medicine at UCLA who were seeing their outpatients in the Medical Ambulatory Care Center.

After receiving explanations of the purpose of the research and signing required consent forms, patients were randomly assigned to one of five groups. Four of the patient groups (Groups I to IV) were screened with the twenty-item Zung

Self-Rating Depression Scale and a ten-item anxiety scale composed of items in the Rand Corporation Health Insurance Study (Ware, Johnston, Davies-Avery, & Brook, 1979). The fifth patient group (Group V) was entered into the study but not screened for depression or anxiety.

The patients in all four screened groups completed both questionnaires before the visit with their physician. When necessary, a research assistant read the questionnaire items to those few patients who could not read or complete them. The scales were scored immediately, and the results were attached with an explanatory note to the front of the patient's chart prior to the visit with the physician. This note clearly specified the patient's adjusted scale score and a key of norms to help the physician interpret the findings. Cues were provided to the physicians in the various groups as follows:

Group I: Information regarding only anxiety scores;
Group II: No information about either of the results of screening;
Group III: Information regarding both anxiety and depression;
Group IV: Information regarding only depression; and
Group V: No prior information.

Chart Audit

Within the three weeks following patient encounters, medical records of the visit were reviewed for notations regarding depression, anxiety, and their treatment (such as notes indicating brief counseling, referral to a mental health professional, or prescribing a psychotropic medication specifically indicated for depression or anxiety). In addition, information about the patient's age, gender, ethnicity, and primary reasons for the clinic visit was recorded. Audits were performed by a research assistant who was blind to the overall objectives of the study.

For a full description of statistical analyses and study results see Linn and Yager (1984).

Summary of Results of Study no. 3

Several limitations of this study must be mentioned. First, the depression and anxiety scales we used were chosen because they could be quickly administered and scored and the screening information could be immediately provided to physicians in a clinically meaningful way. Although the Rand Anxiety Scale has been found to have extremely high internal consistency (reliability), it has not been validated clinically. Similarly, the Zung scale is not a substitute for or equivalent to the clinical diagnosis of an affective disorder. The present study does not suggest that we endorse either of these screening devices as diagnostic instruments. At best, they provide physicians crude information about their parents' clinical status.

Second, when we refer to "anxiety" and "depression," we never intend to imply actual diagnoses of strictly defined depressive or anxiety disorders. Rather, these are self-report symptom complexes and physicians' clinical perceptions of the patients' states. For depression, we made no distinction between syndromes that may be linked to adjustment reactions, secondary depressions, primary affective disorders, or other specific diagnoses.

Third, the assessments of depression and anxiety symptom complexes made here are indicators of prevalence, not of incidence. Therefore, the duration or course of these patients' symptomatic status cannot be determined.

Prevalence of Depression and Anxiety

Almost half of the patients scored within the normal range on the Zung SDS index of depression. About one-fifth had scores indicating minimal depression, one-quarter moderate to marked depression, and the remaining 7% severe depression. Similar to the depression scores, almost half the patients scored within the normal range on the Rand Anxiety Scale. The rest had scores indicating mild, moderate, or severe anxiety in roughly the same proportions as was true for depression. Anxiety and depression scores were highly correlated ($r = .657$). About one-third of patients scored normal on both scales and slightly more than one third scored as both anxious and depressed. When depression or anxiety occurred alone, it tended to be in the mild range, but when they occurred together, both tended to be in the moderate to severe range.

Effect of Screening Information

Unlike the findings in study no. 1, this study did not find significant differences between physician groups who were pre-informed about their patients' anxiety or depression (Groups I and IV) and uninformed physician groups (Groups II and V) on their notation of either anxiety or depression. However, for Group III (patients whose physicians received information about both anxiety and depression), notation about depression and its treatment was very unlikely (11% versus an average 32% for the other groups). The findings regarding Group III strongly suggest that providing certain kinds of information may have a negative or confusing effect, neutralizing or even reversing positive physician behaviors and producing lower than expected notation frequency. In this specific instance, providing physicians with information about both anxiety and depression may have resulted in information overload. These nonpsychiatrists may have experienced some confusion or misunderstanding as to the meaning or significance of patients being both anxious and depressed.

The uninformed physicians had a higher rate of recognition and notation in study no. 3 than in study no. 1. The reason for this is unclear. Perhaps it involves the instruction about depression provided in training, or perhaps a "zeitgeist" more conducive to recognizing depression had, in fact, been created in the clinic.

Appropriateness of Physician Behavior

Although almost half the patients screened scored in the minimal to severe anxiety range, recognition and treatment of anxiety as documented by notations in the record occurred in only 8% to 9% of the cases (versus a 27% notation for depression). However, when recognition did occur, it was appropriate. The apparent difficulty or reluctance of physicians to recognize and treat anxiety may stem from several sources. First, internists may conceptualize anxiety primarily as an isolated symptom rather than as a syndrome, and they may be reluctant to note or treat symptoms in the absence of a more complete explanatory diagnosis. Conceivably, depression is more readily thought of as a complete syndrome warranting intervention. Ambiguity regarding the relationships of anxiety and depression symptoms and disorders reflects the current state of expert dispute in this area (Downing & Rickels, 1974; Kahn et al., 1986; Roth, Gurney, Garside, & Kerr, 1972; Schuman, Kurtzman, Fisher, Groh, & Poston, 1978).

Reluctance to perceive and treat anxiety may also represent a current trend among university-based internists to avoid a negative self-image, according to which primary care physicians are presumed to treat too many anxious people with minor tranquilizers. In the 1980s, recognition and treatment of depressive disorders is often regarded as a more acceptable practice.

Another finding that deserves comment is that anxiety or depression beyond the normal range was rarely noted by the physicians unless the symptoms occurred together. Since among those patients with "anxious depression" both the anxiety and the depression scores were significantly higher than when elevated scores for either occurred alone, these physicians may have been responding to the intensity of the distress. On the other hand, the internists may regard milder anxiety or depression states occurring alone as personality characteristics not requiring attention rather than as pathologic states.

Recommendations for Other Studies

The studies described above and those cited in the literature clearly point to the many areas of ignorance and controversy that remain. In what follows, recommendations for future research are organized within the broad categories of case-finding and intervention.

Case-Finding

Improved Screening and Interview Instruments

There is a clear need for improved screening and interview instruments in primary care settings. Current screening instruments often have adequate sensitivity but inadequate specificity, in that they identify many false positive cases of affective disorder. Changes in the cut-off scores—i.e. evaluating them for case definition—often increases the specificity, but at the same time reduces the sensitivity of the instruments. We see the following specific needs for future screening and clinical research instruments:

Instruments to Better Identify the 25–35% of "Spontaneous Remitters Found in Several Surveys Who Won't Need Drugs for "Depression"

These may be patients whose depressive symptoms are related to acute situational problems or bereavement. For example, Schulberg et al. (1985) showed that many of the false positive diagnoses on the Center for Epidemiologic Studies—Depression Scale (CES-D) included patients who had symptoms for only 4 days or less, not for the 2 or more weeks required for a DSM-III diagnosis of affective disorder. It may also be true that many studies in the contemporary literature may include the bereaved among those diagnosed as depressed.

Instruments to Identify Psychiatric Comorbidity

The concurrence of symptoms of depression (and anxiety) with those of alcohol and substance abuse and/or personality problems and/or organic brain impairment must be correctly identified to achieve accurate diagnoses and appropriate treatment interventions. Screening instruments in medical populations have shown a high prevalence of alcoholism and cognitive impairment, as well as depression. The next generation of screening instruments should address all these dimensions. Physicians recognize these differences clinically on a case-by-case basis and may or may not intervene in certain ways, depending on their assessments of available resources and the effectiveness of interventions. These clinical assessments may influence rates of case finding for depression and of interventions that would seem appropriate for depression per se.

Instruments to Help Factor Out Somatic Symptoms that May Be Due to Medical Illness

Since many of the neurovegetative symptoms of depression may result from physical illness, it has been suggested that screening instruments that omit anorexia and fatigue, for example, would be more appropriate for primary care populations (Bukberg, Penman, & Holland, 1984).

Improved Clinical Research Interviews to Back Up Screening Instruments

Variability among currently available research diagnostic instruments is not trivial, and this variability may in part reflect the inadequacy of some basic conceptualizations about the depressive syndromes. In general, the better we are at diagnosing the affective disorder syndromes in primary care settings with research interviews, the more accurate we can be in ascertaining how appropriate or inappropriate are the treatments used by the primary care physicians. As alluded to above, interviews that pay special attention to the morbidity of medical illness with symptoms of depression are particularly important, including both assessments of the medical illnesses and of the types of treatments they require that may themselves bring about symptoms of depression. Such research interviews would clarify the nature of depressive syndromes currently listed as disorders under Axis III of the American Psychiatric Association's *Diagnostic and Statistical Manuals* (DSM-III and DSM-III-R).

Prevalence and Nature of Depression in Medical Populations

Further studies of the prevalence and specific nature of depressive disorders in high-risk medical populations are needed. Such populations include those in which there is thought to be a high prevalence of "masked depression," such as patients with chronic pain complaints, and the so-called "worried well," with multiple somatic complaints such as fatigue, weakness, and nonspecific gastrointestinal disturbances, frequent and repeated visits to primary care outpatient clinics, and vague, ill-defined neurological problems. Of course, psychiatric problems other than simple depressive disorders, particularly alcohol and substance abuse and personality disorders, and a variety of occult medical problems may be generating these complaints.

Other specific populations deserving close attention include adolescents, cancer patients, (with and without central nervous system impairment due to the cancers and/or therapy), AIDS patients, and patients with coronary and cerebral atherosclerotic diseases.

Mothers of pediatric patients seen in primary care settings represent another potentially high yield population as yet inadequately studied for depression. In these populations the medical complications will be fewer, and interventions may not only help the mothers, but also be of preventive mental health value for the children. Screening for depression among these mothers may uncover a group for whom psychosocial and/or biomedical interventions for depression may be appropriately made, possibly by trained mental health professionals in the pediatric office setting. Using a model of intervention similar to that employed in our studies, potential problems may be identified with screening instruments, feedback could be provided to the pediatricians, and individual and/or group treatment programs could be initiated for mothers identified as depressed or at high risk.

Interventions

Additional studies regarding the extent, nature, and appropriateness of interventions for depression in primary care settings are all needed. Studies such as those of Zung and King (1983), and Zung et al. (1983) suggest that when patients with depression are appropriately identified in primary care settings and appropriately treated with medications, those who are treated do better than either those who are identified but electively not treated and those who are depressed but never identified or treated.

Similarly, Keller et al. (1982) found that among 217 patients with a diagnosis of major depressive disorder treated in primary care settings, even those with the most chronic and severe depressive disorders (e.g., those with psychotic depression) were often not treated adequately. In their study of carefully diagnosed patients, only 34% of the group received tricyclic antidepressants given for 4 consecutive weeks, while only 12% received 150mgs or more of a tricyclic antidepressant equivalent for 4 weeks. Even among those with psychotic depressions, 25% received no somatic therapy, and only 25% received reasonably intensive medication therapy. In this study minor tranquilizers were found to be generally used more than tricyclic antidepressants in the treatment of depression.

However, in a discussion of the Keller et al. (1982) article, Uhlenhuth (1982) argues provocatively that the primary care physicians in that study may in fact have been operating appropriately in relation to the treatment of depression. For example, the physicians may have given benzodiazepines rather than tricyclics because of their concerns with the safety or side effects of the tricyclics. Furthermore, he cites literature providing evidence for some antidepressant effectiveness for some benzodiazepines. He stresses the need for faster and safer tricyclic antidepressants before primary physicians can too quickly be faulted for their intervention practices.

Several other studies in primary care settings suggest that the relationship between intervention for depression and outcome is not necessarily clear-cut, and it is more ambiguous in milder forms of affective disturbance. For example, Catalan, Gath, Edmonds, & Ennis (1984) found that among 91 patients with "minor affective disorder" treated by general practitioners, who randomly assigned them to anxiolytic medications, primarily diazepam or chlordiazepoxide, or counseling without anxiolytics, outcome results were similar across treatments at 1 month and at 7 months.

Cases of depression (based on the General Health Questionnaire) went from 80–86% at entry to 38–46% at one month to 26–28% at 7 months. Of course, all the patients in this study received some treatment, and it also might be argued that since the anxiolytics were probably not effective treatments for depressive disorders anyway, these patients could not be considered to have had adequate trials of an appropriate antidepressant.

Medical record studies may not fully reveal the awareness of primary care physicians about their patients' emotional status. Jencks (1985), using data from the National Ambulatory Medical Care Survey, reported that whereas physicians record psychiatric diagnoses for only about 4.4% of primary care visits, they actually conduct psychotherapy-listening or provide psychotropic medication much more often, perhaps twice as often. Therefore, using a variety of indicators in addition to diagnosis in the medical record (such as a stated mental health reason for a visit or the use of psychotherapy and/or medication), about 11.6% of visits seem to have some indication of significant mental distress. In about 5% of the visits, without any stated mental health reason or psychiatric related diagnosis, psychotherapy or psychotropic medications are given (medications about twice as often as psychotherapy). According to Jencks, reasons for under-recording psychiatric problems in medical records may include the physicians' assessments that the difficulties represent adjustment problems rather than more serious psychiatric diagnoses, concerns about stigmatizing patients with a formal psychiatric diagnosis, concerns with insurance company responses to formal diagnoses, and/or lack of familiarity with Axis III of the DSM-III.

Relatively few studies have examined the belief systems of physicians regarding either the nature of depression or the propriety and efficacy of various interventions for depression in relation to their own practices. Two studies are informative in this regard. Magill and Zung (1982) identified 5 types of clinical decisions made by family physicians in relation to 39 patients who had Zung SDS scores above 55 and who were identified to the physicians as potentially depressed:

1. Patients whom the physicians believed to be depressed and who were treated with antidepressants were primarily those patients who had vegetative symptoms (these patients constituted 31% [$n = 12$] of the group);

2. Eight patients (21%) constituted a group called "probably depressed" for whom the physicians would provide counseling, referral, or follow-up for further evaluation;

3. Two patients (5%) were called "possibly depressed," but further evaluation for treatment of depression was deferred because of more urgent medical problems;

4. Ten patients (26%) were "possibly depressed" but deemed not amendable to therapy because of character disorders and other associated psychiatric problems; and

5. The remaining 7 patients (18%) were not considered to be depressed on clinical grounds in spite of the high Zung SDS scores.

This important study shows that other issues, predominately psychiatric and medical comorbidity and the differential diagnosis of the depressive subtypes, enter into the clinical decisions made by primary physicians and seem reasonably appropriate. These issues clearly require further research.

In the second study, Daniels et al. (1986) asked 282 primary care physicians how they managed patients with depression and how they would manage 10 hypothetical patients presented as case vignettes. The physicians indicated a wide number of different methods. Physician characteristics accounted for about 30% of the variance in their treatment preferences. Predominantly, these characteristics included age, experience with various treatments, and gender. Of note, almost 30% reported that they had never referred a patient to a mental health provider outside of their practice setting, and another 36% utilized referral only rarely. Physicians who recommend medication treatment for depression were likely to be older, male, on the full-time faculty, and to specialize in family medicine. Those recommending referral for the treatment of depression tended to be younger, female, affiliated with internal medicine programs, and residents (perhaps indicating the ease of referral in the medical center). They were also less likely to believe that it was beneficial or efficacious to medicate depressed patients. Those who reported that they would recommend counseling were more likely than others to be affiliated with family medicine programs.

As a result of their findings, the authors suggested that providing physicians with experiences in diverse treatment modalities would likely increase the probability that they would subsequently use or make referrals for such treatments. The further research suggested would examine more precisely how physician and depressive syndrome characteristics and the associated medical and psychiatric problems of the patients interact in determining the types of interventions used.

Finally, the broad issue of how the treatment for depression in primary care settings impact the outcome of depression, the outcome of associated medical problems, related costs, and patient satisfaction needs considerable research. Our own study looked only at cost, not at outcome (Linn & Yager, 1984).

Although it is widely assumed that identification and treatment of depression in primary care settings will reduce the burden of depression and possibly the comorbidity of medical illness as well, few studies have actually tested the assumption. We would suggest further studies along the lines of those conducted by Zung et al. (1983), in which populations at risk for depression are identified, feedback is given to physicians, treatment is instituted, and follow-up assessments are done. Such studies should concern not only the symptoms of depression but also the patient's entire psychiatric and medical status, and the relative costs and benefits of the various medical and psychiatric treatment programs.

References

Blumenthal, M. D., & Dielman, T. E. (1975). Depressive symptomatology and role function in a general population. *Archives of General Psychiatry, 32,* 985–991.

Brody, D. S. (1980). Feedback from patients as a means of teaching nontechnological aspects of medical care. *Journal of Medical Education, 55,* 34–41.

Buckberg, J., Penman, D., & Holland, J. C. (1984). Depression in hospitalized cancer patients. *Psychosomatic Medicine, 46,* 199–212.

Catalan, J., Gath, D., Edmonds, G., & Ennis, J. (1984). The effects non-prescribing of anxiolytics in general practice: I. Controlled evaluation of psychiatric and social outcomes. *British Journal of Psychiatry, 144,* 593–602.

Daniels, M. L., Linn, L. S., Ward, N., & Leake, B. (1986). A study of psychiatric preferences in the management of depression in the general medical setting. *General Hospital Psychiatry*, *8*, 229–235.

Derogatis, L. R., Klerman, G. L., & Lipman, R. S. (1972). Anxiety states and depressive neuroses. *Journal of Nervous and Mental Disease*, *155*, 392–403.

Downing, R. W., & Rickels, K. (1974). Mixed anxiety-depression. Fact or myth? *Archives of General Psychiatry*, *30*, 312–317.

Follette, W., & Cummings, N. A. (1967). Psychiatric services and medical utilization in a prepaid group practice medical program. *Medical Care*, *5*, 25–35.

Francis, V., Korsch, B. M., & Morris, M. J. (1969). Gaps in doctor-patient communication: Patients response to medical advice. *New England Journal of Medicine*, *280*, 535–540.

Goldberg, I. D., Krantz, G., & Locke, S. (1980). Effect of a short-term outpatient psychiatry therapy benefit on the utilization of medical services in a prepaid group practice medical program. *Medical Care*, *8*, 419–428.

Greene, R., & Simmons, J. (1976). Improving physician performance. In R. Greene (ed.), *Assuring quality in medical care* (pp. 173–189). Cambridge, MA: Ballinger Publishing.

Hedlund, J. L., & Vieweg, B. W. (1979). The Zung self-rating depression scale: A comprehensive review. *Journal of Operational Psychiatry*, *10*, 51–64.

Hoeper, E. W., Nycz, G. R., Regier, D. A., Goldberg, I. D., & Hankin, J. (1980). Diagnosis of mental disorders in adults and increased use of health services in 4 outpatient settings. *American Journal of Psychiatry*, *137*, 207–210.

Jencks, S. F. (1985). Recognition of mental distress and diagnosis of mental disorders in primary care. *JAMA*, *253*, 1903–1907.

Katon, W. (1984). Depression: Relationship to somatization and chronic medical illness. *Journal of Clinical Psychiatry*, *45*, 4–11.

Kahn, R. J., McNair, D. M., Lipman, R. S., Covi, L., Rickels, K., Downing, R., Fisher, S., & Frankenthaler, L. (1986). Imipramine and chlordiazepoxide in depressive and anxiety disorder: II. Efficacy in anxious outpatients. *Archives of General Psychiatry*, *43*, 79–85.

Keller, M. B., Klerman, G. L., Lavori, P. W., Fawcett, J. A., Coryell, W., & Endicott, J. (1982). Treatment received by depressed patients. *JAMA*, *248*, 1848–1855.

Lazare, A., Eisenthal, S., & Wasserman, L. (1975). The customer approach to patienthood. *Archives of General Psychiatry*, *32*, 533–558.

Linn, L. S., & Yager, J. (1980). The effects of screening, sensitization and feedback on notation of depression. *Journal of Medical Education*, *55*, 942–949.

Linn, L. S., & Yager, J. (1982). Screening for depression and its relationship to subsequent patient and physician behavior. *Medical Care*, *20*, 1233–1240.

Linn, L. S., & Yager, J. (1984). Recognition of depression and anxiety by primary physicians. *Psychosomatics*, *25*, 593–600.

Magill, M. K., & Zung, W. W. K. (1982). Clinical decisions about diagnosis and treatment for depression identified by screening. *Journal of Family Practice*, *14*, 1144–1149.

Mendels, J., Weinstein, N., & Cochrane, C. (1972). The relationship between depression and anxiety. *Archives of General Psychiatry*, *27*, 649–653.

Moore, J. T., Silimperi, D. R., & Bobula, J. A. (1978). Recognition of depression by family medicine residents: The impact of screening. *Journal of Family Practice*, *7*, 509–513.

Rodin, G. & Voshart, K. (1986). Depression in the medically ill: An overview. *American Journal of Psychiatry*, *143*, 696–705.

Roth, M., Gurney, C., Garside, R. F., & Kerr, T. A. (1972). Studies in the classification of affective disorder: The relationship between anxiety states and depressive illness. *British Journal of Psychiatry, 121,* 147–161.

Schulberg, H. C., Saul, M., McClelland, M., Ganguli, M., Christy, W., & Frank, R. (1985). Assessing depression in primary medical and psychiatric practices. *Archives of General Psychiatry, 42,* 1164–1170.

Schuman, S. H., Kurtzman, S. B., Fisher, J. V., Groh, M. J., & Poston, J. H. (1978). Three approaches to the recognition of affective disorders in family practice: Clinical, pharmacological and self-rating scales. *Journal of Family Practice, 7,* 705–711.

Starfield, B., Steinwachs, D., Morris, I., Bause, G., Seibert, S. & Westin, C. (1979). Patient-doctor agreement about problems needing follow-up visits. *JAMA, 242,* 344–346.

Uhlenhuth, E. H. (1982). Depressives, doctors, and antidepressants. *JAMA, 248,* 1879–1880.

Ware, J. E., Johnston, S. A., Davies-Avery, A., & Brook, R. H. (1979). *Conceptualization and measurement of health for adults.* Health insurance study. (Rand Report R–1987 3-HEW). Santa Monica.

Yager, J., & Linn, L. S. (1981). Physician-patient agreement about depression and its notation in medical records. *General Hospital Psychiatry, 3,* 271–276.

Zung, W. W. K. (1965). A self-rating depression scale. *Archives of General Psychiatry, 12,* 63–70.

Zung, W. W. K. (1968). Evaluating treatment methods for depressive disorders. *American Journal of Psychiatry, 124* (Suppl.), 40–48.

Zung, W. W. K. (1969). A cross-cultural survey of symptoms in depression. *American Journal of Psychiatry, 126,* 154–159.

Zung, W. W. K. (1971). The differentiation of depressive and anxiety disorders: A biometric approach. *Psychosomatics, 12,* 380–384.

Zung, W. W. K. (1972). A cross-cultural survey of depressive symptomatology in normal adults. *Journal of Cross-Cultural Psychology, 3,* 177–183.

Zung, W. W. K., & King, R. E. (1983). Identification and treatment of masked depression in a general medical practice. *Journal of Clinical Psychiatry, 44,* 365–368.

Zung, W. W. K., Magill, M., Moore, J. T., & George, D. T. (1983). Recognition and treatment of depression in a family medicine practice. *Journal of Clinical Psychiatry, 44,* 3–6.

Zung, W. W. K., & Wonnacott, T. H. (1970). Treatment prediction in depression using a self-rating scale. *Biological Psychiatry, 2,* 321–329

10

The Use of Psychiatric Screening Scales to Detect Depression in Primary Care Patients

Richard L. Hough, John A. Landsverk, and Gerald F. Jacobson

Over the last decade and a half, a great deal of concern has been expressed for improving the recognition and treatment of mental disorders in primary care settings. A number of investigators have found that mental disorders are common in such settings (e.g., Goldberg, Hay, & Thompson, 1976; Hoeper, Nycz, Cleary, Regier, & Goldberg, 1979; Locke & Gardener, 1969). Further, some 50% of those who seek help for mental illness are treated exclusively in primary care settings (Regier, Goldberg, & Taube, 1978; Shurman, Kramer, & Mitchel, 1985).

Depressive disorders are the most common mental health problems seen in primary care (Nielsen & Williams, 1980; Wells, 1985). Studies using structured interview schedules (the Schedule for Affective Disorders and Schizophrenia [SADS] [Endicott & Spitzer, 1978] and the Diagnostic Interview Schedule [DIS] [Burke & Regier, 1986; Robins, Helzer, Ratcliff, & Seyfried, 1982]) to assess the mental health status of primary care patients have generally found a prevalence rate of approximately 6% for major depression and an additional 2 to 5% for other affective disorders (Hoeper et al., 1979; Hough, Landsverk, Stone, Jacobson, & McGranahan, 1982; Von Korff et al., 1987). A recent analysis of evidence from the National Institute of Mental Health (NIMH)—funded Epidemiologic Catchment Area Research Program (ECA) (Kessler et al., 1987) suggests that 5.3 to 8.2% of persons using medical services in the last six months exhibit some kind of affective disorder.

Despite its high prevalence in primary care settings, depression and other forms of mental disorder are often not diagnosed or treated (Glass, Allan, Uhlenhuth, Kimball, & Borinstein, 1978; Hankin & Locke, 1983; Hankin & Oktay, 1978; Kessler, Cleary, & Burke, 1985; Nielson & Williams, 1980; Schulberg et al., 1985; Siller, Blascovich, & Lenkei, 1981; Zung, Magill, Moore, & George, 1985).

The use of screening scales has been suggested to improve the recognition and treatment of depression and other mental disorders in primary care settings. To date, data have been mixed on the effectiveness of the such instruments in primary care settings (e.g., Hoeper, Nycz, Kessler, Burke, & Pierce, 1984; Johnstone & Goldberg, 1976; Linn & Yager, 1982). This chapter is concerned with the relative performance of three self-report psychiatric symptom screening scales in recognizing affective disorders in a primary care setting. The research was done on contract with what was then the Clinical Studies Program of the Division of Biometry and Epidemiology of the NIMH. The contract specified that the screening capabilities of three scales be assessed. The Center for Epidemiologic Studies—Depression Scale (CES-D; Radloff, 1977; Radloff & Locke, 1986); the 28-item General Health Questionnaire (GHQ; Goldberg & Hillier, 1979), and the 25-item Hopkins Symptom Checklist (HSCL-25; Hesbacher, Rickels, & Morris, 1980).

The HSCL has been well studied in a variety of clinical and community investigations (Murphy, 1981). It was intended to reflect a wide range of symptomatology: somatization, obsessive-compulsiveness, interpersonal sensitivity (feelings of personal inadequacy and inferiority), depression, and anxiety (Derogatis, Lipman, Rickels, Uhlenhuth, & Covi, 1974). The shortened version used in this research is limited to symptoms of depression and anxiety (Hesbacher et al., 1980).

The original 60-item GHQ was developed by Goldberg (1972) as a screening scale for use in primary care studies that would have acceptable psychometric properties and some capacity to distinguish psychiatric from physical illnesses. In 1978 the 28-item version used in this research was introduced (Goldberg & Hillier, 1979). It was developed, using a factor analytic approach, to yield, in addition to the overall score, subscales of depression, anxiety, and somatic symptoms as well as social dysfunction.

The Center for Epidemiologic Studies—Depression Scale (CES-D) was developed to serve as a case-finding instrument for epidemiologic studies of depressive illness. It yields a single score that can be used to indicate the likelihood of having one of a range of depressive illnesses and the cut-off can be set high enough to provide some certainty that the subject is likely to meet clinical standards for needing a definitive evaluation for treatment. It was designed to have face validity among primary care physicians (Radloff, 1977; Radloff & Locke, 1986).

Although all these questionnaires have been widely used and have had acceptable performance demonstrated in relation to other instruments or clinical diagnoses, none of them has been tested extensively in comparison to standardized diagnostic interviews that apply American Psychiatric Association *Diagnostic and Statistical Manual-III* (DSM-III) criteria (American Psychiatric Association, 1980).

As designed by program officers at NIMH,[1] this study was designed to compare the results of the three screens with those obtained by the NIMH DIS. The DIS is a highly structured diagnostic interview schedule developed under the auspices of the National Institute of Mental Health to allow collection of standard symptomatological data by carefully trained, nonclinical interviewers. The data, in turn,

---

[1] The program officers for the NIMH were J. D. Burke, Jr., and L. G. Kessler.

allow computer generation of psychiatric diagnoses based on DSM-III criteria. The validity of the DIS has been explored in a series of recent publications (Anthony et al., 1985; Burke & Regier, 1986; Helzer et al., 1985; Robins, 1985; Robins, Helzer, Croughan, & Ratcliff, 1981; Robins et al., 1982).

The investigators in this study had considerable experience in administering the DIS in both English and Spanish as part of the Los Angeles ECA research effort (Hough, Karno, Burnam, Escobar, & Timbers, 1983). The Spanish language DIS used in this study was developed under contract with NIMH (Karno, Burnam, Escobar, Hough, & Eaton, 1983), and the reliability of the translation was carefully assessed in a study that included English-Spanish as well as Spanish-Spanish comparisons (Burnam, Karno, Hough, Escobar, & Forsythe, 1983). Version III of the DIS was used and diagnoses were made without exclusion criteria.

The Study Design and Procedures

The Design

The overall study design is summarized in Table 10.1. A sample of approximately 500 subjects was to be drawn from a primary care population and given the three screens prior to, and the DIS following, a clinical visit. In this particular report, we focus only on the affective disorder portions of the DIS.

The Study Setting and Sample

A sample of 525 respondents was recruited from a Maxicare ambulatory care center in Los Angeles. At the time of the study, Maxicare was a federally qualified health maintenance organization (HMO) with an enrollment of approximately 108,000 members. The Hawthorne facility in which the study was done served approximately 43,000 enrollees including Medical and Medicare patients and individuals and groups representing a number of industries and occupations. The center provided a full range of primary care and medical specialty services.

Table 10.1. Study Design

Target Population	Prior to Clinical Visit	Clinical Visit	After Clinical Visit
Primary Care Patients (N = 500)	GHQ-28 HSCL-25 CES-D		Diagnostic Interview Schedule
	Patient Report Form		Physician Report Form

Of the total number of physicians practicing at the center, twelve had practices predominantly in primary care. Patients of these physicians constituted the study population. Table 10.2 provides an overview of the respondent recruitment process. At step 1, respondents were sampled from appointment logs and initially recruited for the study by telephone. First-time users, private patients who were neither Hispanic nor Anglo, and those of less than 18 years of age were excluded. As can be seen in the table (step 2), some 62% of those screened were eligible. At step 3, 27% of the eligibles were sampled. Sampling was by appointment time frames rather than by individuals in order to spread the interviews evenly across the day. Telephone contacts were then used (step 4) to contact members of the sample. The research team had approximately 36 hours in which to make contact between the completion of the appointment logs and the time the respondents would be coming in for their appointment. Within this time frame, some 52% of the sample was contacted. Of those, approximately 30% was declared ineligible when the telephone contact determined they were not Anglo or Mexican American. Note that some 155 potential subjects (9.4%) refused the telephone interview.

The telephone contacts attempted to recruit the respondent into the project, asking them to appear for their appointment approximately fifteen minutes early and to plan, if possible, on remaining after their appointment about an hour to finish a longer interview. Some 28% of those contacted by telephone refused to

Table 10.2. Recruitment Process

1	Primary Care Appointments: 18,552	Not Eligible: 7,060 (38.1%)[1]
2	Eligible: 11,492 (61.9%)	Not Sampled: 8,343 (72.6%)
3	Sampled: 3,149 (27.4%)	Not Contacted: 1,499 (47.6%)[2]
4	Contacted: 1,650 (52.4%)	Ineligible: 498 (30.2%)[3]
5	Eligible: 997 (60.4%)	Refused: 155 (9.4%)
6	Accepted Screening: 716 (71.8%)	Refused Screening: 281 (28.2%)
7	Participated in Study: 525	Did Not Participate: 191 (26.6%)[4]

[1] "Not eligibles" included new patients (1,458), private patients (4,460), too young (277), and previous contacts (865)

[2] "Not contacted" included those with no phone (324), with no answer after repeated attempts (653), and those not available at time of phone calls (520)

[3] "Ineligibles" were non-Hispanic or Anglo

[4] "Did not Participate" included
No-shows for appointments: 70
Physician cancelled appointment: 8
Refused to complete screening instruments: 35
No shows or unable to schedule for DIS interview: 43
No shows for the study: 24
Refused to complete the DIS: 11

participate in the study, but 716 agreed to participate (step 6). Of those, another 191 (26.6%) either did not show for their appointment or elected not to participate when they did appear. This resulted in our final N of 525. Hispanics were oversampled and the final data are weighted to take that into account.

Once they were recruited into the study, each respondent completed the three screens and a patient report form before his or her clinical visit. Following the appointment, the physician completed a brief report form and the client was given the DIS. Most of the DIS interviews were completed during the initial office visit, and all were completed within a week following the gathering of the screening data.

The screening instruments were self-administered. The DIS interviews were administered by carefully trained interviewers who had at least a master's degree in a mental health discipline and some clinical experience. All interview materials were available in both Spanish and English and were administered in the language chosen by the respondent.

Evaluating Screens for Use in Primary Care Populations

Before the findings of the study are presented, it is appropriate to comment on what characteristics of screens one might wish to maximize to make them most useful in a primary care setting. A full description of our suggestions has been presented elsewhere (Hough, Landsverk, & Burke, 1985). The portion of that argument most directly relevant to the primary care situation is summarized here.

Table 10.3 presents a general paradigm for identifying screening scale characteristics. Though the rates noted at the bottom of the figure may seem obvious to researchers who regularly deal with questions of validity, their definition here will make sure the results to follow will be appropriately interpreted. The most often reported screen characteristics are their *sensitivity* (the percentage of criterion positives who are positive on the screen—D/B+D) and *specificity* (the percentage of criterion negatives who are negative on the screen—A/A+C).

Table 10.3. General Paradigm for Screening Scale Evaluations

		Criterion		
		−	+	
Screen	−	A	B	A + B
	+	C	D	C + D
		A + C	B + D	

Sensitivity Rate = D/D + B
Specificity Rate = A/A + C
Positive Misclassification Rate = C/C + D
Negative Misclassification Rate = B/A + B

False-Negative Rate = B/B + D
False-Positive Rate = C/A + C
Positive Predictive Power = D/C + D
Negative Predictive Power = A/A + B

Positive and *negative predictive power* refer, respectively, to the percentage of screen positives who are criterion positives (B/B+D) and the percentage of screen negatives who are criterion negatives (A/A+B).

We call the proportion of screen positives who are criterion negatives (C/C+D) the *positive misclassification rate* and the proportion of screen negatives who are classified as cases by the criterion (B/A+B) the *negative misclassification rate*. The proportion of criterion negatives who are identified by the screen as positive is labeled the *false-positive rate* (C/A+C) and the proportion of criterion positives who are identified by the screen as negative, the *false-negative rate* (B/B+D).

For the ideal screen, all of these rates would approach 100. That is, they would be nearly perfectly sensitive and specific and would have nearly perfect positive and negative predictive power. We know, however, that screens with anything approaching these kinds of characteristics are not yet in the realm of possibility. This means that those responsible for clinical policy in a primary care setting must decide whether or not to use screens to identify clients with affective disorders on the basis of the relative strengths and weaknesses of specific screens.

Unfortunately, there is no universal agreement on the question of what characteristics one might wish to maximize in a screen to be used in a primary care setting. However, two major concerns would probably determine whether or not to employ a screen. First, a screen would be useful if it would improve clinical care by identifying populations with treatable disorders that, without the screen, would go undiagnosed and untreated. A quality screen would, therefore, correctly identify most of those with a need for care (sensitivity). The use of a highly sensitive screen would be particularly cost effective if it encouraged the treatment of depressives who consume a disproportionate amount of primary care resources. This assumes, of course, that treated depressives will limit their use of other primary care. The second major consideration in whether or not to use a screen in a primary care setting would be what proportion of the patients it identifies as positive will, in fact, be negatives in terms of diagnosable disorder (positive misclassification rate). If most of those positively identified were diagnosably mentally disordered, the use of a screen would entail little secondary cost. If, however, a large proportion of those so identified are not diagnosably disordered and are not in need of treatment, then a great deal of expensive, professional time would have to be spent in secondary, clinical evaluations of clients, a large proportion of whom may not really need careful assessment. If the positive misclassification rate is high, the use of a screen would, in effect, create exorbitant new costs for the primary care system (secondary evaluation) which may not be matched by the benefits.

The sensitivity and positive misclassification rates of specific screens are usually reported only for cutpoints (identifying those with significant numbers of symptoms) that are most commonly used in the research literature. However, the cutpoints can obviously be changed if sufficient evidence exists that better sensitivity and positive misclassification rates can be obtained in a primary care setting by doing so. Unfortunately, lowering the cutpoint to increase sensitivity increases the number of positive misclassifications and upping the cutpoint to decrease the number of positive misclassifications decreases sensitivity. The degree to which this is true in the Maxicare sample described above is explored in the following section.

Findings

Overall, the sample was relatively young, predominantly Anglo, disproportionately female, and on average, of moderate educational and socioeconomic status (Table 10.4).

In terms of screening scale scores (Table 10.5), as one would expect, higher

Table 10.4. Characteristics of Sample

	N	%
Age:		
18—24	80	15.3
25—44	257	49.1
45—64	170	32.5
65 and over	16	3.1
Race/Ethnicity:		
Hispanic	162	30.9
Anglo	363	69.1
Sex:		
Male	175	33.3
Female	350	66.7
Education:		
Some high school	101	19.3
High school graduate	159	30.4
Some college	173	33.1
College graduate	90	17.2
Employment:		
Full time	372	71.1
Part time	38	7.3
Unemployed	15	2.9
Retired	20	3.8
Housekeeping	61	11.7
Student	8	1.5
Disabled	9	1.7
Socioeconomic Status[1]:		
7—23	122	24.0
24—48	124	24.4
49—62	167	32.8
63—93	96	18.9

[1] Duncan Socioeconomic Index Scores with housewives and students excluded

Table 10.5. Scale Characteristics for the CES-D, GHQ-28, and HSCL-25

	CES-D	GHQ-28	HSCL-25
Usual Cutpoint	16/17	51/52	43/44
Percent Above Usual Cutpoint	25.2	36.3	20.4
Mean	11.3	46.2	36.6
Mode	5.0	39.0	31.0
Standard Deviation	9.2	10.9	10.1
Median	9.0	43.0	33.0
Range	46.0	64.0	56.0

proportions scored above established cutpoints than had positive DIS diagnoses. In the primary care site, 25% of the respondents were positive on the CES-D (using the standard cutpoint of 16/17), 20% on the HSCL-25 (using the standard cutpoint of 43/44), and 36% on the GHQ-28 (using the standard cutpoint of 51/52).

Some 19% of the respondents met criteria for at least one DIS/DSM-III diagnosis in the last month (Table 10.6), while 11% were diagnosable for some form of affective disorder, including 5.6% with major depression and 8.6% with dysthymia. (Note that with the DIS, dysthymia can be diagnosed only on a lifetime basis.)

The most prevalent diagnoses were major depression, alcohol abuse and dependence, and phobia.

The central question addressed by the study was how accurately the three screens classified caseness compared to DIS/DSM-III diagnosis for affective disorder. Table 10.7 examines the screens' abilities, using established cutpoints, to detect one-month DIS affective diagnosis. The first column in the table presents the data on identification of affective disorder without dysthymia, including mania, bipolar disorder, and major depression. The data in the second and third columns are for dysthymia and for all affective disorders combined.

The most dramatic finding was the great difference in sensitivity rates for dysthymia and severe affective disorder—the more serious affective disorders. Sensitivities for dysthymia ranged from .546 to .644 across the three scales, while for more severe depression, they ranged from .821 to .857. Of the three scales, the HSCL-25 was the most sensitive to severe depression (sensitivity = .857) and the least sensitive to dysthymia (.546). However, we should note that the differences between scales in sensitivity rates are not of sufficient magnitude to strongly recommend the use of one as opposed to another.

We suggested above that the second major criterion for the selection of a screen for use in primary care would be a low positive misclassification rate. As might be expected, the positive misclassification rates were highest in regard to severe depression (.774 to .830) across the three scales. One of the concomitants of the high sensitivities observed for this disorder is that the great majority of screen positives are misclassified. The positive misclassification rates for dysthymia are

Table 10.6.   Distribution of One-Month DIS/DSM-III Diagnosis

	N *	%
Affective Disorders		
Mania	4	0.8
Bipolar disorder	7	1.9
Major depression	29	5.6
Dysthymia (lifetime)	45	8.6**
Affective disorders combined	58	11.1***
Substance Abuse Disorders		
Alcohol abuse/dependence	13	2.5
Drug abuse/dependence	5	1.0
Substance abuse disorders combined	17	3.3
Anxiety Disorders		
Obsessive-compulsive	4	0.8
Phobia	35	6.8
Panic	7	1.4
Anxiety disorders combined	41	8.0
Other Disorders		
Schizophrenia	4	0.8
Schizophreniform	1	0.2
Somatization	3	0.6
Antisocial personality	1	0.2
Any DIS/DSM-III Diagnosis	99	18.9

* N refers to the number of persons reaching criteria for the diagnosis

** Lifetime diagnoses are reported for dysthymia since recency data was not collected.

*** Including dysthymia

slightly lower (.774 to .794), but the great majority of screen positives are still DIS/DSM-III negatives. Again, there are no differences between the three screens large enough to suggest the use of one as opposed to the other.

Although they are of less importance to the immediate concerns of this paper, the specificity and negative misclassification rates for the three screens in relationship to DIS/DSM-III affective disorders are also presented in Table 10.7. In general, there is not a great deal of variation in specificity across scales or disorders. Specificity rates range between .759 (the GHQ-28 in relationship to severe depressive disorder) and .849 (the HSCL-25 in relationship to affective disorders including dysthymia). Negative misclassification rates are the lowest for severe depression (.010 to .013) and the highest for affective disorders including depression (.048 to .049).

The analysis next examined whether the characteristics of the screens might vary if the cutpoints were modified. Table 10.8 presents sensitivity and positive misclassification rates for the three screens with three cutpoints. The first set of rates is simply a repeat of the standard cutpoint data from Table 10.7, made for comparison's sake. The second set of rates is for the cutpoints necessary to

Table 10.7. Summary of the Characteristics of the CES-D, HSCL-25, and GHQ-28 to DIS/DSM-III Affective Disorder Diagnosis

	Severe Depressive Disorder[1]	Dysthymia[2]	Any Affective Disorder[3]
Sensitivity			
CES-D	.821	.614	.667
HSCL-25	.857	.546	.649
GHQ-28	.828	.644	.690
Specificity			
CES-D	.783	.784	.802
HSCL-25	.832	.826	.849
GHQ-28	.759	.761	.778
Positive Misclassification			
CES-D	.822	.791	.705
HSCL-25	.774	.774	.651
GHQ-28	.830	.794	.716
Negative Misclassification			
CES-D	.013	.044	.049
HSCL-25	.010	.049	.049
GHQ-28	.013	.043	.048

[1] "Severe Depressive Disorder" includes mania, bipolar disorder, and major depression in the last month.

[2] "Dysthymia" is lifetime.

[3] "Any Affective Disorder" includes the severe disorders and dysthymia.

Table 10.8. Summary of Screening Abilities of the CES-D, HSCL-25, and GHQ-28 in Relationship to DIS/DSM-III One-Month Severe Depressive Diagnosis with Varying Cutpoints

Scale	Cutpoint	Sensitivity	Positive Misclassification
CES-D	16/17	23/28 (.821)	106/129 (.822)
HSCL-25	43/44	24/28 (.857)	82/106 (.774)
GHQ-28	51/52	24/29 (.828)	113/141 (.830)
With Cutpoints Set to Achieve 90% Sensitivity			
CES-D	9/10	27/28 (.964)	222/249 (.892)
HSCL-25	38/39	26/28 (.929)	150/176 (.852)
GHQ-28	47/48	27/29 (.931)	160/187 (.856)
With Cutpoints Set to Minimum Positive Misclassification			
CES-D	28/29	17/28 (.607)	18/35 (.514)
HSCL-25	60/61	8/28 (.286)	10/18 (.556)
GHQ-28	63/64	16/29 (.552)	26/42 (.619)

achieve at least 90% sensitivity. Ideally, one might wish for a cutpoint that would lower the positive misclassification rate to 10% or less. However, that was impossible to achieve. Instead, the characteristics for the scales at the cutpoints that yielded the lowest positive misclassification rate are reported.

Given that the scales appeared to be more sensitive to severe affective disorders, the dysthymia diagnoses are excluded from these analyses.

Murphy (1981) has suggested that 90% is a desirable level of sensitivity for screens. The cutpoints for the three scales can be modified to make sure nine of ten patients with diagnosable severe affective disorders are correctly classified. In order to achieve this level of sensitivity, the cutpoints on the scales had to be lowered from 16/17 to 9/10 for the CES-D, from 43/44 to 38/39 for the HSCL-25, and from 51/52 to 47/48 for the GHQ-28. The consequence of this is an increase in the positive misclassification rates to a point that 85 to 89% of the screen positives would not be diagnosable. The specific positive misclassification values for the screens were .852 for the HSCL-25, .856 for the GHQ-28, and .892 for the CES-D.

Positive misclassification rates were not so amenable to change. The cutpoints had to be raised to 28/29 for the CES-D, 60/61 for the HSCL-25, and 63/64 for the GHQ-28 to achieve the minimum misclassification rates of .514, .556, and .619, respectively. At their best, over half of the screen positives on each scale would not meet diagnostic criteria for affective disorder.

In order to achieve positive misclassification rates this low, sensitivity rates were dramatically decreased from those obtaining at the standard cutpoint level: .821 to .607 for the CES-D, .857 to .286 for the HSCL-25, and .828 to .552 for the GHQ-28.

Table 10.9 presents a summary of sensitivities of screening scales using established cutpoints for caseness and DIS/DSM-III diagnosis for major diagnostic groupings. Table 10.10 presents a summary of sensitivities of screening questionnaires with established cutpoints for caseness to DIS one-month affective disorder diagnoses by sociodemographic characteristics.

Table 10.9. Summary of Sensitivities of Screening Scales Using Established Cutpoints for Caseness and DIS/DSM-III Diagnosis for Major Diagnostic Groupings

	Affective Disorders		Anxiety Disorders		Substance Abuse		Any Disorders	
	SN	SP	SN	SP	SN	SP	SN	SP
CES-D	.857	.746	.455	.725	.534	.722	.558	.758
HSCL-25	.857	.832	.465	.817	.454	.804	.543	.854
GHQ-28	.838	.666	.558	.653	.466	.643	.630	.685

SN = Sensitivity

SP = Specificity

Table 10.10. Summary of Sensitivities of Screening Questionnaires with Established Cutpoints for Caseness to DIS One-Month Affective Disorder Diagnoses by Sociodemographic Characteristics

	CES-D	HSCL-25	GHQ-28
Sex:			
Male	.690*	.690*	.690*
Female	.878	.878	.855
Age:			
18—25	1.000*	1.000*	1.000*
26—40	.866	.866	.944
40+	.818	.818	.634
Education:			
High school or less	.947	.947	.851
More than high school	.698	.698	.812
Socioeconomic Status Index:			
0—46	.925	.925	1.000
47—100	.773	.773	.622
Ethnicity			
Hispanic	.857	.857	1.000
Non-Hispanic	.857	.857	.762

* Based on fewer than five DIS/DSM-III diagnosed cases

Conclusions and Discussion

This chapter has explored the suitability of three instruments, the CES-D, the HSCL-25, and the GHQ-28, for use as screens for affective disorders in primary care settings. Data were obtained on the correspondence of screen scores and DIS/DSM-III affective disorder diagnoses on 525 patients in a large HMO in Los Angeles.

The characteristics of screens regarded to be of greatest potential concern to a primary care practice were their sensitivity and their positive misclassification rates. On the former, the three screens, when used with standard cutpoints, identified an average of some 84% of those with DIS/DSM-III diagnosable severe depression (mania and bipolar and major depressive disorders) and 60% of those with dysthymia. Though the screens were not particularly sensitive to the milder affective disorder reflected by dysthymia, the largest proportion of patients needing more careful assessment and possible referral or treatment for more severe depression could be identified. Further, cutpoints could be lowered to get the sensitivity levels above 90%.

The major problem with the screens is the high positive misclassification rate. In order to get 90% sensitivity, one has to tolerate misclassification of 85 to 90% of the screen positives. The practical costs of using screens become untenable: the screens are identifying one-third (HSCL-25) to one-half (CES-D) of all patients as positive. If the screen results were taken seriously in the primary care practice, all screen positives would have to be given expensive secondary diagnostic procedures on which the vast majority would turn up as negatives.

At the lower established cutpoints, 77 to 83% of the screen positives would still be misclassified. The possibility was explored of raising cutpoints to minimize positive misclassification. At the best, 51 to 62% of the screen positives are DIS/DSM-III negatives. These positive misclassification rates are not as costly as lower sensitivity rates. The screens only identified 18 to 42 positives out the sample of 525, as compared to the 176 to 250 identified as positive at the 90% sensitivity level cutpoint. Financially, it would be possible to give 40 persons a follow-up psychiatric examination even if only 15 are true positives.

However, by lowering the rate of positive misclassification, the sensitivity of the scales was also lowered. At the minimum misclassification level, sensitivities were .61 for the CES-D, .55 for the GHQ-28, and only .29 for the HSCL-25. A screen that only picks up just over one-half of the true positives is not very satisfactory from a clinical perspective of maximizing effectiveness of treatment. It is also not desirable from a cost-benefit perspective in terms of reducing the costs of primary treatment by identifying and treating the depressed and thereby decreasing their use of the general medical care program.

In sum, it does not appear, at least from the data produced by this study, that enough of an advantageous balance of sensitivity and positive misclassification rates of these screens can be achieved at this time to enthusiastically recommend them for use in screening for affective disorders in primary care populations. No one of the three instruments appears to have significant advantages over the others.

However, these results do not suggest that the notion of introducing screens to primary care settings in order to improve the recognition and appropriate treatment of affective disorders ought to be abandoned. In an analysis of the effectiveness of the instruments in screening for six-month anxiety and affective disorders, Hough et al. (1983) found that they were more effective for females, the young, and those with less education and lower socioeconomic status. This suggests that perhaps the instruments could be useful for screening within certain populations of primary care patients. However, the sample size is not large enough in the study being reported here to explore that possibility in relationship to one-month severe depressive disorders.

The reader should also keep in mind that these are the results of a single study and that they may reflect the particulars of its research design, measurement, or sampling. For example, it can be argued that the DIS/DSM-III depression measures are not perfect for this kind of study. Though there is no reason to assume that studies employing psychiatric diagnoses as the criterion variable would produce different results, replication with that sort of measurement procedure would be informative. Replication in other primary care settings with different client populations is also needed.

The results do suggest, however, that there is a need for another generation of screening instruments that can more perfectly mimic DSM-III diagnostic criteria before we can strongly advocate the use of any given instrument in primary care settings. Further, the stronger performance of the screens in relationship to relatively severe depression, as opposed to dysthymia, suggests that future developmental work might concentrate on screens for the former.

References

American Psychiatric Association (1980). *Diagnostic and statistical manual of mental disorders* (3rd ed.). Washington, D.C.: American Psychiatric Association.

Anthony, J., Folstein, M., Romanoski, M., Von Korff, M., Nestadt, G., Chahal, R., Merchant, A., Brown, C., Shapiro, S., Kramer, M., & Gruenberg, E. (1985). Comparison of lay D.I.S. and a standardized psychiatric diagnosis: Experience in eastern Baltimore. *Archives of General Psychiatry, 42,* 667–675.

Burke, J. D., & Regier, D. A. (1986). Assessing performance of the Diagnostic Interview Schedule. In J. Barrett (ed.), *Diagnostic categorizing by the Diagnostic Interview Schedule (DIS): A comparison with other methods of assessment* (pp 255–285). New York: Guilford Press.

Burnam, M. A., Karno, M., Hough, R. L., Escobar, J. I., & Forsythe, A. B. (1983). The Spanish Diagnostic Interview Schedule reliability and comparison with clinical diagnoses. *Archives of General Psychiatry, 40,* 1189–1196.

Derogatis, L. R., Lipman, R. S., Rickels, K., Uhlenhuth, E. H., & Covi, L. (1974). The Hopkins Symptoms Checklist (HSCL): A self-report symptom inventory. *Behavioral Science, 19,* 1–15.

Glass, R., Allan, A., Uhlenhuth, M., Kimball, C., & Borinstein, D. (1978). Psychiatric screening in a medical clinic. *Archives of General Psychiatry, 35,* 1189–1195.

Goldberg, D. P. (1972). *The Detection of psychiatric illness by questionnaire: A technique for the identification and assessment of non-psychotic psychiatric illness.* London: Oxford University Press.

Goldberg, D., Hay, C., & Thompson, L. (1976). Psychiatric morbidity in general practice and the community. *Psychological Medicine, 6,* 565–570.

Goldberg, D. P., & Hillier, V. F. (1979). A scaled version of the General Health Questionnaire. *Psychological Medicine, 9,* 139–145.

Hankin, J., & Locke B. (1983). Extent of depressive symptomatology among patients seeking care in a prepaid group practice. *Psychological Medicine, 13,* 121–129.

Hankin, J., & Oktay, J. S. (1978). *Mental disorder and primary medical care: An analytical review of the literature* (National Institute of Mental Health Series D, No.5) (DHEW Publication No. ADM 78–661). Washington, D.C.: U.S. Government Printing Office.

Helzer, J. E., Robins, L. N., McEvoy, L. T., Spitznagel, E. L., Stoltzman, R. K., Farmer, A., & Brockington, I. F. (1985). A comparison of clinical and diagnostic interview schedule diagnoses: Physician reexamination of lay-interviewed cases in the general population. *Archives of General Psychiatry, 42,* 657–666.

Hesbacher, P., Rickels, K., & Morris, R. J. (1980). Psychiatric illness in family practice. *Journal of Clinical Psychiatry, 41,* 6–10.

Hoeper, E., Nycz, G., Cleary, P., Regier, D. A., & Goldberg, I. D. (1979). Estimated prevalence of RDC mental disorder in primary medical care. *International Journal of Mental Health, 8,* 6–15.

Hoeper, E. W., Nycz, G. R., Kessler, L. G., Burke, J. D. Jr., & Pierce, W. E. (1984). The usefulness of screening for mental illness. *Lancet,* January, 33–35.

Hough, R. L., Karno, M., Burnam, M. A., Escobar, J. I., & Timbers, D. M. (1983). The Los Angeles Epidemiologic Catchment Area Research Program and the epidemiology of psychiatric disorders among Mexican Americans. *Journal of Operational Psychiatry, 14,* 42–51.

Hough, R. L., Landsverk, J. A., & Burke, J. D. (September 1985). Multiple uses of psychiatric screening instruments in community and clinical settings. Paper presented at the meeting of the Section on Epidemiology and Community Psychiatry of the World Psychiatric Association, Edinburgh, Scotland.

Hough, R. L., Landsverk, J. A., Stone, J. D., Jacobson, G. F., & McGranahan, C. (1982). *Comparison of psychiatric screening questionnaires for primary care patients.* (Contract No. 278–81–0036). Los Angeles: Didi Hirsch Community Mental Health Center.

Johnstone, A., & Goldberg, D. P. (1976). Psychiatric screening in general practice. *Lancet, March 20,* 605–608.

Karno, M., Burnam, M. A., Escobar, J. I., Hough, R. L., & Eaton, W. W. (1983). The development of a Spanish language version of the NIMH Diagnostic Interview Schedule. *Archives of General Psychiatry, 40,* 1183–1188.

Kessler, L. G., Burns, B. J., Shapiro, S., Tischler, G. L., George, L. K., Hough, R. L., Bodison, D. & Miller, R. H. (1987). Psychiatric diagnoses of medical service users: Evidence from the Epidemiologic Catchment Area Program. *American Journal of Public Health, 77,* 18–24.

Kessler, L. G., Cleary, P. D., & Burke, J. D., Jr. (1985). Psychiatric disorders in primary care: Results of a follow-up study. *Archives of General Psychiatry, 42,* 583–587.

Linn, L. S., & Yager, J. Y. (1982). Screening of depression in relationship to subsequent patient and physician behavior. *Medical Care, 20,* 1233–1240.

Locke, B. Z., & Gardener, E. A. (1969). Psychiatric disorders among the patients of general practitioners and internists. *Public Health Reports, 84,* 167.

Murphy, J. M. (1981). *Psychiatric instrument development for primary care research: Patient self-report questionnaire.* (Contract No. DBE–77–0071). Rockville, MD: National Institute of Mental Health.

Nielson, A., & Williams, T. (1980). Depression in ambulatory medical patients. *Archives of General Psychiatry, 37,* 999–1004.

Radloff, L. S. (1977). The CES-D Scale: A self-report depression scale for research in the general population. *Applied Psychological Measurement, 3,* 385–401.

Radloff, L. S., & Locke, B. Z. (1986). The community mental health assessment survey and the CES-D Scale. In M. M. Weissman, J. K. Myers & C. E. Ross (eds.), *Community surveys of psychiatric disorders* (pp. 177–190). New Brunswick, NJ: Rutgers University Press.

Regier, D. A., Goldberg, I. D., & Taube, C. A. (1978). The de facto U.S. mental health service system. *Archives of General Psychiatry, 35,* 685–693.

Robins, L. N. (1985). Epidemiology: Reflections on testing the validity of the psychiatric interviews. *Archives of General Psychiatry, 42,* 918–924.

Robins, L. N., Helzer, J. E., Croughan, M. D., & Ratcliff, K. S. (1981). The National Institute of Mental Health Diagnostic Interview Schedule, its history, characteristics and validity. *Archives of General Psychiatry, 38,* 381–389.

Robins, L. N., Helzer, J. E., Ratcliff, K. S., & Seyfried, W. (1982). Validity of the Diagnostic Interview Schedule, Version III: DSM-III diagnosis. *Psychological Medicine, 12,* 855–870.

Schulberg, H. C., Saul, M., McClelland, M., Ganguli, M., Christy, W., & Frank, R. (1985). Assessing depression in primary medical and psychiatric practices. *Archives of General Psychiatry, 42,* 1164–1170.

Shurman, R., Kramer, P. & Mitchell, J. (1985). The hidden mental health network: Treatment of mental illness by non-psychiatric physicians. *Archives of General Psychiatry, 42,* 89–94.

Siller, R., Blascovich, J., & Lenkei, E. (1981). Influence of stereotypes in the diagnosis of depression by family practice residents. *Journal of Family Practice, 12,* 849–854.

Von Korff, M., Shapiro, S., Burke, J., Teitlebaum, E. A., German, P., Turner, R. W., Klein, L., & Burns, B. (1987). Anxiety and depression in a primary care clinic: Comparison of the Diagnostic Interview Schedule, General Health Questionnaire, and practitioners assessments. *Archives of General Psychiatry, 44* (2), 152–156.

Wells, K. B. (1985). *Depression as a tracer condition for the National Study of Medical Care Outcomes: Background review.* Santa Monica: Rand Corporation.

Zung, W., Magill, M., Moore, J., & George, D. (1985). Recognition and treatment of depression in a family medicine practice. *Journal of Clinical Psychiatry, 44,* 3–6.

11

Screening for Depression in General Medical Care

William W. K. Zung and
Kathryn Magruder-Habib

Significant numbers of patients in medical and surgical clinics are suffering from mental disorders that go undiagnosed or untreated (Regier, Goldberg, & Taube, 1978). Furthermore, even those receiving a psychiatric diagnosis often are not treated in a timely, appropriate manner (Keller et al., 1982; Zung, Magill, Moore, & George, 1983). Such is the case with depression, despite its prevalence as a major disorder. For example, Nielson and Williams (1980), in a medical chart review, found that 50% of the depressed patients in an ambulatory medical clinic were not so diagnosed by their primary physicians. Even when diagnosed, however, depressives are often not treated adequately (Keller et al., 1982; Ketai & Hull, 1978).

A major contributing factor to the low detection and treatment rates for depression is the fact that most mentally ill patients are in the care of nonpsychiatric physicians (Regier et al., 1978). In these medical and surgical settings, patients are more likely to present with somatic complaints and symptoms reflecting organic diseases, and physicians are more likely to have an organic illness orientation. Other physician factors include inadequate training in psychiatric disorders, the lack of knowledge specifically concerning depression, and negative attitudes toward mentally ill patients and their treatment.

The reasons for the low rates of detection and adequate treatment of depression are many and complex. Clinical decision-making regarding any disease is a complicated process that involves not only the physician's attitudes, knowledge, and skills, but also the prevalence and severity of the disease, the nature of diagnostic information, the testing available, and the characteristics of the patient (Eddy & Clanton, 1982; Parker & Kassirer, 1975). Obviously, the physician plays a pivotal role in the diagnosis and treatment of any disease. The physician also influences health services utilization: it is the physician who prescribes medications, orders x-rays, laboratory tests, and diagnostic procedures, and admits patients to the hospital.

Depression is the most prevalent of the major mental illnesses and is so debilitating that it is the leading cause of hospital admissions for mental illness in the United States (Fauman, 1981; Teuting, Koslow, & Hirschfeld, 1981).

Persons who are depressed or otherwise emotionally ill have higher utilization rates of all kinds of health care services such as emergency room and inpatient admissions, outpatient visits, diagnostic laboratory tests, and surgical procedures (Broskowski, Marks, & Budman, 1981; Hankin & Shapiro, 1980; Hankin et al., 1982; Hillard, Ramm, Zung, & Holland, 1983; Waxman, Carner, & Blue, 1983; Widmer & Cadoret, 1978).

Not only do depressed persons use more medical and other health care services, but Widmer and Cadoret found that patients increase their utilization of medical services with the development of their depression. The medical records of 154 depressed patients were compared with 154 nondepressed patients, matched by age, sex, and season of the year in which they were treated. Compared with matched controls, the depressed group had more patient-initiated home and office visits, hospitalizations, and somatic complaints. Furthermore, while the control group showed no change in the number of home or office visits over the 19-month period, the mean number of visits for the depressed group doubled in the 7-month period immediately prior to diagnosis compared with the period a year prior. This was a retrospective study, however, and did not allow for causal inferences and with no information regarding the medical severity of the control group.

Early recognition and appropriate treatment for depression has been shown to have an "offset effect" and can reduce medical and other health care utilization, particularly of unnecessary, costly, and potentially harmful diagnostic procedures (Jones & Vischi, 1979). In addition, Barsky (1981) has pointed out that chronic disease patients who have "an unaccountably prolonged convalescence or unduly slow rehabilitation in spite of apparently adequate treatment" may have an unde-tected emotional disorder. One possible explanation for the lack of medical improvement of these patients is that various symptoms of depression can interfere with the patient's compliance with the medical regimen. Difficulty concentrating, restlessness, and lack of self-concern, for example, might cause the patient to misunderstand or ignore the physician's prescription or advice. Furthermore, benefits from adequate treatment for depression include not only improved overall health status for the patient and satisfaction with medical care, but also improved physician-patient relationships.

Physician resistance to diagnosing depression was studied by Hoeper, Nycz, Kessler, Burke, Jr., and Pierce (1984), and two psychiatric referrals by Steinberg, Torem, and Saravey (1980). Steinberg et al. found the following specific reasons for physician resistance given by physicians: that there was no psychiatric problem (38%), that the patient would resist psychiatric treatment (20%), that psychiatry cannot help (12%), that the patient had real reasons to be depressed or upset (10%), that the doctor-patient relationship would be impaired (8%), and other reasons (12%).

Several of the issues relating to low diagnosis and treatment rates for depression have been studied, including the effect of psychiatric training, the use of screening instruments, and patient sociodemographic characteristics. Physicians can no longer argue the uselessness of diagnosing the condition based on the unavailability of effective therapy. The efficacy of drug treatment and of psychotherapy for depression has been established in controlled clinical trials (Weissman et al., 1979). Furthermore, diagnosed and treated depressives have been found to improve regardless of type of therapy compared with untreated depressives (Zung, 1980).

Much research has been devoted to developing screening instruments and to monitoring their use in various settings in order to test a variety of hypotheses. Of particular interest are those studies that used self-administered scales with feedback to the physicians. Results of such studies have demonstrated significant increased recognition rates for depression (Johnstone, 1976; Linn & Yager, 1980; Zung et al., 1983). Not all studies have shown increased diagnosis and treatment rates with informational feedback to the physician (Shapiro, 1983). Screening results by themselves are not sufficient. In the clinical decision-making process, the physician must decide what information to seek, use, and emphasize. This process is common to both psychiatric and nonpsychiatric diagnostic procedures. Indeed, studies have shown that even clinical laboratory findings and nonpsychiatrically oriented screening instruments have been ignored by physicians (Krieg, Gambino, & Galen, 1975; Schneiderman, DeSalvo, Baylor, & Wolf, 1972). Both timing and the type of information are important in determining physician agreement on diagnosis (Linn & Yager, 1982) and treatment (Fisch, Hammond, Joyce, & O'Reilly, 1981; Popkin, Mackenzie, Hall, & Callies, 1980).

Two studies have dealt with the kinds of information used by the diagnostician in determining a psychiatric case. A comparison of 300 new patient symptom checklists with their independently assessed diagnostic rating forms showed that the interviewers varied in their clinical evaluation of the diagnostic importance of psychiatric symptoms (Conover & Climent, 1976). This result was consistent with the more rigorous experimental study of the clinical judgment of general physicians in evaluating and prescribing for depression (Fisch et al., 1981).

Linn & Yager (1982) examined the effect on subsequent physician diagnostic behavior when feedback on screening results from the Zung Self-Rating Depression Scale was given to the physician either before or after the physician's own examination. Patients identified before the examination were more likely to be diagnosed as depressed than either the unscreened or the screened after physician examination groups. Furthermore, patients identified afterward as depressed had more diagnostic procedures ordered. The study, however, did not assess utilization outside of the facility in their year of follow-up, did not examine whether there was any improvement in the patient's depressive symptomatology or overall health status, and did not determine whether the patients received any treatment for their depression.

This paper reports findings of a randomized clinical trial designed to improve physician recognition and treatment of depression in general medical care. Specifically, the aims of the project were: (a) to determine the prevalence of depression (both detected by providers and undetected); (b) to evaluate the effects of a simple screening feedback procedure on physicians' recognition of previously unrecognized depression; (c) to evaluate the effects of screening feedback on the probability of treatment; and (d) to determine the effects of treatment on patient outcomes.

Methods

The setting for the study was the General Medical Clinic (GMC) at the Veterans Administration Medical Center in Durham, North Carolina. The GMC is comprised of approximately 1600 veterans who are followed longitudinally by 8 physicians with faculty appointments in the Division of General Internal Medicine at Duke University. There are also 3 physician assistants and 2 fellows who provide care.

The GMC was considered a good setting for the study for a number of reasons:

1. The patient population is extremely stable (it has often been said that the only attrition from the clinic is through death);

2. There is very little turnover among health care providers in the clinic (all are permanently assigned to the GMC except the fellows, who change annually);

3. A wide range of services (including psychiatric services) is available on site;

4. Cost of the services (including medications) is not a consideration for patients in the VA system; and

5. VA medical records provide evidence of all services (including consultations, referrals, and prescription received under VA auspices).

The protocol called for a double screening process: consenting eligible patients were first administered the Zung Self-Rating Depression Scale (SDS) (an adjusted score of ≥ 50 was considered depressed); SDS positive patients were then given the DSM-III criteria for depression in checklist format. Those screening positively on both criteria were then randomly assigned to one of two groups: Group A, primary physician informed of depression screening results, or Group B, primary physician not informed of depression screening results. The depression feedback sheet was prominently placed on top of the visit note so that the physician was aware of the results as he or she opened the chart. It was pink, in contrast with other chart materials. A random sample of those who screened negatively by both criteria became Group C; no feedback was given to their physicians.

All study patients (Groups A, B, and C) were then followed for 12 months. The protocol called for reinterviewing patients at 6 weeks, 3 months, 6 months, 9 months, and 12 months after the index visit in order to assess depression status. Also during the follow-up period, patient medical records were blindly audited to assess recognition and treatment for depression, health services utilization, and medications prescribed. Recognition was defined as notation of depression in the medical record, significant listing of depressive symptoms, or referral to mental health services. At the most stringent level, only a specific notation of depression was considered sufficient evidence of recognition (level 1). At the next level, a significant listing of depressive symptoms without notation of depression was considered as recognition (level 2), and at the least exclusive level, referral to mental health services (without a notation of depression or listing of symptoms) was considered (level 3). Treatment was defined as an antidepressant prescription, mental health clinic visit, or mental health consultation. Medications prescribed were obtained from a computerized listing of all prescriptions, their dosages, refill authorizations, fill dates, and prescribing physician.

Results

A total of 1,586 patients was seen in the GMC during the 13 months of enrollment. Of these patients, 516 were not eligible for the study for the following reasons: already recognized as depressed (153), 90 years or older (32), female (51), hospital employee (39), too physically disabled to participate (101), on another protocol (6), or patient of a physician who was part of the study team (134). Those 90 and older were screened anyway in order to estimate prevalence of depression in the clinic for all age groups. Of the remaining 1,070 patients, 190 (17.7%) were not interested in participating, leaving 880 who signed consent forms. Information on age and service-connection status was available for nonresponders. Their average age was 63.1 years, compared to 59.1 years for study participants; the difference was statistically significant ($t = 3.4666$, $p < .01$). Service-connected status was not statistically different, with 42.7% of the nonresponders claiming a service-connected disability rated at 50% compensation or higher, compared to 44.0% of the responders ($chi^2 = 1.4292$, $p < .50$).

Of the 880 eligible patients screened, 112 (12.7%) met both screening criteria and were considered "unrecognized" depressed patients. Combining the unrecognized depressed patients and the previously recognized depressed patients, a 28.2% prevalence of all depression (excluding patients 90 years old) was obtained—16.1% previously recognized and 12.1% unrecognized.

Of the 112 potential study patients, twelve scored so high (≤ 75) on the SDS that it was considered unethical to randomize them; their physicians were informed immediately on the pink sheet of their screening results and they were followed as Group E. Physicians were not aware that this group was different from other patients about whose depression status they were informed. The remaining 100 were randomly assigned to Group A—physician informed ($n = 48$),—or Group B—physician not informed ($n = 52$).

Table 11.1 shows descriptive characteristics of Groups A, B, C, and E at the

Table 11.1. Descriptive Statistics (Index Visit)

	Group A Depressed	Group B Depressed	Group E Depressed (SDS ≥ 75)	Group C Not Depressed
	MD Informed ($n = 48$)	MD Not Informed ($n = 52$)	MD Informed ($n = 12$)	MD Not Informed ($n = 60$)
Sociodemographic Information				
Age	57.9(±1.5)	61.9(±1.5)	56.8(±2.7)	58.1(±1.4)
White	68.8%	67.3%	41.7%*	67.7%
Married	72.9%	66.7%	41.7%*	75.0%
Svc. Connect.>49%	45.7%	45.8%	36.4%	42.6%
Retired	77.1%	75.5%	77.8%	62.7%
Know MD ≥1 yr	56.3%	67.3%	33.3%*	65.0%
No non-VA help	60.4%	68.6%	50.0%	61.7%
No non-VA hosp	91.7%	92.2%	91.7%	88.3%
Test Scores				
SDSX	60.4+	61.6	78.6++	37.4**
SASX	62.6+	64.7	74.9++	39.8**
KAS:SE	59.6+	62.4	70.1++	51.5**
KAS:FT	63.8+	67.3	77.6++	60.6**
Poor Health (self)	58.3%+	68.6%	90.9%	15.0%**

*   p <.05 A & B vs. E

** p <.01 A & B vs. C

\+   p <.01 A, B, & E vs. C

\+\+ p < .01 A & B vs. E

index visit. The average age of all groups was close to 60 years, with Group B being slightly older. Groups A, B, and C were approximately two-thirds white and mostly married, while Group E had less than half married and were predominately black. Slightly less than half in all of the groups had a service-connected disability rated at higher than 49% (meaning they were entitled to all ambulatory care on a space available basis). Most were retired (more in Groups A, B, and E), and most reported having known their primary care physicians for a year or more, except for Group E, where only one-third so reported. Most reported receiving no help outside the VA, and about 90% reported no use of hospitals other than the VA. Self-rated poor health was the main factor that distinguished the groups, with 90.9% of the severely depressed patients (Group E) reporting poor health compared to 58.3% in Group A, and 68.6% in Group B reporting poor health, compared to only 15.0% in Group C.

Table 11.1 also shows mean scores at the index visit for the four groups for depression (Self-Rating Depression Scale), anxiety (Self-Rating Anxiety Scale), performance of socially expected activities (KAS-SE), and performance of free-time activities (KAS-FT) as measures of activities of daily living. There are no significant differences between Groups A and B except for a marginal difference on performance of free-time activities (Group B doing slightly worse). Group C was significantly different from Groups A and B on all variables except for free-time activities in Group A. Group E was significantly worse off on all scores. Anxiety and depression appear to be closely linked with these patients, and the socially expected and free-time activities also are associated with the depression categorizations.

Table 11.2 shows ambulatory health services utilization data for the year prior to the index visit for each of the four groups. Clearly this is a group of fairly high use patients. Groups A and B did not differ on any use variables, while Group C was significantly lower than Groups A and B combined on the average number of clinics visited and the depressed patients (Groups A, B, and E combined) on average number of visits and clinics. Of note is the trend for Group E (the most depressed patients) to have consistently higher utilization patterns and for Group C (the not depressed patients) to have consistently lower utilization patterns.

Table 11.3 (also Figure 11.1) shows the cumulative percentage of (previously unrecognized) patients recognized as depressed by their physicians during the 12-month study period. At the index visit, 33.3% of patients in the experimental group (A) were recognized at levels 1, 2, and/or 3 (the most inclusive categorization) by their physicians as depressed, compared to 11.5% in the natural history group (B) ($chi^2 = 6.9, p < .01$). At levels 1 and/or 2 (at least symptom notation), 31.2% in the informed group were recognized compared to 11.5% in the unin-

Table 11.2. Retrospective (One-Year) Chart Review

	Group A Depressed	Group B Depressed	Group E Depressed (SDS ≥ 75)	Group C Not Depressed
Mean	MD Informed ($n = 45$)	MD Not Informed ($n = 49$)	MD Informed ($n = 12$)	MD Not Informed ($n = 59$)
Visits	7.1+	8.3	8.7	6.1
Clinics	7.8+	8.9	9.2	6.6**
Laboratory	10.4	11.3	13.3	9.8
Psychiatric Consults	0.1	0.1	0.2	0.03
Other Consults	0.7	0.9	1.2	1.0
Psychiatric Referrals	0.1	0.1	0.0*	0.02
Other Refs.	0.6	0.8	0.5	0.8

* p < .01 A & B vs. E

**p < .05 A & B vs. C

+ p< .05 A, B, & E vs. C

Table 11.3. Cumulative Percentage of Patients Recognized Over Time

	At Index	By 6 wks	By 3 mos	By 6 mos	By 9 mos	By 12 mos
Level 1:						
A (n = 48)	25.0%	29.2%	31.3%	35.4%	41.7%	41.7%
B (n = 52)	7.7%	15.4%	17.3%	19.2%	19.2%	21.2%
E (n = 12)	33.3%	33.3%	50.0%	50.0%	50.0%	50.0%
C (n = 60)	5.0%	6.7%	6.7%	6.7%	6.7%	6.7%
Levels 1, 2:						
A	31.2%	35.4%	39.6%	43.7%	54.2%	54.2%
B	11.5%	19.2%	23.1%	25.0%	26.9%	28.8%
E	33.3%	41.6%	58.3%	66.6%	66.6%	75.0%
C	8.3%	10.0%	11.6%	13.3%	15.0%	15.0%
Levels 1, 2, 3:						
A	33.3%	37.5%	41.7%	45.8%	56.2%	56.2%
B	11.5%	19.2%	25.0%	28.8%	30.8%	34.6%
E	41.7%	50.0%	66.7%	75.0%	75.0%	83.3%
C	8.3%	11.7%	15.0%	18.3%	21.7%	21.7%

formed group; and at level 1 (an explicit notation of depression), 25.0% of Group A were recognized compared to only 7.7% of Group B. The results at these levels were also statistically significant. Clearly, the differences among the groups persist regardless of the levels of recognition.

By 6 weeks, 37.5% of the patients in Group A were recognized cumulatively (levels 1, 2, and/or 3), compared to 19.2% in Group B (chi^2 = 3.9, p < .05). By 3 months, 41.7% were recognized (levels 1, 2, and/or 3) in Group A and 25.0% in Group B, and by 12 months this had increased to 56.2% in Group A and 34.6% in Group B (all differences were statistically significant).

In general, throughout the 12-month period, there was a gradual increase in recognition, but the difference among the groups was fairly constant. Using Gehan-Wilcoxon survival curve analysis, we found that the two curves were significantly different at the .005 level (chi^2 = 7.83, 1 df).

Group E patients (SDS ≥ 75) were consistently more often recognized at all levels and over all times than Groups A or B, and Group C patients were less often recognized. (Over the 12-month study period only 6.7% of Group C patients were labeled depressed. The remainder that were considered "recognized" in Table 11.3 were due to symptom listing and mental health referrals.) Thus, overall, recognition was related to level of severity of depression (SDS S score), and between groups A and B, to the intervention.

In terms of the treatment data (see Table 11.4 and Figure 11.2) at the index visit, 27.9% of Group A were treated, compared to 3.8% of Group B. By 6 weeks, 33.3% in Group A were treated compared to 21.2% in Group B; by 3 months 37.5% in Group A and 26.9% in Group B were treated; and skipping to 12 months, 56.2% in Group A versus 42.3% in Group B were treated. Thus, as

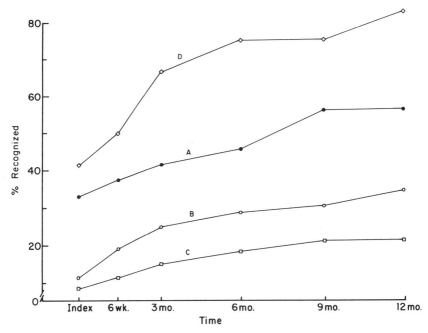

Figure 11.1. Cumulative Percentage of Patients Recognized over Time

with recognition, the difference among the groups was fairly constant across all measurement points; although cross-sectionally only the difference at index was statistically significant, the two curves were different by the Gehan-Wilcoxon survival test (chi^2 = 3.88, 1 df, p = .0489).

Group E patients were consistently more likely to be treated than Group B, but not until 3 months were they more often treated than Group A. Group C patients were consistently less apt to be treated than any of the groups.

In order to examine the effect of treatment on depression symptoms, SDS scores over the six study time points were "realigned" for those patients who were treated so that the SDS score closest to the time of treatment was used as the baseline score and the following scores were used to chart patient progress. Table 11.5 and Figure 11.3 show these average scores over the 12-month study

Table 11.4. Cumulative Percentage of Patients Treated over Time

	At Index	By 6 wks	By 3 mos	By 6 mos	By 9 mos	By 12 mos
A (n = 48)	27.9%	33.3%	37.5%	45.8%	52.1%	56.2%
B (n = 52)	3.8%	21.2%	26.9%	30.8%	38.5%	42.3%
E (n = 12)	16.7%	33.3%	58.3%	83.3%	83.3%	83.3%
C (n = 60)	5.0%	6.7%	8.3%	11.7%	11.7%	11.7%

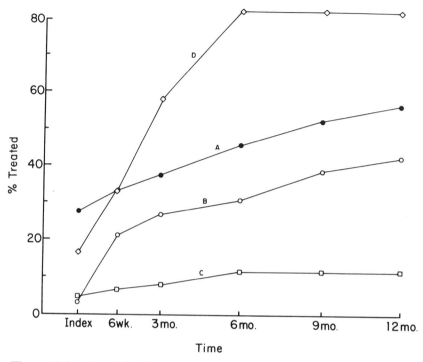

Figure 11.2. Cumulative Percentage of Patients Treated over Time

period. Using these "realigned" scores for treated patients, a repeated measures analysis of variance was performed with SDS scores at the various time points (6 weeks, 3 months, 6 months, 9 months, and 12 months) as the dependent variable, group (A, B, C, or E) and treatment status (treatment, no treatment) as independent variables, SDS index score as a control variable, and appropriate interaction terms. In this model, there were no significant findings concerning treatment status. A second model was attempted with treatment trichotomized (drug treatment, other treatment, no treatment). Treatment status approached significance ($p = .086$) at 3 months, but was insignificant at other times and in the overall model. Thus, despite the apparently greater decreases in SDS score for treated patients than for untreated patients, the trend is not statistically significant. There were significant group effects (due to the extreme differences of the C and E groups); however, the specific contrast between groups A and B was not significant.

Discussion

The results of this clinical trial answer some questions as well as raise a number of important issues. We find evidence that feedback to physicians of SDS scores

Table 11.5. Average SDS Score over Study Period By Treatment Status and Group

		Index	6 wks	3 mos	6 mos	9 mos	12 mos
A	Treated*	62.16	57.00	59.50	57.53	56.50	54.00
	Not Treated	59.05	58.26	57.89	55.69	59.40	55.94
B	Treated*	61.89	61.40	55.93	54.36	55.60	56.67
	Not Treated	60.77	55.93	59.69	59.52	61.12	58.55
E	Treated*	75.80	75.20	64.00	57.89	67.50	73.33
	Not Treated	76.00	74.50	78.00	73.00	73.00	80.00
C	Treated*	39.43	39.00	36.14	37.71	40.50	35.00
	Not Treated	36.98	36.72	38.23	35.65	36.76	36.57

* Treated scores have been "realigned" to correspond more closely to time of treatment.

of previously unrecognized depressed patients can make a significant difference in higher rates of recognition and treatment of depression and at earlier times. This difference is most apparent at the index or screening visit when feedback actually takes place and persists over time. Although we used the SDS strictly as a screener in this study, perhaps our results would have diverged more over time had we continued to feedback SDS results to the physicians of the intervention group. The SDS would have been used as a thermometer, and physicians might have learned more about the effectiveness (or ineffectiveness) of treatments they prescribed. Thus, we find the possibility of these screening tools being used as lab tests over time intriguing.

As expected, in our study SDS scores for all patients decreased over time. Although treated patients' scores consistently decreased more than untreated patients' scores, the difference between treated and untreated patients did not reach statistical significance. This raises the issue of what constitutes appropriate

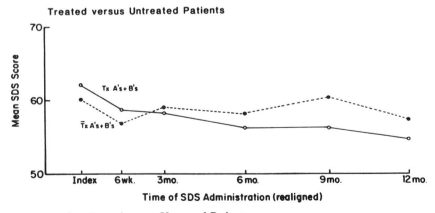

Figure 11.3. Treated versus Untreated Patients

and effective treatment of depression for primary care as opposed to psychiatric patients. Should these patients be prescribed dosages of antidepressants consistent with psychiatric recommendations, or might they respond to lower doses? Is antidepressant treatment the most appropriate and effective form of treatment for these patients or would they respond as well or better to other forms of treatment such as counseling?

Is depression in primary care even the same as depression in psychiatric settings? Certainly there are overlapping features, but also there are differences. In our own patients, depression and anxiety were clearly linked, and we are in the process of examining the question of whether treatment for one decreases the other or merely unmasks it. Depression and physical health were clearly related—both in terms of self- and physician-rated health status and health services utilization. For the relationships of depression to both anxiety and physical health, the question of cause and effect is open. The answer is important in terms of treatment priority in primary care where depression is only one of a number of problems listed.

In summary, although this research answers a number of questions regarding the efficacy of screening on rates of recognition and treatment in primary care, it also generates the next iteration of questions.

References

Barsky, A. J. (1981). Hidden reasons some patients visit doctors. *Annals of Internal Medicine, 94*, 492—598.

Broskowski, A., Marks, E., & Budman, S. H. (1981). *Linking health and mental health.* Beverly Hills: Sage Publications.

Conover, D., & Climent, C. E. (1976). Explanations of bias in psychiatric case finding instruments. *Journal of Health and Social Behavior, 17*, 62—69.

Eddy, D. M., & Clanton, C. H. (1982). The art of diagnosis: Solving the clinicopathological exercise. *New England Journal of Medicine, 306*, 1263—1268.

Fauman, M. A. (1981). Psychiatric components of medical and surgical practice: A survey of general hospital physicians. *American Journal of Psychiatry, 138* (10), 1298—1301.

Fisch, H. U., Hammond, K. R., Joyce, C. R. B., & O'Reilly, M. (1981). An experimental study of the clinical judgement of general physicians in evaluating and prescribing for depression. *British Journal of Psychiatry, 138*, 100—109.

Hankin, J. R., & Shapiro, S. (1980). The demand for medical services by persons under psychiatric care. In L. Robins, P. Clayton, & J. Wind (eds.), *Social consequences of psychiatric illness* (pp. 17—32). New York: Brunner/Mazel.

Hankin, J. R., Steinwachs, D. M., Regier, D. A., Burns, B. J., Goldberg, I. D., & Hoeper, E. W. (1982). Use of general medical care services by persons with mental disorders. *Archives of General Psychiatry, 39*, 225—231.

Hillard, J. R., Ramm, D., Zung, W. W. K., & Holland, J. M. (1983). Suicide in a psychiatric emergency room population. *American Journal of Psychiatry, 140*, 459—462.

Hoeper, E. W., Nycz, G. R., Kessler, L. G., Burke, J. D., Jr., & Pierce, W. E. (1984). The usefulness of screening for mental illness. *Lancet, January 7,* 33—35.

Johnstone, A. (1976). Psychiatric screening in general practice: A controlled trial. *Lancet, March 20,* 605—608.

Jones, K. R., & Vischi, T. R. (1979). Impact of alcohol, drug abuse and mental health treatment on medical care utilization. *Medical Care, 17* (suppl. 12), 1—82.

Keller, M. B., Klerman, G. L., Lavori, P. W., Fawcett, J. A., Coryell, W., & Endicott, J. (1982). Treatment received by depressed patients. *Journal of the American Medical Association, 248,* 1848—1855.

Ketai, R. M., & Hull, A. L. (1978). Tricyclic antidepressant prescribing habits: A comparison of family physicians and psychiatrists. *Journal of Family Practice, 7,* 1011—1014.

Krieg, A. F., Gambino, R., & Galen, R. S. (1975). Why are clinical laboratory tests performed? When are they valid? *Journal of the American Medical Association, 233,* 76—78.

Linn, L. S., & Yager, J. (1980). The effect of screening sensitization and feedback on notation of depression. *Journal of Medical Education, 55,* 942—949.

Linn, L. S., & Yager, J. (1982). Screening for depression in relationship to subsequent patient and physician behavior. *Medical Care, 20,* 1233—1240.

Nielsen, A. C., & Williams, T. A. (1980). Depression in ambulatory medical patients: Prevalence by self-report questionnaire and recognition by nonpsychiatric physicians. *Archives of General Psychiatry, 37,* 999—1004.

Parker, S. G., & Kassirer, J. P. (1975). Therapeutic-decision making, a cost-benefit analysis. *New England Journal of Medicine, 293,* 229—234.

Popkin, M. K., Mackenzie, T. B., Hall, R. C. W., & Callies, A. L. (1980). Consultees' concordance with consultants' psychotropic drug recommendations. *Archives of General Psychiatry, 37,* 1017—1021.

Regier, D. A., Goldberg, I. D., & Taube, C. A. (1978). The de facto U.S. mental health services system. *Archives of General Psychiatry, 35,* 685—693.

Schneiderman, L. J., DeSalvo, L., Baylor, S., & Wolf, P. L. (1972). The "abnormal" screening laboratory result. *Archives of Internal Medicine, 129,* 88—90.

Shapiro, S. (November 1983). Secondary prevention with adult patients in primary care settings. Paper presented at the Annual Meeting of the American Public Health Association, Dallas.

Steinberg, H., Torem, M., & Saravey, S. M. (1980). An analysis of physician resistance to psychiatric consultations. *Archives of General Psychiatry, 37,* 1007—1012.

Teuting, P., Koslow, S. H., & Hirschfeld, R. M. (1981). *Special report on depression research* (DHHS Publication No. 81-1085). Washington, D.C.: National Institute of Mental Health.

Waxman, H. M., Carner, E. A., & Blue, A. (1983). Depressive symptoms and health service utilization among the community elderly. *Journal of the American Geriatrics Society, 31*(7), 417—420.

Weissman, M. M., Prusoff, B. A., Dimascio, A., Neu, C., Goklaney, M., & Klerman, G. L. (1979). The efficacy of drugs and psychotherapy in the treatment of acute depressive episodes. *American Journal of Psychiatry, 136,* 555—558.

Widmer, R. B., & Cadoret, R. J. (1978). Depression in primary care: Changes in pattern of patient visits and complaints during a developing depression. *Journal of Family Practice, 7,* 293—302.

Zung, W. W. K. (1980). The clinical course of undiagnosed depression. *Journal of Clinical Psychiatry, 41,* 186—190.

Zung, W. W. K., Magill, M., Moore, J., & George, T. (1983). Recognition and treatment of depression in a family medicine practice. *Journal of Clinical Psychiatry, 44,* 3—6.

12

Methodological Issues Associated with the Use of Depression Screening Scales in Primary Care Settings

Paul D. Cleary

Depression is prevalent among primary care patients and is often associated with serious morbidity, but many relatively serious mental health problems go undetected (Goldberg, Roghmann, McInerny, & Burke, 1984; Hankin & Oktay, 1979; Hoeper, Nycz, Cleary, Regier, & Goldberg, 1979; Jacobson et al., 1980; Kessler, 1984; Kessler et al., 1986; Manderscheid & Witkin, 1983; Regier et al., 1982; Schlesinger, Mumford, Glass, Patrick, & Sharfstein, 1983; Shepherd, 1983; Westhead, 1985; Wilkinson, 1986). To facilitate the detection of mental health problems such as depression, researchers have developed and evaluated numerous screening tests that can identify patients at high risk of having a psychiatric disorder (e.g. Cleary, Goldberg, Kessler, & Nycz, 1982; Goldberg, 1972; Schulberg et al., 1985). However, since the majority of studies uses only one of these scales, it is often difficult to evaluate the relative accuracy of different measures. In this chapter, I review some of the techniques for evaluating the performance of screening scales and review some of the methodological issues involved in such evaluations.

Ideally, a screening instrument should be short and easy to administer, and it should be accurate. *Accuracy,* or *validity,* refers to the extent to which a test reflects the condition it is meant to detect and only that condition. There are many ways of quantitatively describing the accuracy of a test, but the parameters most frequently used by clinical epidemiologists are sensitivity and specificity. *Sensitivity* refers to the proportion of cases with test results that meet the criterion for caseness, and *specificity* refers to the proportion of noncases that have test results below the specified criterion. Sensitivity and specificity are useful statistics for evaluating validity because when the criterion variable is measured without error, they are independent of the prevalence of disease, unlike many other measures of concordance (Swets, 1986). However, they are dependent on the cutpoint chosen and tend to be inversely related. The choice of cutpoint for virtually all mental health screening scores is arbitrary, and so it is difficult to make comparisons among scales using one estimate of sensitivity and specificity for each scale.

ROC Curves

Since neither the choice of criteria nor the marginal distribution of the variables is an integral aspect of test performance, researchers in signal detection theory developed *receiver operating characteristic* (ROC) graphs to describe the ability of a test to discriminate between two states. ROC curves are based on the relationship between the probability of a true-positive (sensitivity) versus a false-positive result (1-specificity) over all possible scale cutpoints. Originally developed as a mathematical theory of the processes of detecting radar signals, signal detection theory was soon applied in studies of human perception and later to other discrimination and diagnostic tasks (Peterson, Bridsall, & Fox, 1954; Swets, 1986). There have been numerous applications of ROC theory in psychology (Green & Swets, 1966; Swets, 1973), as well as in medicine (Swets & Green, 1978; Weinstein & Fineberg, 1980). Surprisingly, however, ROC analysis has not been used often to evaluate psychiatric screening scales (Bridges & Goldberg, 1986; Mari & Williams, 1985; Mari & Williams, 1986; Murphy et al., 1987). ROC curves are well suited to the evaluation of depression screening scales, and available microcomputer software makes them easy to compute. They are especially useful because they can be used to evaluate the relative performance of mental health screening scales for different subsets of patients as well as the relative performance of different scales among the same patients.

An ROC curve can be derived in several ways (Cleary, Bush, & Kessler, 1987; Swets, 1986), but the approach used in most applications is to assume that the shape of the curve is the empirical probability of a true positive plotted as a function of the probability of a false positive for all possible criteria. There are several parameters that can be used to describe ROC curves, but in most applied situations, Swets (1986) recommends use of an index that is equivalent to the proportion of the area of the ROC graph that lies below the curve. When the ROC curve lies on the diagonal of the graph, the proportion of the area under the curve is 0.5 (chance discrimination), and when an ROC point is observed in the upper left corner of the graph, the area is 1.0 (perfect performance). In general, the larger the area under the ROC curve, the better the test performs. There are several computer programs available for estimating the area under an ROC curve (Dorfman & Alf, 1969; Swets & Pickett, 1982), and researchers evaluating depression scales can easily use these techniques to facilitate comparison among studies.

The area under an empirical ROC curve is equivalent to the probability that a detection instrument will be able to discriminate correctly between randomly paired normal and sick patients (Hanley & McNeil, 1982). The Wilcoxon statistic represents an equivalent aspect of the curve, and Hanley and McNeil (1982) present an efficient method of calculating both the statistic and its approximate standard error. When comparing different scales in the same sample, the standard error of the difference between estimates of the areas under two curves must incorporate a term representing the covariance of the estimators. Hanley and McNeil (1983) present a table of the correlation between two areas that can be used in the standard formula for testing differences between paired observations.

Making comparisons within populations can be extremely informative. For example, in chapter 10, Dr. Hough and his colleagues noted that the sensitivity of their screening scales, one of which was the General Health Questionnaire (GHQ), tended to be higher among women. We have also recently compared the performance of the GHQ (Goldberg, Rickels, Downing, & Hesbacher 1976) among men and women (Cleary et al., 1982). To test for an overall difference in performance, we first calculated the number of patients meeting any Research Diagnostic Criteria (RDC) (Spitzer, Endicott, & Robins, 1978) for each GHQ score and plotted the empirical ROC curves separately for men and for women. The area under the empirical ROC for men was 0.79 ($s.e.$ = .06); for women it was 0.80 ($s.e.$ = .04). Using standard formulae for testing the differences between means, we found that these areas were not significantly different (Z = .12). Although the overall shape of the curves was similar, the GHQ tends to be more sensitive and less specific for psychiatric disorders among women across a wide range of scale cutpoints. For example, using a score of four or more on the scale as the criteria for mental health problems (Cleary et al., 1982; Goldberg et al., 1976; Mann, 1977), we found that the sensitivity and specificity of the GHQ in this study for men were 0.58 and 0.87 and that the comparable figures for women were 0.74 and 0.75. In this small sample, these differences are not statistically significant, but they could be substantively important.

These results indicate that the interpretation of test results may vary substantially by patient group, even when the overall validity is comparable. The data from this study, as well as the data presented by Dr. Hough and his colleagues (ch. 10), suggest that in screening situations, there will be more true positives as well as false positives among women. That is, for any particular cutpoint, the GHQ will falsely identify more women as at risk of having a psychiatric disorder and will miss more men with a disorder.

Age Differences

When patients under 33 years of age from the study described above (Cleary et al., 1982) were compared to other patients, the areas under the empirical curves were 0.81 (.04) and 0.78 (.05), and the maximum likelihood estimates were 0.82 (.04) and 0.79 (.05), respectively. Although the area under the curve was somewhat greater for younger patients, the difference was not significant. However, younger patients were slightly more likely to meet criteria for at least one diagnosis (27.8% vs. 27.0%) and were more likely to have a positive screening score on the GHQ (35.3% vs. 27.0%). Furthermore, at the standard cutpoint, the GHQ was more sensitive (0.76 vs. 0.56) and less specific (0.80 vs. 0.84) among younger patients.

Our post hoc explanation for these findings is that among persons with a higher prevalence of symptoms, expression of those symptoms is more socially acceptable, and as a group, they will be more likely to report symptoms. Mari and Williams (1986) report data consistent with this explanation. They analyzed the correlates of misclassification on the GHQ and the Self-Report Questionnaire (SRQ) and found that men had about a five times greater risk of being misclassified as negative by the SRQ than women in the study. Sex apparently was not a significant predictor of false positives, and only the interaction of sex and education is reported for the analysis of false negatives on the GHQ.

However, there are at least two other possible explanations for why screening tests have higher sensitivity and lower specificity among subgroups with a higher prevalence of disorder. One is measurement error in the criterion for caseness. In subgroups with a higher prevalence of disorder, it is likely that there will be a lower proportion of false positives on the criterion measure and consequently, a screening scale is likely to identify fewer false positives in that population.

For example, let us assume that the sensitivity and specificity of the schedule for (SADS-L) using a perfect criterion, are 0.90 and that the sensitivity and specificity of the GHQ evaluated against a perfect criterion are 0.80. Further assume that we conduct a study using the SADS-L against which to evaluate the GHQ in two populations, one with a prevalence of 10% and the other with a prevalence of 50%. In this case, even though the validity of the GHQ is the same in the two populations, the apparent sensitivity in the low prevalence population would be 0.50, and in the high prevalence population it would be 0.74. A third explanation for higher sensitivity in a subgroup with a higher prevalence is that the spectrum of disease in that group is more serious and hence more likely to be detected by the screening test (Ransohoff & Feinstein, 1978).

Predictive Value

Although epidemiologists most often use sensitivity and specificity to evaluate screening tests, the predictive value of the test may provide information that is more relevant to clinical applications. *Positive predictive value* refers to the probability that a person with a positive test is actually a case. Conversely, *negative predictive value* is the probability that a person with a negative screening score will not be a case. These statistics are especially important because they describe how useful a scale will be to a clinician. For example, let us assume that we have a population in which 8% of the patients has severe depression and 50% has mild depression. If we assume that the sensitivity and specificity of the screening scale are 0.85 and 0.70, respectively, then the positive predictive value for severe disease is 19.8%, and for the mild disease it is 73.9%. If a scale is equally likely to detect mild and severe cases, the predictive value of the test is inversely related to the prevalence of the disorder. One obvious implication of this tendency is that if we focus our efforts on more narrowly defined and less prevalent conditions, nonspecific scales will probably have less predictive accuracy.

Validity of Criteria

It is extremely difficult to assess the validity of a diagnostic instrument, but since the validity of an instrument is limited by its reliability, one way of assessing the maximum validity is to evaluate its reliability. One measure of reliability is consistency. Below, I examine consistency of diagnosis of depression in the Epidemiologic Catchment Area (ECA) studies. The ECA project was a five-site, multiwave study of the incidence of the prevalence of major psychiatric disorders and the use of health and mental health services. Each of the ECA studies involved face-to-face interviews with approximately 3,000 noninstitutionalized persons over the age of 18. The persons interviewed in each community represented a probability sample of noninstitutionalized adults, but the exact nature of the sampling frame varied from site to site (Eaton & Kessler, 1985). Assessment of psychiatric conditions was done using the Diagnostic Interview Schedule (DIS), a structured interview designed for use by lay interviewers. Data collected using the DIS can be used to classify respondents in terms of DSM-III or Feighner criteria, or RDC. All analyses of psychiatric diagnoses presented in this chapter are based on DSM-III criteria calculated in the four sites for which longitudinal data were available.

The ECA project collected interview data at least two points in time, and so it is possible to examine how consistent responses to the DIS were. To do this, I first calculated the number of persons in different age groups who reported symptoms that met DSM-III criteria for major depression at the first interview, but who did not meet criteria at the second interview, approximately one year later. The results of these analyses are presented in Table 12.1. The data in this table are quite striking for a couple of reasons. First, it is surprising how high a percentage of all respondents who had a diagnosis at the first interview did not report enough symptoms at the second interview to meet the DSM-III criteria at

Table 12.1. Percentage of Lifetime Cases Reported at the First Interview That Were Not Reported at the Second Interview

Age Group	Percentage of Cases Not Reported
18—24	52.7%
25—34	44.5%
35—44	26.4%
45—54	39.7%
55—64	52.5%
65—74	31.6%
75 or older	33.3%

any point in their lives. Between approximately one-quarter and one-half of all respondents with an initial diagnosis changed their status at the second interview. Anyone who reported an episode of depression at the second interview was considered to have reported a lifetime episode, and, if we were to remove all the persons who reported an episode in the previous year at the one-year follow-up but who did not report a previous episode, these figures would be even higher.

The second noteworthy aspect of the data in Table 12.1 is that the proportion of cases not reported at the second interview varies by age, from a high of about 53% to a low of about 26%. In order to assess the possible impact on analyses of the relationship between age and rates of disorder, I recalculated the lifetime prevalence rates for all those completing the first interview and then recalculated the rates excluding cases from the numerator that were not also reported at the one-year follow-up. The results of these calculations are presented in Table 12.2. The most striking feature of Table 12.2 is that eliminating the cases that were not remembered at the second interview dramatically reduces the age differential in rates of major depression.

One possible explanation for the age differences in rates is that recall is likely to be related to whether one is currently experiencing an episode of depression. It may be, for example, that younger persons move in and out of episodes more frequently than older persons and have a higher probability than older persons of not being in an episode at the second interview. For example, Aneshensel (1985) examined data from five administrations of the Center for Epidemiologic Studies—Depression Scale (CES-D) and found that persons over the age of 50 were

Table 12.2. Rates of Major Depression by Age Group with and without Forgotten Cases Included

Age Group	Number of Respondents*	Rate Excluding Cases Not Reported	at Overall Rate
18—24	1390	5.3%	
2.5%			
25—34	2479	8.4%	
4.7%			
35—44	1518	9.5%	
2.5%			
45—54	1098	5.7%	
3.5%			
55—65	1600	3.7%	
1.8%			
65—74	2416	1.6%	
1.1%			
75 or older	1371	1.5%	
1.0%			

* Persons with an episode in an unknown period excluded.

more than three times as likely as persons under the age of 30 to have scores 16 at all five administrations. She also analyzed data for all respondents who were symptomatic at the first interview and calculated the probability that the person would be symptomatic at all subsequent interviews. The figure for those between the ages of 18 and 30 was 4.8%, for respondents aged 31 to 49 the figure was 9.4%, and for those over the age of 50, more than 24% were symptomatic at all subsequent administrations.

To examine this issue in the ECA data, I calculated the proportion of persons who met criteria for a lifetime episode at the first interview who reported an episode within the past month. The results of these calculations are presented in Table 12.3. This table shows that older respondents and those under 24 tended to report a higher proportion of episodes within the past month. For those over the age of 75 the figure was 70.8%.

These results indicate that although it is useful to evaluate screening scales against some standardized assessment, some of the most widely used assessment instruments are subject to substantial amounts of measurement error and that error may seriously compromise one's ability to accurately evaluate the performance of screening scales, especially when one is interested in subgroup comparisons. One major limitation of the DIS is that it is conducted by lay interviewers. In most clinical studies it would be possible to incorporate clinical assessments into an evaluation protocol. Using clinician assessments may improve the reliability and validity of assessments, but measurement error is still likely to be an important confound in studies of this type.

The Appropriate "Gold Standard"

Researchers and clinicians should always be concerned about reliability and validity of assessments, but a larger issue concerns what the most appropriate criterion for screening studies is. As Dr. Barrett points out in ch. 4, different classification systems have different goals. The goal of screening programs in

Table 12.3. Proportion of Episodes within Past Month among Respondents Reporting Any Lifetime Episode at First Interview

Age Group	Number of Respondents*	Rate of Recent Episodes (Past Month)
18—24	74	51.4%
25—34	210	41.4%
35—44	134	32.1%
45—54	62	43.6%
55—65	59	67.8%
65—74	38	44.7%
75 or older	24	70.8%

* Persons with an episode in an unknown period excluded.

clinic settings is almost always to identify those persons in need of care. However, different persons may have substantially different concepts of what constitutes "need." In a large number of cases, patients, providers, and epidemiologists would agree about whether a person needs services, but there are also a substantial number of cases in which there would be disagreement.

Leaf and colleagues (Leaf, Livingston, & Tischler, 1985) examined the distribution of four alternative indicators of need in a thirteen-town area in south-central Connecticut using data from the ECA study . The indicators of need examined were whether or not the respondent met DSM-III criteria for a psychiatric disorder, the extent of the person's symptoms, subjective appraisal of mental health, and reported disability due to mental or emotional problems. In the representative sample of community residents, the prevalence of these different types of need were 15.4%, 16.2%, 2.8%, and 3.3%, respectively. There was substantial overlap among these different indicators, but there were also many respondents who had one type but not others. For example, 6.2% of the respondents met criteria for a diagnosis, but were not high on the measure of symptoms, and 7.1% had many symptoms, but did not meet criteria for a diagnosis. Perceived need was only weakly related to whether or not the person met criteria for a diagnosis; only 9.7% of those with a diagnosis reported need, for example.

Similarly, Von Korff and coworkers (Von Korff et al., 1987) evaluated the mental health of a sample of primary care patients using the assessment of the primary care provider, the GHQ, and the DIS. The GHQ and practitioner assessment indicated that over 30% of the patients had a disorder, but the DIS identified only about 8% of the patients as having a disorder. All three assessments were positive in only about 5% of the patients.

Scope of Evaluation

Studies that evaluate screening programs for depression and other mental health problems tend to focus on the overall impact of the program. However, in applied research, the multiple possible goals of a program are often confused. When thinking about what reasonable expectations for a screening program are, it is useful to distinguish between efficacy trials and effectiveness trials. *Efficacy trials* provide tests of whether a technology, treatment, procedure, or program does more harm than good under optimum conditions. *Effectiveness trials* address similar questions, but in real world conditions.

It is important to keep this distinction in mind when evaluating whether screening programs are effective. For a screening program to have an impact on patient outcomes, patients must seek care, patients who would not otherwise be detected must acknowledge problems on the screening instrument, the scale should discriminate between those who are and are not in need, physicians must attend to the data, respond, and the responses must work. I would characterize the studies that evaluate primarily the discriminate performance of a screening scale, without addressing the other steps described, as efficacy trials. I would characterize studies that look at the ultimate effect of the program in terms of patient outcome as effectiveness trials. It is important to conduct effectiveness trials, but I think that most of these trials have been too narrow in their focus. Good effectiveness trials require assessment of program implementation, availability of the program to patients, and acceptability to both patients and physicians. A variety of factors, such as physician-patient communication, physicians' and patients' attitudes, physician training, availability of an effective treatment or referral source, and reimbursement could all affect the outcome of a screening study. "Screening" studies that examine the effect on patient outcomes often evaluate only the screening process and don't adequately assess a variety of other processes that are likely to affect whether screening leads to better outcomes.

Future Research

I think that our failure to take into account all the variables affecting outcome in effectiveness trials is one of the major reasons that screening studies often show no impact. I also think that we now have very good screening scales that perform quite well in clinical settings. If we had a treatment with demonstrated efficacy and a well-defined population for whom that treatment is efficacious, then screening scales would be widely used.

Our research agenda should address the questions that need to be answered before such a situation can exist:

1. Define the conditions for which we have efficacious treatments. For example, Dr. Barrett (ch. 4) has suggested that bipolar and major depression, panic, agoraphobia, schizophrenia, anorexia, and alcohol and drug abuse are all conditions for which we have treatments. This implies that when considering depression, we should focus our screening efforts on bipolar and major depression.

2. Develop a screening *and* diagnostic protocol. I mentioned earlier that a practical screening scale should be short, easy to use, and accurate. The data in other chapters in this volume indicate that there are numerous screening scales with adequate accuracy for use in primary care settings. However, it is probably possible to shorten many of these scales without greatly affecting their accuracy. Unfortunately, we know very little about what types of scales are acceptable to both patients and physicians. Although many of the evaluations in the literature can best be characterized as effectiveness trials, few studies evaluated patient or physician reactions to the screening process. Screening is only the first step in the diagnostic process, but in outcome studies, clinicians are rarely given explicit directions concerning how to make a final diagnosis.

3. Specify the treatment regimen for the defined conditions. Screening will lead to better outcomes only if an efficacious treatment is used.

4. Define the array of possible ways of organizing and financing care.

5. Conduct demonstration and efficacy trials that focus on a wide array of outcomes. These studies should investigate not only psychiatric status, but also evaluate functioning in terms of activities of daily living, role functioning, and social functioning.

6. Study the acceptability and diffusion of these programs.

7. Continue to conduct basic research on the detection and treatment of specific diseases and syndromes. This should include basic research on nosology and the way in which factors such as age, gender, and culture affect both the experience of psychiatric disease and the expression of illness.

Conclusion

The psychometric properties of screening scales are an important topic, and short, easy to use screening scales are a necessary condition for an effective screening program for depression. However, a review of the extensive literature on screening scales suggests that the narrow focus on developing better instruments may have distracted us from the broader issues of what our ultimate "gold standard" is, whether we have efficacious treatments for the conditions we are detecting, and how the organization and financing of care as well as medical training affect the treatment patients receive. It is only by addressing these broader issues that we will ultimately meet the unmet needs that currently exist in primary care.

References

Aneshensel, C. S. (1985). The natural history of depressive symptoms: Implications for psychiatric epidemiology. In J. R. Greenley (ed.) *Research in community and mental health* (pp. 45–75). New York: JAI Press.

Bridges, K. W., & Goldberg, D. P. (1986). The validation of the GHQ-28 and the use of the MMSE in neurological in-patients. *British Journal of Psychiatry, 148,* 548–553.

Cleary, P. D., Bush, B. T., & Kessler, L. G. (1987). Evaluating use of mental health screening scales in primary care settings using Receiver Operating Characteristic curves. *Medical Care, 25* (Suppl.), S90–S98.

Cleary, P. D., Goldberg, I. D., Kessler, L. G., & Nycz, G. R. (1982). Screening for mental disorder among primary care patients. Usefulness of the General Health Questionnaire. *Archives of General Psychiatry, 39,* 837–840.

Dorfman, D. D., & Alf, E., Jr. (1969). Maximum likelihood estimation of parameters of signal-detection theory and determination of confidence intervals–Rating method data. *Journal of Mathematical Psychology, 6,* 487–496.

Eaton, W. W., & Kessler, L. G. (eds.) (1985). *Epidemiologic field methods in psychiatry: The NIMH Epidemiologic Catchment Area Program.* Orlando: Academic Press.

Goldberg, D. P. (1972). *The detection of psychiatric illness by questionnaire.* London: Oxford University Press.

Goldberg, D. P., Rickels, K., Downing, R., & Hesbacher, P. (1976). A comparison of two psychiatric screening tests. *British Journal of Psychiatry, 129,* 61–67.

Goldberg, I. D., Roghmann, K. J., McInerny, T. K., & Burke, J. D., Jr. (1984). Mental health problems among children seen in pediatric practice: Prevalence and management. *Pediatrics, 7,* 278–293.

Green, D. M., & Swets, J. A. (1966). *Signal detection theory and psychophysics.* New York: Krieger.

Hankin, J. R., & Oktay, J. S. (1979). *Mental disorder and primary medical care: An analytical review of the literature* (Publication No. ADM 78–661). Washington, D.C.: National Institute of Mental Health Series D, U.S. Dept. of Health, Education, and Welfare.

Hanley, J. A., & McNeil, B. J. (1982). The meaning and use of the area under a receiver operating characteristic (ROC) curve. *Radiology, 143,* 29–36.

Hanley, J. A., & McNeil, B. J. (1983). A method of comparing the areas under receiver operating characteristic curves derived from the same cases. *Radiology, 148,* 839–843.

Hoeper, E. W., Nycz, G. R., Cleary, P. D., Regier, D. A., & Goldberg, I. D. (1979). Estimated prevalence of RDC mental disorder in primary medical care. *International Journal of Mental Health, 8,* 6–15.

Jacobson, A. M., Goldberg, D., Burns, B. J., Hoeper, E. W., Hankin, J. R., & Hewitt, K. (1980). Diagnosed mental disorder in children and use of health services in four organized health care settings. *American Journal of Psychiatry, 137,* 559–565.

Kessler, L. G. (1984). Treated incidence of mental disorders in a prepaid group practice setting. *American Journal of Public Health, 74,* 152–154.

Kessler, L. G., Burns, B. J., Shapiro, S., Tischler, G. L., George, L. K., Hough, R. L., Bodison, D., & Miller, R. H. (1986). Psychiatric diagnoses of medical service users: Evidence from the Epidemiologic Catchment Area Program. *American Journal of Public Health, 77,* 18–24.

Leaf, P. J., Livingston, M. M., & Tischler, G. L. (August, 1985). *Can we live by diagnosis alone? The necessity of alternative indicators of caseness in studies of need.* Proceedings of the Second International Conference on Illness Behavior, Toronto, Ontario, Canada.

Manderscheid, R. W., & Witkin, M. J. (1983). The specialty mental health services–United States (DHHS Publication No. ADM 83-1275). In C. A. Taube, & S. A. Barrett (eds.), *Mental health, United States* (pp 3–40). Rockville, MD: National Institute of Mental Health.

Mann, A. H. (1977). The psychological effect of a screening program and clinical trial for hypertension upon the participants. *Psychological Medicine, 7,* 431–438.

Mari, J. J., & Williams, P. (1985). A comparison of the validity of two psychiatric screening questionnaires (GHQ–12 and SRQ–20) in Brazil, using Relative Operating Characteristic (ROC) analysis. *Psychological Medicine, 15,* 651–659.

Mari, J. J, & Williams P. (1986). Misclassification by psychiatric screening questionnaires. *Journal of Chronic Diseases, 39,* 371–378.

Murphy, J. M., Berwick, D. M., Weinstein, M. C., Borus, J. F., Budman, S. H., & Klerman, G. L. (1987). Performance of screening and diagnostic tests: Application of receiver operating characteristic (ROC) analysis. *Archives of General Psychiatry, 44,* 550–555.

Peterson, W. W., Bridsall, T. G., & Fox, W. C. (1954). The theory of signal detectability. *Transactions of the IRE Professional Group on Information Theory, 4,* 171–212.

Ransohoff, D. F., & Feinstein, A. R. (1978). Problems of spectrum and bias in evaluating the efficacy of diagnostic tests. *New England Journal of Medicine, 299,* 926–930.

Regier, D. A., Goldberg, I. D., Burns, B.J., Hankin, J., Hoeper, E. W., & Nycz, G. R. (1982).

Specialist/generalist division of responsibility for patients with mental disorders. *Archives of General Psychiatry, 39,* 219–224.

Schlesinger, H. J., Mumford, E., Glass, G. V., Patrick, C., & Sharfstein, S. (1983). Mental health treatment and medical care utilization in a fee-for-service system: Outpatient mental health treatment following the onset of a chronic disease. *American Journal Public Health, 73,* 422–429.

Schulberg, H., Saul, M., McClelland, M., Ganguli, M., Christy, W., & Frank, R. (1985). Assessing depression in primary medical and psychiatric practices. *Archives of General Psychiatry, 42,* 1164–1172.

Shepherd, M. (1983). Mental disorder and primary care in the United Kingdom. *Journal Public Health Policy, 4,* 83–88.

Spitzer, R., Endicott, J., & Robins, E. (1978). *Research criteria (RDC) for a selected group of functional disorders.* New York: New York State Psychiatric Institute.

Swets, J. A. (1973). The relative operating characteristic in psychology. *Science, 182,* 990–1000.

Swets, J. A. (1986). Indices of discrimination or diagnostic accuracy: Their ROCs and implied models. *Psychological Bulletin, 99,* 100–117.

Swets, J. A., & Green, D. M. (1978). Applications of signal detection theory. In H. L. Pick, Jr., H. W. Leibowitz, J. E. Singer, A. Steinschneider, & H. W. Stevenson (eds.), *Psychology: From research to practice* (pp. 311–331). New York: Plenum Press.

Swets, J. A., & Pickett, R. M. (1982). *Evaluation of diagnostic systems: Methods from signal detection theory.* New York: Academic Press.

Von Korff, M., Shapiro, S., Burke, J. D., Teitlebaum, M., Skinner, E. A., German, P., Turner, R. W., Klein, L., & Burns, B. (1987). Anxiety and depression in a primary care clinic. Comparison of diagnostic interview schedule, general health questionnaire, and practitioner assessments. *Archives of General Psychiatry, 44,* 152–156.

Weinstein, M. C., & Fineberg, H. V. (1980). *Clinical decision analysis.* Philadelphia: W. B. Saunders.

Westhead, J. N. (1985). Frequent attenders in general practice: Medical, psychological, and social characteristics. *Journal of the Royal College of General Practitioners, 35,* 337–340.

Wilkinson, G. (1986). *Mental health practices in primary care settings: An annotated bibliography, 1977–1984.* New York: Tavistock Publications.

Part III
Special Population Issues in Screening for Depression

Contributors to this section examine the characteristics of special populations that may affect the utility of various depression screening methods in primary care. There are several important reasons for understanding age-related, gender, ethnic, cultural, and socioeconomic differences. Such knowledge (a) assists researchers in constructing screening instruments that are maximally sensitive to the full range of medical patients suffering from depression, (b) helps clinicians detect depressed patients more rapidly and reliably in their practices, and (c) helps researchers design services research studies that focus on efficacy of treatment and referral options. Failure to appreciate special population differences can lead to misdiagnosis or delimit detection and appropriate treatment of depression in important subgroups of medical patients.

Robert E. Roberts examines the phenomenology of depression as a function of culture. He gives special attention to measurement issues, the relationship between mood and somatic illness, and likely sources of bias which may compromise screening outcomes. Following Roberts' chapter are several chapters reporting empirical studies involving special populations. Anna E. Barón, Spero M. Manson, Lynn M. Ackerson, and Douglas L. Brenneman examine depressive symptomatology in older American Indians with chronic disease. Barón et al. are particularly interested in the validity of the widely used Center for Epidemiologic Studies—Depression (CES-D) scale and report support for use of the CES-D as a screening tool for preventive interventions with American Indians. However, their research indicates that the scale operates quite differently with older and chronically ill American Indians than it does within general population studies.

The third paper in this section, by Jeanne Miranda, Ricardo F. Muñoz, and Martha Shumway reports on the use of depression screening instruments to select high-risk patients who might benefit from depression prevention programs. In addition to examining the results of a depression prevention clinical trial with a multi-ethnic sample, Miranda et al. examine the utility of the CES-D within ethnic and language subgroups.

In the concluding chapter John Matthew, a primary care physician practicing in Vermont, views clinical depression from the perspective of a practitioner who has daily contact with patients across the age range, from urban to rural, and who range from the well-educated to those who are illiterate. Many of Matthew's patients have been in his practice through numerous life transitions and others are more recent additions to a growing practice. Matthew emphasizes the need to screen for depression in ways that are respectful of the patient-doctor relationship and recognize the patient's individual needs and style. Although opposed to questionnaires, Matthew advocates that physicians screen for depression, insofar as possible, during every patient encounter.

13

Special Population Issues in Screening for Depression

Robert E. Roberts

A discussion addressing the topic of special populations is potentially as broad as the range of attributes that can make any human group distinct from another. My focus is considerably more circumscribed. The issue that I wish to explore is screening for depression and related conditions across different cultural contexts. My specific objective is to raise questions about reliability and validity of procedures for screening for psychological dysfunction (in this case depression) in a highly pluralistic society such as that of the United States.

I would like to organize consideration of this topic around five central themes: (a) culture and ethnicity in the United States, (b) the phenomenology of depression from a cross-cultural perspective, (c) measurement of depression, (d) the relationship between mood and somatic illness, and (e) sources of bias which may compromise screening outcomes.

Ethnicity

Ethnic groups are collectives that are distinguishable in terms of their class position, their cultural traits, and their physiognomy (Marden & Meyer, 1962) and that have varying amounts of power, privilege, and prestige (Lenski, 1966). Schermerhorn (1969) stresses ethnicity as a function of shared experiences that focus on such symbolic elements as kinship patterns, physical contiguity, religious affiliation, languages or dialect forms, tribal affiliation, nationality, phenotypic features, or any combination of these. Yancey, Ericksen, and Juliani (1976) argue that ethnicity depends not so much on historical origin as on conditions of residential stability and segregation, common occupational positions, and dependence on local institutions and services. Ethnicity is essentially a manifestation of the way populations are organized in terms of interaction patterns, institutions, personal values, attitudes, lifestyles, and presumed consciousness of kind. In addition, ethnicity, and particularly minority group status, is also a manifestation of the way the larger society perceives and interacts with its subnations. Two somewhat different kinds of ethnic manifestations have been observed, referred to variously as "old" and "new" ethnicity (Novak, 1977), "behavioral" and

183

"ideological" ethnicity (Stein & Hill, 1977), or in terms of a contrast between "cultural groups" and true "ethnic groups" (Patterson, 1975). The fundamental differences relates to (a) the degree to which group members in fact share cultural standards, and (b) the range of social situations in which ethnic identity is expressed. As Harwood (1981) notes, in behavioral ethnicity, the ethnic culture is learned by members as part of the socialization process, and culture serves as the fundamental basis for interaction within the group as well as interaction with other groups and the larger society. On the other hand, ideological ethnicity is based largely on customs that are neither central to social life nor necessarily intrinsic to the socialization process.

Drawing upon reformulations of the traditional concept of culture (see Hannerz, 1969; Keesing, 1974), Swidler (1986) presents a definition of culture that focuses on how culture influences behavior. Ethnic culture, according to Swidler, consists of symbolic vehicles of meaning, including beliefs, ritual practices, art forms, and ceremonies, as well as informal cultural practices such as language, gossip, stories, and rituals of daily life. Swidler argues that culture provides "strategies of action," persistent ways of ordering action through time, a "repertoire" for constructing action. These strategies of action incorporate and thus depend upon moods, habits, sensibilities, and views of the world (Geertz, 1973). People construct chains of action beginning with at least some prefabricated links. Culture influences action through the shape and organization of those links.

The ethnic and cultural mosaic of the United States stems from immigration. Archdeacon (1983) has described in detail how foreign peoples and cultures have transformed the United States during the past four centuries. In particular, he notes the contemporary impact of the interaction of diverse cultural traditions from Europe, Asia, and Africa with the indigenous peoples of the Western Hemisphere. There are literally hundreds of ethnic or cultural groups in the United States, and their numbers are growing. The 1980 census counted over 14 million foreign-born persons in the United States, over half of whom had immigrated within the previous decade (U.S. Bureau of the Census, 1984) from virtually every country in the world.

My point in raising this issue is that there are many diverse ethnic groups in our society, particularly in large urban areas, with equally diverse cultural repertoires regarding recognition, interpretation, and labeling of signs and symptoms of illness and help-seeking, all of which have implications for detection of depression in primary care settings.

Culture and Depression

A number of authors (Akiskal & McKinney, 1975; Friedman, 1974; Robins & Guze, 1972; Whybrow & Palatore, 1973) have noted the heterogeneity of depressive phenomena. For example, Akiskal (1979) has distinguished four types of depressive phenomena: (a) normal depression, (b) situation or reactive depression, (c) secondary depression, and (d) primary depression or melancholia. The first two phenomena are subclinical mood disturbances, differing from each other in terms of severity and duration. *Normal depression* is seen as a universal adaptive response to stress, frustration, or loss, ordinarily lasting a few hours to a few days. *Situational* or *reactive depression* is more severe, usually lasting from several weeks to several months. Grief in response to loss of a love object or pronounced nostalgia are examples of this type of depressive phenomena. Primary and secondary depressions are examples of clinical depression. *Secondary depressions* are analogous to situational depressions, except that they are more severe and are sequelae of other serious medical or psychiatric disorders. The dysphoria usually parallels the course of the primary disorder (Guze, Woodruff, & Clayton, 1971; Woodruff, Murphy, & Herjanic, 1967) and rarely reaches melancholic proportions (Winokur, 1972). Contrasted with situational and secondary depressions, *primary depressions,* or melancholias, either arise without preexisting or concurrent nonaffective disorder or seem out of proportion to life changes preceding them. Akiskal points out that primary depression is where one finds the development of the full syndrome that has many attributes of a disease state, such as disruption of psychomotor and vegetative functions, considerable morbidity and mortality, autonomous course, and favorable response to specific pharmacologic agents (see also Prange, 1973). DSM-III (and also DSM-III-R) is quite explicit about what constitutes depression. The overriding feature is dysphoria, accompanied by other symptoms, chief among which are (a) disturbed appetite or weight change, (b) insomnia or hypersomnia, (c) psychomotor agitation or retardation, (d) anhedonia, (e) loss of energy or fatigue, (f) feelings of worthlessness, self-reproach, or guilt, (g) diminished ability to think or concentrate, and (h) recurrent thoughts of death and suicide ideation or gestures (American Psychiatric Association, 1980, pp. 205–224).

Acknowledging that there are criticisms of DSM-III diagnostic criteria on a variety of issues, what can we say about this particular diagnostic system vis-à-vis its utility in screening and/or diagnosing primary care patients from diverse ethnic and cultural origins? Recent extensive reviews of the literature (Kleinman & Good, 1985; Marsella, 1980) conclude unequivocally that there is no universal conception of depression. Many non-Western cultures do not even have a concept of depression equivalent to Western definitions (such as operationalized in DSM-III). Even dysphoria, the central feature of our construct "depression," is either not a prominent feature (sometimes it is not even present), or it has dramatically different manifestations and meanings in different cultures. In addition to cross-cultural variations in dysphoria, there also are wide variations in other symptoms of depressive illness, in particular, feelings of worthlessness, self-reproach, or guilt (Marsella, 1980). In fact, Marsella concludes that assessment of depression by affect descriptors has limited crosscultural validity, since affective states in many cultures are not even labeled.

While it is true that the most divergent data on the phenomenology of depression emanate from crossnational studies, the findings in no way are limited to that context. A number of studies comparing different ethnic populations in the United States provide additional evidence.

Boyer (1964) has reported finding no concept representing depression as either a disease symptom or syndrome among American Indians. Johnson and Johnson (1965) have reported a pattern of disorder among Sioux Indians that translates as "totally discouraged," involving feelings of helplessness, thoughts of death, and preoccupation with ideas of ghosts and spirits. Manson, Shore, and Bloom (1985) present data indicating that 93% of their Hopi informants reported no Hopi equivalent for our concept of depression. However, 50% of their patient sample had chronic and major depression according to Research Diagnostic Criteria (RDC). One form of Hopi indigenous illness category (*uu nung mo kiw ta*) was composed of symptoms of weight loss, disrupted sleep, fatigue, and psychomotor retardation as well as agitation, loss of libido, sinfulness, shame, not being likable, and trouble thinking clearly. Of relevance for DSM-III criteria, Hopi often reported dysphoria for one week, but rarely for two weeks.

Kinzie and Manson (1987) report development of a fifteen-item depression screening scale suitable for use with Vietnamese in the United States (it correctly identified 91% of the clinically depressed). Of interest for this discussion is that the scale consists of items from three sets of symptoms: physical symptoms commonly associated with depression in the Western concept; psychological symptoms related to lowered dysphoric mood in the Western concept; and symptoms that seemed unrelated to the Western notion of depression. The authors conclude that some symptoms that reliably define depression among Vietnamese do not fit the Western idea of depression, but rather reflect Vietnamese ideas concerning cognitive, affective, and behavioral indicators of mood disturbance.

Of interest here is a paper by Beiser and Fleming (1986). They used items drawn from a number of measures of psychopathology, including several developed specifically for crosscultural studies, to study three Southeast Asian refugee groups—Chinese from Vietnam, ethnic Vietnamese, and Laotians. Four distinct measures emerged, relating to panic, depression, somatization, and well-being. Beiser and Fleming report that in addition to being culturally sensitive, the scales have good reliability, concurrent validity, and stability of structure across ethnic groups.

Tanaka-Matsumi and Marsella (1977) report very different semantic structures (implying different connotations) for the construct "depression" among Japanese nationals, Japanese Americans, and Anglos. In an earlier paper (Marsella & Tanaka-Matsumi, 1976) they report differences in frequency, duration, and severity of symptoms of depression among these same three groups.

Marsella, Kinzie, and Gordon (1973) report that Japanese Americans evidence a strong interpersonal component to depression (e.g., dislike being around others, not talking to others, not caring for appearance), that Chinese Americans show a strong somatic component (e.g., stomach pains, sleep difficulty, weakness), and that Anglos show more traditional depressive symptoms (e.g., despair, loss of purpose, hollow and empty feelings). Based on a subsequent study, Marsella and his associates (Marsella, Brennan, Kameoka, & Shirzuru, 1974; Marsella, Shirzuru, Brennan, & Kameoka, 1974) report that body image satisfaction and self-concept discrepancy may be important aspects of depression across Anglo, Chinese, and Japanese groups.

Studies of depressive symptomatology among black Americans have generally emphasized predominance of somatic complaints (Carter, 1974; McLaughlin, Rickels, Abidi, & Toro, 1969; Simon, Fleiss, Gurland, Stiller, & Sharpe, 1973) in contrast to an emphasis on cognitive disturbances and depressed mood in whites. Tonks, Paykel, and Klerman (1970) and Hanson, Klerman, and Tanner (1973) have concluded, however, that differences between black and white depressed patients are minimal and that similarities between the two groups are far more prominent than differences. Simon et al. (1973) report no differences between black and white patients on depressed mood, but report anxiety, irritability, worry, and somatic complaints among the former. Unlike the Klerman studies, this study did not control for status differences between the two groups. Helzer (1975) reports that black and white inpatients with a diagnosis of bipolar depression differed only with respect to a higher incidence of initial insomnia among the former. There were no differences in terms of euphoria, irritability, hyperactivity, flight of ideas, grandiosity, or other symptoms. In one of the more carefully controlled studies of the phenomenology of depression among blacks, Raskin, Crook, and Herman (1975) report that black and white patients were remarkably similar on the core symptoms of depression (e.g., depressed mood, sleep disturbance, guilt, etc.).

I would like to conclude this part of my discussion by examining an ethnic group that has been the focus of much of my research: persons of Mexican origin. Although the existence of culturally specific symptoms and syndromes such as *susto, mal puesto, ataque de nervios, pena, dolor de cerebro,* and *embrujado* are well-documented in the literature, there have been few systematic studies of the phenomenology of mental disorders in this group. There have been a few studies, and the data from these are both provocative and equivocal.

Fabrega, Swartz, and Wallace (1968a; 1968b) found that when Mexican-American schizophrenics who had been hospitalized for less than two years were compared with Anglo and black schizophrenics, based both on psychiatrists' ratings and on ward observations made by nurses, the Mexican-American group showed significantly more regressed behavior, social disorganization, and psychoticism. Pokorny and Overall (1970) found that the observed mean scores of Mexican-American patients were significantly higher on five of eight symptom sets derived from the Brief Psychiatric Rating Scale—mental disorganization, mental distortion, withdrawal, retardation, motor distortion, and depression—even after controlling for demographic and socioeconomic differences among blacks, Anglos, and Mexican Americans.

Meadow and Stoker (1965) analyzed the medical records of matched samples of Anglo and Mexican-American inpatients and found a significantly higher frequency among Mexican Americans on agitation, alcoholism, auditory and visual hallucinations, crying spells, depression, eating difficulty, threats and attempts to hurt others, mutism, poor orientation, sleeplessness, slow thoughts and movements, withdrawal, postpartum psychosis, belief in witches, and visits to curers. In a second study, Stoker, Zurcher, and Fox (1968–69) report that compared to Anglos, Mexican-American women had significantly higher frequencies of many symptom categories: agitation, crying, dependency, depression, eating difficulty, hostility, hyperactivity, overtalkativeness, sleeplessness, somatic complaints, suicide attempts, temper tantrums, visual hallucinations, and staying in bed.

Heiman and Kahn (1977) report that Mexican-American patients were judged significantly more bizarre, to have delusions and hallucinations more often, and to have a tendency to be more depressed and more likely to have a thought disorder. However, after controls were implemented for differences in sex and social class, most of the initial contrasts disappeared. In a more recent study, Lawson, Kahn, and Heiman (1982) compared Anglo and Mexican patients admitted to the inpatient unit of a mental health center, using both the Minnesota Multiphasic Personality Inventory (MMPI) and clinical diagnoses. The two groups did not differ significantly.

There have been several attempts to examine dimensionality of various screening scales when used with persons of Mexican origin. Roberts (1980) reports results of confirmatory factor analysis of the Center for Epidemiologic Studies—Depression Scale (CES-D) items in which the same general structure emerges in different ethnic contexts (Anglo, black, Mexican origin) and this structure reflects the dimensions originally attributed to the scale—that is, depressed affect, positive affect, somatic and retarded activity, and interpersonal relations. Aneshensel, Clark, and Frerichs (1983) also examined dimensionality of the CES-D across Anglos, blacks, and Mexican Americans and found that the same four factors emerged and that these factors were invariant across these population groups. Vernon and Roberts (1981) report that eighteen of the Psychiatric Epidemiology Research Interview (PERI) psychopathology scales developed by Dohrenwend and his colleagues (Dohrenwend, Shrout, Egri, & Mendelsohn, 1980) yield equivalent results when used in these same three ethnic groups and, furthermore, that results for the PERI were similar to those for the CES-D and Bradburn scales. Codina and Roberts (1987) report mixed results in their attempt to confirm for a sample of U.S. and foreign-born persons of Mexican origin the dimensionality of nineteen items indicative of mood and somatic disturbance used in a previous national survey (Veroff, Douvan, & Kulka, 1981). Originally, these items were reported to form three distinct subscales, indicative of ill health, anxiety, and immobilization. I could not replicate these results. I did find some support for a two-factor structure, whose items were somewhat parallel to those falling into the anxiety domain (trouble sleeping, nervousness, headaches, loss of appetite, upset stomach, difficulty getting up, and weight loss) and ill health domain (shortness of breath, limitation of activity, heart beating hard, and dizziness) in the original study. In general, comparability of dimensionality declined as one moved from non-Hispanic, nonblacks, at one extreme, to foreign-born persons of Mexican origin assessed in Spanish at the other extreme.

There have been several studies of the role of language in psychopathology among Hispanics. Ruiz (1975) reports that feelings reported in a native language are more likely to be expressed with more emotion. History provided in the patient's primary language may not appear as bizarre as when the patient provides the same history in a secondary language (Philippus, 1971). Disclosure of interpersonal relationships, feelings, and general health also have been found to be significantly greater in Spanish than in English for Spanish-dominant bilinguals (Price & Cuellar, 1981). Such factors as self-disclosure, history presented, expression of feelings, and degree of affect are not minor variables in diagnostic formulation. As a whole they are potentially capable of "coloring" the clinical picture presented by Spanish-speaking patients. Del Castillo (1970) reports clinical experiences in which Spanish-speaking patients appeared psychotic during native-tongue interviews but seemed much less so when the interview was conducted in English, sometimes without any overt psychotic symptoms. Marcos, Urcuyo, Kesselman, and Alpert (1973) report, in contrast, that the psychiatric rating of ten schizophrenic patients, whose native language was Spanish, disclosed more psychopathology when they were interviewed in English than when they were interviewed in Spanish. Gonzales (1978) also studied ten bilingual Hispanic schizophrenic patients and found that Spanish-language interviews lasted longer and appeared to contain different material. However, the difference was not that more pathology was reported in Spanish, but that pathology was presented more intensely. For example, the patients displayed significantly more discomfort from their symptoms when interviewed in Spanish compared to English. None of these studies had as its focus depression, and, in fact, there are no data on the role of language in the manifestation of depression or other forms of psychopathology among Hispanics or any other major ethnic minority in the United States.

There currently are three studies that collected data permitting rigorous examination of the phenomenology of depression among persons of Mexican origin. The Los Angeles Epidemiologic Catchment Area (ECA) project (Burnam, Karno, Hough, Escobar, & Telles, 1987) used the full Diagnostic Interview Schedule (DIS) with 1,200 Anglos and 1,200 Mexican-origin persons sampled from the community. The study also included the CES-D. The Hispanic Health and Nutrition Examination Survey included the depression section from the DIS and the CES-D with a sample of 3,341 Mexican origin adults from the Southwestern United States. I am currently analyzing data from a sample of 210 Anglo and 349 Mexican origin patients from public mental health facilities in San Antonio,

Texas, all of which were administered the DIS and the CES-D. Thus far, none of these studies has published analyses that have had as their focus the phenomenology of depression and whether its presentation varies by language, ethnic status, or place of birth. Taken together, these data sets should provide more knowledge about the manifestation of depression in this important ethnic group than all previous research efforts combined.

There are, as I noted earlier, increasing numbers of individuals in American society who have immigrated from countries with very different cultural traditions, both Western and non-Western. There also have been studies of depression in a number of these societies, although few of immigrants. For good discussions of crossnational research on depression, excellent sources are Singer (1975), Marsella (1980), and Kleinman and Good (1985).

Measuring Depression

In terms of a discussion of strategies appropriate for screening for depression in primary care settings, Akiskal's fourfold classification can be reduced to a dichotomy: clinical depression and nonclinical depression. The rationale for this reduction is straightforward. Classifying depressive phenomena as clinical or nonclinical gives us the advantage of having a disease classification that closely mirrors measurement approaches extant in psychiatric epidemiology, i.e., clinical and psychometric (Dohrenwend & Dohrenwend, 1982).

The most frequently used screening devices are nonclinical in nature, primarily because they are more economical and feasible to use (Seiler, 1973). A variety of measures of nonclinical psychopathology have been developed over the years by mental health researchers (see Boyd & Weissman, 1981; Dohrenwend, Oksenbeg, Shrout, Dohrenwend, & Cook, 1981; Link & Dohrenwend, 1980; Vernon & Roberts, 1981). Although there seems to be a common universe of content to which the items in these various measures refer, there is still substantial diversity in actual item content. Furthermore, there is considerable conceptual confusion concerning what exactly is being measured. Constructs used to describe the phenomenon being measured have included mental illness, psychological impairment, psychophysiological distress, psychological distress, nonspecific psychological well-being, psychiatric symptoms, and other variations of these themes (see Seiler, 1973, for example). Some measures have been developed specifically to measure depressive symptoms and are so labeled. Perhaps three of the better known examples are the twenty-item Zung Self-Rating Depression Scale (Zung, 1965), the twenty-one-item Beck Depression Inventory (Beck, Ward, Mendelsohn, Mock, & Erbaugh, 1961), and the twenty-item CES-D (Radloff, 1977), although there are others. The overriding disadvantage of measures of nonclinical impairment, as Weissman and Klerman (1978) succinctly point out, is that impairment ratings are independent of diagnosis. Indeed, studies have demonstrated that the relationship between nonclinical measures and specific diagnoses is not strong (Myers & Weissman, 1980; Roberts & Vernon, 1981, 1983). Thus, while symptom checklists may provide estimates of "expressed distress," they do not permit classification of subjects into discrete disease categories (see Spiro, Siassi, & Crocetti [1972] for a discussion of the requirements for a psychiatric screening instrument). In fact, it has been argued that, in the absence of other, more diagnosis-specific information, nondiagnostic measures are of limited use in assessing mental health service needs or identifying etiologic factors since recent research demonstrates that different psychiatric disorders have differing clinical manifestations, natural histories, family aggregation, and responses to treatment (Weissman & Klerman, 1978).

On the other hand, recent investigations suggest brief symptom checklists may be useful from at least two perspectives: as measures of nonspecific psychological distress and as the initial assessment procedure used in two-stage case-identification in psychiatric screening.

Dohrenwend et al. (1980) report that all symptom checklists are similar in content, have properties that meet the requirements for being collectively defined as a dimension, have reliabilities in the range of .80–.85, and tend to correlate with each other about as highly as their reliabilities permit. They argue that these attributes indicate that the various indexes are all measures of the same thing and that this phenomenon is "nonspecific psychological distress," or what others have referred to as "demoralization" (Frank, 1973) or "expressed distress" (Roberts, 1981). The items in the scales are generally related to affective distress but are not specific to any particular psychiatric disorder. Dohrenwend and his colleagues suggest further that these global measures function much as a thermometer does in physical diagnosis. Elevated scores indicate something is wrong, but do not, by themselves, permit a differential diagnosis. Dohrenwend and his colleagues (Dohrenwend et al., 1980; Link & Dohrenwend, 1980) argue that what these instruments measure is best defined using Frank's (1973) concept of "demoralization." The central features of this phenomenon are low self-esteem, helplessness-hopelessness, sadness, and anxiety. Frank posits that this condition is a major factor leading people to seek help and is also the condition that psychotherapy attempts to relieve (p. 278). Link and Dohrenwend (1980) argue that demoralization is a condition that is likely "to be experienced in association with a variety of problems, including severe physical illness, particularly chronic illness, stressful life events, psychiatric disorders, and perhaps conditions of social marginality as experienced by minority groups and persons such as housewives and the poor whose social positions block them from mainstream strivings" (p. 115). A measure of demoralization even has been developed (Dohrenwend et al., 1980) incorporating the central features of Frank's concept. Work by Link and Dohrenwend (1980) and by Vernon and Roberts (1981) provides additional support for this interpretation. Several authors (Akiskal, 1979; Klein, 1974) have also noted that a state of demoralization is commonly observed in chronic psychiatric disorder, presumably stemming from the episodic and unpredictable exacerbations of the disease, ambiguities about etiology and outcome, as well as the social and interpersonal costs incurred.

In view of these considerations, brief psychiatric symptom scales may prove useful as screening instruments, since the rationale for most disease-screening procedures is to provide a fast, economical method of detecting cases of suspected or potential illness in the general population (Roberts, 1981). Because these techniques select out subjects with a high probability of being a case (i.e., the false-negative rate is low), they can increase efficiency in community surveys (Weissman & Klerman, 1978). But few screening tests are sufficient to establish a definitive diagnosis (due primarily to their low specificity). Thus, it is not surprising that Cooper and Morgan (1973) argue that a two-stage process of case identification is virtually essential to generate valid epidemiologic results. Shrout and Fleiss (1981) have demonstrated that multimethod procedures are essentially mandatory if accurate case ascertainment is to be achieved. In their discourse on this topic, Dohrenwend and Dohrenwend (1982) argue for the use of symptom scales (with their strong psychometric properties and economy of administration) as initial assessments, followed by assessments using clinical diagnostic procedures. Such a two-stage process clearly is critical in establishing sensitivity and specificity of the screening instrument, since a prerequisite for evaluating the discriminant power of a screening test is the existence of a criterion classification, based on some independent and more definitive procedure, against which the test results can be judged (Mausner & Bahn, 1974). The definitive criterion used for validation is usually a clinical psychiatric examination. Unfortunately, the sensitivity and specificity of most screening instruments in psychiatric epidemiology are essentially unknown (see Myers & Weissman, 1980).

Even though some research might suggest that brief psychiatric symptom scales may provide adequate operational measures of demoralization of nonspecific psychological distress, we still have very little knowledge concerning their utility as first-stage screening instruments in epidemiologic surveys. In fact, the evidence concerning the efficacy of one of the more widely used of these scales, the CES-D, is mixed at best (Myers & Weissman, 1980; Roberts & Vernon, 1983; Schulberg et al., 1985), as is the evidence concerning other scales of this type (Roberts & Vernon, 1981; Wheaton, 1982). In general, we still know very little about how such scales operate in two-stage screening procedures or factors that affect their operating characteristics. I suggest, nevertheless, that we do know enough about specific scales to cause us to use them with extreme caution.

In recent analysis of the effects of gender on responses to items in the CES-D scale, Clark, Aneshensel, Frerichs, and Morgan (1981) found gender differences in interitem and interscale correlation coefficients and in factor loadings. These findings suggest that the scale may not measure the same phenomenon in men and women. As the authors point out, if the objective is to compare subgroups in order to study etiologic factors, the scale must be constructed so as to measure this phenomenon similarly in all groups. Newmann (1984) also reports a distinct gender bias in the demoralization subscale of the PERI (Dohrenwend et al., 1980). Codina and Roberts (1987) analyzed data on persons of Mexican origin using the same set of nineteen items on psychological functioning used in the 1957 and 1976 surveys on the mental health of Americans (Veroff et al., 1981) and found that the dimensionality of the items was different for subjects of Mexican origin, particularly those born in Mexico.

There also is indirect evidence that the order of administration of the CES-D affects the resulting prevalence rates generated by the instrument when it is used in combination with a diagnostic instrument such as the Schedule for Affective Disorders and Schizophrenia (SADS), RDC, or DIS. Roberts (1987a) points out that the prevalence rates in studies in which the CES-D follows clinical assessment are only about one-half the rates in studies that use the CES-D alone or in which the CES-D precedes the clinical assessment. Furthermore, personal communication from researchers who have used the CES-D and other nonclinical measures in prospective studies indicates that over a twelve-month follow-up period the overall prevalence declines 20 to 30% between T_1 and T_2 assessments.

Evidence from studies of primary care settings also indicates that mixed symptoms of depression and anxiety are common among such patients (Goldberg, 1979; Goldberg & Bridges, 1985; Goldberg & Huxley, 1980; Von Korff et al., 1987). In a recent examination of this issue, Goldberg, Bridges, Duncan-Jones, and Grayson (1987) use latent trait analysis to examine the relationships among psychiatric symptoms that constitute common psychological dysfunctions encountered in primary care settings. Two highly correlated symptom dimensions of anxiety and depression appear to underlie these disorders, based on the evidence from this study. The issue of the relationship between anxiety and depression assumes added importance in view of recent discussions of panic disorder, generalized anxiety disorder, and major depressive disorder (Breier, Charney, & Heninger, 1985; Breslau, 1985; Breslau & Davis, 1985; Breslau, Davis, & Prabucki, 1987). A consensus seems to be emerging in which panic disorder and depression are considered valid diagnostic categories, but generalized anxiety disorder is not. Rather, generalized anxiety is considered a concomitant of depression, either as distress associated with being psychiatrically ill or perhaps a subtype of depression defined by the presence of associated anxious symptoms (Breslau & Davis, 1985). The relevance for this interpretation of screening is provided in a provocative paper by Breslau (1985), who reports that the utility of the CES-D for detecting major depression was equal to its utility for detecting generalized anxiety and that the two disorders had additive effects on the CES-D. This study did not identify any individual CES-D symptom as specific to either major depression or generalized anxiety disorder. The implications for screening seem obvious: To what extent do our screening instruments need to elicit symptoms of depression and anxiety specifically, and to what extent will combination screening scales increase our ability to detect depression in primary care settings? Beyond these more general questions, there is the issue of the extent to which symptoms of depression and anxiety covary or occur somewhat independently across different cultural contexts, as Mirowsky and Ross (1984) have suggested is the case for persons of Mexican origin.

Recognition of the limitations of brief symptom checklists in psychiatric epidemiology has been a major factor in researchers' attempts to operationally define psychiatric disorder with specific inclusion and exclusion criteria for a variety of nosological groups, thereby increasing the reliability of psychiatric diagnosis (see Weissman & Klerman, 1978). Three of these attempts to date seem to have demonstrated some initial success in this regard. Collaboration of investigators principally from Columbia University and Washington University have developed the RDC and an interview guide, the SADS which have been demonstrated to have adequate reliability and validity (at least in patient populations) for research purposes (see Spitzer, Endicott, & Robins, 1978). More recently, collaboration between Washington University and the National Institute of Mental Health has resulted in the DIS, which incorporates DSM-III, the Feighner criteria, and RDC diagnoses in a form suitable for use by lay interviewers in community studies (Robins, Helzer, Croughan, & Ratcliff, 1981). A parallel and related thrust by English researchers is the Present State Examination (PSE), a diagnosis-specific instrument that has been used in both clinic and community settings (see Wing, Cooper, & Sartorius, 1974). One of the latest entries to this area of clinical assessment is the Structured Clinical Interview for DSM-III (SCID), developed at the New York State Psychiatric Institute (Spitzer & Williams, 1983). A major difficulty is using such structured diagnostic instruments in screening is the time demand involved. Depending on the degree of impairment, the DIS or SADS may take one to two hours to complete. This demand characteristic can be reduced considerably by using only the sections on depression, for example. This in fact was done in the Hispanic Health and Nutrition Examination Survey. The survey included the CES-D and the depression component from the DIS.

However, there are other problems as well. Even though there is some evidence on the reliability and validity of these diagnostic instruments, the issue is far from settled. Two recent papers illustrate this point. Anthony et al. (1985) report that prevalence estimates based on the DIS one-month diagnoses were significantly different from those based on independent diagnoses by psychiatrists in the Baltimore ECA sample. Helzer et al. (1985) report somewhat better results, but the concordance between lay-administered DIS and psychiatrist examinations was only modest for most diagnoses and quite low for several. Thus far, these are the only two community studies of the concordance between the DIS and independent psychiatric examinations. Clearly the DIS administered by lay interviewers yields different results, in some instances markedly different, than does examination by psychiatrists.

In her commentary on these two articles, Robins (1985) identifies still another problem that involves issues of reliability and validity vis-à-vis the DIS. She notes that in the four ECA sites that had completed both waves of data collection to that point, respondents in the second interview frequently failed to report symptoms they reported (on a lifetime basis) in the first interview. I have obtained some preliminary ECA data that illustrate this findings. Unpublished data from the ECA program (Charles E. Holzer, III, personal communication) indicate this T_1–T_2 decay in prevalence may range from 10 to 20%, depending upon the diagnostic category. Aneshensel, Estrada, Hansell, and Clark (1987) report finding a substantial decline in reports of lifetime episodes of depression in subsequent waves of a prospective study in Los Angeles. At T_1 and T_5 a depressive episode was described and respondents were asked if they had ever had such an episode for a period of at least two weeks. The overall error rate at T_5 was 24%; 86% of the error was failure of subjects at T_5 to report an episode reported at T_1. Those positive at both T_1 and T_5 comprised only 32% of those positive at either time. As Robins points out, psychiatric symptoms are not socially desirable and consequently, few subjects would be expected to report symptoms they never had. Thus, the drop in lifetime prevalence between T_1 and T_2 probably indicates less validity at T_2 than at T_1. The problem of response error in follow-up studies using the DIS is further illustrated in a study by Pulver and Carpenter (1983). Their study had as its focus the feature of the DIS permitting estimates of lifetime prevalence of psychiatric disorders. Pulver and Carpenter (1983) report that their data suggest that the DIS seriously underestimates the lifetime experience of psychotic symptoms. For example, a third of the patients with a well-documented episode of hospitalization for a psychotic illness were not identified by the DIS as ever having a history of psychotic illness. The DIS failed to elicit from 12 to 80% of seven specific symptom dimensions of psychotic illness.

Schulberg and his colleagues (1985) used the DIS in a multistage depression screening project in both primary medical and psychiatric settings and report low concordance with diagnoses of depression by medical practitioners and by psychiatric practitioners. For example, primary care providers diagnosed depression in only 44% of the medical patients so diagnosed using the DIS, while psychiatric providers assigned 164% more diagnoses of depression among mental patients than did the DIS. Nor is the problem specific to the DIS. For example, Bromet, Dunn, Connell, Dew, and Schulberg (1986) report poor test-retest reliability of the SADS over an eighteen-month follow-up period. Only 38% of the subjects (all women) consistently reported RDC episode of depression at both interviews. In fact, of those reporting a lifetime episode of major depression at T_1, only 48% reported a lifetime episode at T_2, a substantial decay in lifetime prevalence. Bromet et al. (1986) found that while clinical status during the eighteen-month follow-up interval influenced reliability of SADS-RDC diagnoses, demographic, psychosocial, and interviewer characteristics did not. In general, those women who reported episodes of depression prior to T_1 and T_2 and who had not previously reported any episode were more likely to have experienced psychiatric difficulties in the T_1–T_2 interval. Conversely, those women who reported lifetime episodes at T_1 but not at T_2 were less likely to have experienced difficulties in the T_1–T_2 interval. Thus far there have been three studies of the reliability/validity of the DIS in Hispanic populations, and the results are not encouraging for those interested in crosscultural studies. Burnam, Karno, Hough, Escobar, and Forsythe (1983), using data from Hispanic patients in Los Angeles, report very low concordance between the DIS and independent clinical diagnosis. The average kappa for Spanish language assessments was .31. Canino, Bird, Shrout, Rubio-Stipec, & Bravo, (1987), using data from a study in Puerto Rico, report average kappas of .56 for lay and clinician administered DIS, but only .42 for the lay DIS versus independent clinical diagnosis (all assessments were in Spanish). Our own research (Roberts, Vernon, & Rhoades, 1988) indicates good test-retest reliability for the DIS administered by lay interviewers in English and Spanish. However, the concordance between the lay DIS and two other sources of clinical diagnosis—hospital records and independent clinical assessment—was quite poor (generally below .30).

Evidence indicating limited reliability and validity is now emerging from research on diagnostic instruments for children as well. Edelbrock, Costello, Dulcan, Kalas, & Conover (1985) report a decline in mean level of reported symptoms of 23% over a three- to four-week period using the Diagnostic Interview Schedule for Children (DIS-C). There was a distinct age effect with a decline of 32% for children aged 6 to 9 and 16% for those aged 14 to 18. Test-retest reliability was .62 overall, and .64 for depression. However, for those aged 14 to 18 the reliabilities were higher, .71 overall and .81 for depression. Chambers et al. (1985) report that the test-retest reliability of the Schedule for Affective Disorders and Schizophrenia for School Aged Children (K-SADS) with children aged 6 to 17 was generally lower than for comparable studies of adults using the SADS, for symptoms, scales, and diagnoses. The reliability of anxiety disorders was unacceptably low; the reliability of depression was only moderate.

Although there is growing interest in the issue of depression among children and adolescents in primary care settings (National Institute of Mental Health, 1987), there are few screening instruments available with demonstrated efficacy in detecting depression in these populations. There are no data on reliability and validity of instruments to detect depression in minority children and adolescents in primary care settings.

Depression and Somatic Illness

The relationship between psychic and somatic distress is well documented. For purposes of the discussion here, two points merit particular attention. One concerns somatization and the other somatic disease as a risk factor for depression.

Kleinman and Kleinman (1985) argue that somatization, the expression of personal and social distress in the form of an idiom of bodily complaints and medical help-seeking, is the predominant expression of mental illness in the non-Western world (see also Marsella, 1980). They note that somatization is common in Western societies as well. A number of studies have demonstrated that somatization cases account for substantial proportions of patient visits to primary care physicians in the United States and the United Kingdom (Collyer, 1979; Goldberg, 1979; Hankin & Oktay, 1979; Hoeper, Nycz, Cleary, Regier, & Goldberg, 1979; Katon, Ries, & Kleinman, 1984; Kessler, Cleary, & Burke, 1985; Regier, Goldberg, & Taube, 1978; Widmer, Cadoret, & North, 1980). Studies in the West also find that somatization is associated with lower socioeconomic and educational level, rural origins, active and traditional religious affiliation, and behavioral ethnicity (Harwood, 1981).

Somatization is an illness behavior that can be associated with depression, anxiety, and other psychiatric disorders but that also occurs in the absence of mental illness as a coping style, a form of social communication, or a cultural symbol and its interpretation. The Kleinmans distinguish between *acute somatization,* in which psychophysiological reactions become defined and experienced primarily as a physical health problem and help is sought for treatment of what is construed as somatic disease, and *chronic somatization,* which results from physical symptoms and disability in the course of chronic medical disorders. Chronic somatization also results from conversion of illness behavior to sick-role behavior, as in chronic pain syndrome, and in the absence of psychiatric or medical disorder as a habitual coping style or "idiom of distress" (p. 473) shaped by the particular cultural context and experiences of those exhibiting the behavior. Singer (1975), on the other hand, has sounded a cautionary note regarding existing evidence on somatization and depression across cultural contexts. Singer points out that virtually all data bearing on this subject have emanated from studies of patients, and the results thus may be at least partially the product of self-selection for treatment, referral patterns, or accessibility of treatment, as well as the product of a somatic orientation to disease and interpretation of the sick role that may be a function of social class as much as culture per se.

In the study by Beiser and Fleming (1986) cited earlier, the structural similarity of scales between Caucasians and the three Asian refugee groups suggests that Asians experience psychic symptoms of depression and have little difficulty in expressing them. Beiser and Fleming also note that depression and somatization emerged as orthogonal factors in both the Caucasian and Asian groups, suggesting that rather than being substitutes for each other, depression and somatization represent alternative ways of expressing distress. It also should be noted that an increased risk of depression has been found to be associated with the presence of a variety of other medical and psychiatric disorders, such as substance abuse, anxiety, cancer, myocardial infarction, stroke, and childbirth (see, for example, Boyd & Weissman, 1982; Hirschfeld & Cross, 1982; Roberts, 1987b).

There is overwhelming evidence that the postpartum period (up to six months) carries an excess risk for more serious disorders (Paffenberger & McCabe 1966; Pugh, Jerath, Schmidt, & Reed, 1963; Weissman & Klerman, 1977), and most of this excess is depression. Pitt (1982) reviews a number of studies, almost all based on patients, and reports that the prevalence of moderate to severe depression is about 10% in these studies and that of nonclinical depression (or the "blues") about 50%. He also expresses doubt that there are clinical features that distinguish depression associated with childbirth from that occurring at other times.

Although there is no clear consensus on the relationship between anxiety and depression (see Downing & Rickels, 1974; Gersh & Fowles, 1979), there have been at least three recent papers suggesting that the prevalence of secondary depression in persons suffering from anxiety disorders may be in the range of 30 to 40% (Clancy, Noyes, Hoenk, & Slymen, 1978; Dealy, Ishiki, Avery, Wilson, & Dunner, 1981; Noyes, Clancy, Hoenk, & Slymen, 1980). Petty and Nasrallah (1981) review clinical studies of the association between alcoholism and depression and conclude that the relationship appears to be unidirectional—i.e., alcoholism predisposes to depression but not the reverse.

Another disease in which researchers have studied depression is cancer. Petty and Noyes (1981), based on an extensive review of the literature, estimate that 17 to 25% of patients hospitalized with neoplastic disease suffer from depression severe enough to warrant psychiatric intervention. Petty and Noyes also point out a number of methodologic problems that compromise much of the research on the psychological impact of cancer, as do Freidenbergs, Gordon, Hibbard, Levine, Wolf, & Diller (1981–82). Still, the consensus seems to be that, compared to the general population, cancer patients are at increased risk of both clinical depression and demoralization. There is also evidence for a relationship between cardiovascular disease and depression. For example, there is a higher prevalence of both demoralization (Huapaya & Onanth, 1980) and clinical depression (Rabkin, Charles, & Kass, 1983) among hypertensives than among nonhypertensives, although an etiologic explanation for this association is not yet available. A high prevalence of depression has also been reported among stroke patients (Storey, 1967), although Robins (1976) has argued that depression in stroke patients is a nonspecific affective response to the complex physical and psychological stresses imposed by severe illness. This interpretation doubtless is applicable to the psychological impact of severe illness experience generally. To illustrate this point further, a number of investigators (Cassem & Hackett, 1971; Wishnie, Hackett, & Cassem, 1971; Wynn, 1967) have reported that symptoms of anxiety and depression are quite common among patients who have experienced a myocardial infarction. Cassem and Hackett (1971) report prevalences of 32% for anxiety and 30% for depression.

The bulk of the research on physical health and depression has come from studies of patients. However, there are community studies documenting this relationship as well. My colleagues at the Human Population Laboratory and I (Kaplan, Roberts, Camacho-Dickey, & Coyne, 1987) have found that after prior depression, the strongest predictor of future depression is physical health status, in particular chronic disease conditions and physical disability. Aneshensel and Huba (1984) also report that physical illness is a strong predictor of future depression in a prospective study. They report that there is a reciprocal relationship as well, with depression increasing slightly the risk of subsequent physical illness. Kolody, Vega, Meinhardt, and Bensussen (1986) have examined the relationship between depressive symptoms and severity of somatic complaints, contrasting Anglos with U.S.–born and foreign-born persons of Mexican origin. They report a direct, linear relationship between depression and somatic distress within each ethnic group, and this relationship was found not to change significantly with multivariate controls. Of interest, there was evidence that the relationship was stronger for Mexican Americans than for Anglos.

At this time, however, we do not have data from rigorously designed studies that permit us to disentangle the effects of somatization, somatic disease, and depressive disorder in primary care patients, regardless of their cultural background. Until we have carefully controlled studies of this type, the role of two often closely related syndromes—somatization and depression—in the help-seeking process and in primary health care settings will remain poorly understood.

Other Measurement Issues

There have been a number of recent articles on the subject of response error and its effect on research outcomes (Austin, Criqui, Barrett-Connor, & Holdbrook, 1981; Criqui, 1979; Greenland, 1977; Greenland & Criqui, 1981). *Response error* refers to misrepresentation of the target population's risk factor and/or disease experience by the respondents due to differential response rates or loss to followup (Greenland & Criqui, 1981). This circumstance obviously introduces a potentially important source of bias into all types of surveys and is only one source of invalidity. There are a number of other potential sources of response error related to survey questionnaires and the interview process that also may result in misrepresentation of a population's risk factor and/or disease experience. Weiss (1975) has enumerated in some detail sources of response error that may be either random or systematic. While random misreports reduce reliability and increase variation, systematic bias poses a serious treat to the validity or results obtained.

Based on their exhaustive review of the literature (over five hundred references through 1980), Marquis, Marquis, and Polich (1986) found thirty-one full-design criterion validity studies dealing with factual versus attitudinal data. The focus of these studies was diverse, covering welfare, income, drug use, criminal history, and embarrassing medical conditions (including mental illness). The results were not encouraging for alcohol, drugs, and health. Marquis and his colleagues used the index of reliability to assess the outcomes of the studies, defining anything below 70% as problematic. The index varied from 17 to 56 for five health studies, from 18 to 80 for seven drug use studies, and 36 to 71 for three studies of alcohol use. Marquis and his coworkers suggest that special steps are needed to protect users of survey data on sensitive topics from making seriously distorted estimates from their data. They suggest that it is critical that we begin to test hypotheses and design features that reduce response unreliability. These researchers estimate, for example, that reliabilities below 70% imply that the correlation of sensitive variables with other more accurately measured variables will be attenuated by more than 20%, and regression coefficients on the sensitive topic measures by more than 30%.

Concern about problems of recall, judgment, and understanding during the administration of questionnaires involves questions on the cognitive aspects of survey methodology (Jabine, Straf, Tanur, & Tourangeau, 1984). Because queries about signs and symptoms of psychological dysfunction require answers from people, because survey respondents are people, and because people use comprehension, recall, and judgment to provide these answers, there is a common set of problems involving these cognitive tasks that besets virtually all surveys. Many anomalous effects have been demonstrated—variation across interviewers, the mode of interview, context of questions, ordering of response alternatives, sensitivity, saliency, reference period, repeated measurements, and many others (Jabine, 1985; Lessler & Sirken, 1985).

A critical problem in virtually all health interview studies, including mental health studies, is that much of the focus is on past health experiences (past month, past year, lifetime). Retrospective—or memory-based—responses provide important views of the past. However, there is increasing evidence that substantial portions of memory-based data are flawed not only by temporal confusion, forgetting, and confabulation, but are systematically influenced by respondents' current emotional state and beliefs about life and self (see Bradburn, Rips, & Shevell, 1987). The memory process is basically reconstructive (Bartlett, 1932). According to Dawes and Pearson (1986), response to questions on health (for example) requiring retrospective responses are probably best considered as global judgments based on a memory that is organized by current "theory-based" schemas about self and society. For example, there is experimental evidence that recall of past experiences occurring during a particular mood is facilitated by creation of that mood (Bower, 1981), as research on depression illustrates nicely. Lewinsohn and Rosenbaum (1987) report that currently depressed subjects recall their parents as having been more rejecting and as having used more negative control than normal control subjects, whereas the remitted depressed did not differ in their recall of parental behavior. Other researchers also report that recall and current reporting of previous depressive episodes are dependent upon the experience of psychological distress subsequent to those prior episodes (Bromet et al., 1986; Aneshensel et al., 1987). Findings such as these create severe problems for mental health researchers, since much of what we do involves determining the antecedents of particular mood states by gathering data on a retrospective basis, for the mood itself may in large part determine what is recalled. Even prospective studies do not solve the problem, since in subsequent waves questions involve recall for the time elapsed since the previous assessment.

Certain types of bias seem particularly likely to occur when psychiatric symptoms form the subject of the interview because such symptoms are generally more subjective than other types of medical diagnostic criteria and because psychiatric conditions, particularly if they result in institutionalization, still carry a social stigma (Steadman, 1981). One type of bias that has received attention from survey researchers, particularly among those interested in the study of mental disorders, is an attribute of respondents called "response tendency or style." Response tendencies are predispositions or attitudes of the respondent that introduce a noncontent source of variance in answers to questions and thus may constitute a source of bias if they are related systematically to the dependent and/or independent variables under study.

The principal effects of response tendencies (Greenland, 1977) are classification error that results in inaccurate estimates of incidence or prevalence and (Criqui, 1979) alterations of observed associations between presumed risk factors and mental status. *Classification error,* resulting in false positives and false negatives, occurs when response tendencies are related to mental status, while spurious associations may be produced when response tendencies are related systematically both to risk factors and to mental status. For example, Klassen, Hornstra, and Anderson (1975) concluded that estimates of prevalence using the Langner twenty-two-item index of psychiatric morbidity (Langner, 1962) ranged from 6% for persons scoring high on a certain response tendency to 21% for those scoring low. More recently, Linden, Paulhus, and Dobson (1986) report that measures of response tendencies or styles account for up to one-fifth of the variance in physical health inventories and up to 60% of the variance in psychological screening inventories. Prevalence estimates for population subgroups may be affected differentially since response tendencies have been shown to vary systematically across factors such as age, gender, ethnicity, and socioeconomic status (Dohrenwend, 1966; Gove & Geerken, 1977; Klassen et al., 1975; Vernon, Roberts, & Lee, 1982).

Another problem is posed by the measurement of response tendencies. Conventional measures such as the ones used in most studies are subject to the same problems of reliability and validity that beset the measurement of psychiatric constructs such as depression. Vernon (1980) reports that, in general, measures of acquiescence, need for approval, and trait desirability operated in a similar manner in three ethnic groups. Thus, the differential effects by ethnicity of response tendencies on CES-D scores probably are not explained by subgroup differences in the operating characteristics of such measures. However, the results of these analyses confirmed our suspicion that more attention needs to be directed towards establishing the reliability and validity of measures of response tendencies if they are to be useful as indicators of potential bias (see, for example, Bradburn, Sudman, & Associates 1979; Paulhus, 1984).

A promising approach has been developed by Paulhus and his colleagues (Paulhus, 1984; Linden, Paulhus, & Dobson, 1986), who subsume tendencies such as defensiveness, repression, denial, and social desirability under two constructs: impression management and self-deception. According to Paulhus and his coworkers, the best available measure of impression management is the Other-Deception Questionnaire (Sackheim & Gur, 1978), comprised of twenty questions about desirable and undesirable behaviors, and the best available measure of self-deception is the Self-Deception Questionnaire (Sackheim & Gur, 1978), also consisting of twenty items. The two scales have been reworded and combined into one instrument, the Balanced Inventory of Desirability Responding (BIDR), in which both scales are balanced for direction of keying. The two components of the BIDR have acceptably high internal consistency reliability and high scores predict attenuated reports of symptoms, both somatic and psychological. For example, 18% of the variance in the Beck Depression Inventory was accounted for by the combined ODQ and SDQ scales. These results are particularly impressive since there is little apparent overlap in the content of the BIDR and most psychological symptom scales, a criticism that has been made of other measures of response styles.

Consideration of response styles in screening for depression in primary care settings is salient from several perspectives. First, most of the research on response styles has been conducted in nonclinical settings; none in fact has been done in primary care settings. Second, there is evidence that response styles affect the reporting of both somatic and psychological complaints (Linden et al., 1986; Parkes, 1980). Third, the work by Paulhus and his coworkers represents an advance, both theoretically and methodologically, in the study of response styles as a source of error in screening for psychological dysfunction.

As previously mentioned, there are a number of other possible sources of systematic error related to predispositions of the interviewer, the interaction between respondent and interviewer, and procedures used in the study (Weiss, 1975). For example, Riessman (1979) found that gender differences in symptom reports appeared to be related to status factors, with women reporting less symptom information to identified physicians while men reported more symptoms to identified physicians. This finding not only has implications for reported gender differences on self-report symptom measures but also suggests another way of measuring social desirability bias. If the latter is the case, social desirability bias may operate differently by gender, a possibility for which there was some support in our previous studies.

The importance of the cognitive aspects of health survey methodology recently has been acknowledged formally by the National Center of Health Statistics (NCHS), which has implemented a research program on the Cognitive Aspects of Survey Methodology (CASM). Two types of collaborative research efforts are underway. The first has as its focus the use of the cognitive research laboratory for designing and testing NCHS questionnaires; the second will investigate cognitive issues associated with specific survey response tasks (Lessler & Sirken, 1985). However, as noted by Fienberg, Loftus, and Tanur (1985), most surveys conducted by NCHS do not assess mental health conditions or problems, and, not surprisingly, survey questions on psychiatric morbidity are not part of the initial CASM program.

The need for accurate data on the extent of depression and other mental disorders in primary care populations and on the association of these disorders with identifiable risk factors clearly requires that we continue to assess potential sources of inaccuracy and develop ways of reducing their influence on scientific results. Taken together, the data thus far suggest that there are significant unresolved measurement problems in contemporary psychiatric research. The principal effects of these problems are: (a) classification error that results in inaccurate estimates of incidence and prevalence, and (b) almost certain bias in observed associations between presumed risk factors and psychiatric disorders. The problem is that we do not know the contexts under which these conditions obtain, nor do we have available well-established strategies for their resolution.

Concluding Remarks

Depressive phenomena are relatively common (Roberts, 1987b; Weissman, 1987), whether defined in terms of demoralization or clinical depression. I submit that screening in primary care should focus on both of these manifestations as outcome measures. I suggest this for several reasons. First, clinical depression is fairly prevalent, represents a behavioral disorder with life-threatening implications, and in the case of chronic forms of the disorder, is a disease with considerable illness burden at the individual, familial, and societal levels. Failure to screen for clinical depression ignores the more serious forms of the disease. Second, demoralization is extremely prevalent and is also the source of considerable suffering. Third, there is apparently a relationship between these two psychic states, although at this juncture we are not sure about what this relationship is. I believe we should reconsider how we conceptualize and measure these two constructs. The lack of agreement observed between measures of demoralization and clinical depression may represent more than a measurement problem. The measurement issue remains, as we have noted, a thorny one. An equally important issue may be theoretical—i.e., what is the role of demoralization in depression? That is, to what extent do demoralized individuals become clinically depressed, and to what extent do the clinically depressed manifest demoralization during or after the depressive episode has remitted? From an epidemiologic perspective, does demoralization increase the risk of clinical depression and, if so, in whom and under what circumstances? In order to examine these questions, we need a research design that permits us to partition a particular population into four groups (Link & Dohrenwend, 1980): (a) those manifesting clinical depression and demoralization, (b) those having only clinical depression, (c) those having only demoralization, and (d) those having neither. I suggest this strategy would be useful for studying the occurrence of depressive phenomena in primary care populations, as well as the consequences of such phenomena. To do so, however, we will need reliable and valid indicators of our constructs. At present, the evidence suggests that our measures may be suspect, in particular where ethnic and minority populations are concerned.

How our measures are suspect and to what extent they are remain empirical questions at this point. How can we achieve some resolution of this issue? Part of the answer lies in expanding our knowledge base. The available evidence does not permit us to answer the question of whether there are cultural variations in the prevalence of depression or demoralization, or whether there are cultural variations in how depressive phenomena are manifested in contemporary American society. Very few crosscultural studies of depression in primary care have been conducted among American ethnocultural groups. The problem goes beyond issues of quantity, however; part of the problem is the type of research that has been done.

In general, our research designs have not permitted us to partition the variance in our assessment procedures attributable to the independent as well as the joint effects of minority status, ethnic culture, and social class (Roberts, 1987a; Kessler & Neighbors, 1986). A major unresolved issue, as a consequence, is that we do not know whether there is a unique disease experience vis-à-vis depression associated with membership in an ethnic group above and beyond that attributable to risk factors for depression identified in studies of other populations (such as age, gender, income, education, social support, physical illness, or life strains [see Roberts, 1987b]).

Part of the problem involves sampling, from at least two perspectives—representativeness and comparability. Representativeness also is an issue from two perspectives: (a) the extent to which the sample adequately depicts the characteristics of the ethnic group or groups in a particular primary care setting and (b) the extent to which it adequately depicts the characteristics of the larger ethnic population from which the care-seekers emanate. The former question concerns the validity of our inferences about the group's illness profile in that primary care setting, while the latter involves validity of inferences concerning the illness experience of the larger ethnic collective in society. Comparability is an issue that affects our ability to attribute observed outcomes to the effects of ethnic culture.

Singer (1975) as well as others (Dohrenwend, 1966; Roberts, 1987a) have cautioned about the dangers of attributing ethnic differentials in psychological dysfunction to cultural factors when in fact the primary causal factor may be social class. Given the confounding of social class and ethnicity in the United States, if we wish to examine whether either the prevalence or the phenomenology of depression has a unique cultural component, we must have a design that permits us to compare prevalence or phenomenology between ethnic groups, controlling for the effects of social class (Dohrenwend, 1966; Roberts & Vernon, 1984). This is particularly critical in studies of primary care populations. The bulk of primary medical care services for many minorities is delivered in public health clinics or hospitals. The bias in studying treatment populations in general, and public health facilities more specifically, is well known. The work of Dutton (1978) is instructive in this regard. She found that culturally based practices and values played a significant role in determining use of medical services. However, she found that neither cultural factors nor socioeconomic factors explained use of medical services as well as variables measuring how the medical services were organized and delivered. Following this line of reasoning, a more rigorous examination of the effect of ethnic culture on screening for depression in primary care would require us to employ designs permitting assessment of the relative effects of socioeconomic, cultural, and delivery system variables on our outcome measures. Marsella (Marsella, 1980; Marsella, Sartorius, Jablensky, & Fenton, 1985) suggests that one way to overcome the sampling problem is to employ "matched sample" designs in which patients from different cultural groups are matched for key variables such as age, gender, socioeconomic status, and so forth. Given our earlier discussion of somatic illness and depression, this strategy for maximizing comparability should also be extended to physical health diagnosis (including type, duration, and severity). Regardless of whether matching, sampling disproportionate to size, or multivariate statistical controls is the method of choice, it is imperative that we be able to assess the effect of culture, independent of other effects.

Measurement problems quite obviously are not unique to screening for mental health problems in primary care, but the unique historical and cultural experiences of many ethnic groups (such as those of Mexican origin) does create additional methodologic burdens for researchers. A number of these issues have been discussed already, such as reliability and validity of current assessment procedures, the possible role of cognitive factors (particularly response styles), the role of physical illness and somatization in depression, the relationship between symptom checklists and clinical diagnosis, and the phenomenology of depression in different cultural groups. An additional problem is the lack of assessment procedures that are adequately translated and standardized and for which equivalency in English and another ethnic dialect or language has been demonstrated (Cuellar & Roberts, 1984). Brislin (1976) has outlined a number of strategies for ensuring adequate rendition of an instrument into a different language. Another measurement issue that remains relatively unexplored regarding screening for depression in different ethnic groups concerns the emic-etic distinction in cross-cultural research (Berry, 1969; Brislin, Lonner, & Thorndike, 1973; Lonner, 1980). That is, to what extent are there symptoms that are manifested in a universal (*etic*) manner and to what extent are there culturally specific (*emic*) symptom patterns? Other than a few studies of culture-specific syndromes or a few studies of specific ethnic groups we have little knowledge about how the cultural backgrounds of American ethnic groups shape psychopathology in unique ways.

Clarification and resolution of the issues raised in this discussion obviously will require more attention to the crosscultural utility of existing procedures for depression screening in primary are. I submit it also will require a different research strategy than we typically employ, one that draws more heavily upon medical anthropology, crosscultural psychology, and ethnopsychiatry than in the past (Kleinman & Good, 1985). Recent discussions by Hui and Triandis (1985), Marsella et al. (1985), and Good & Kleinman (1985) outline a rationale for, as well as the need for, greater focus on crosscultural aspects of depression, the properties of culturally relevant measures, and research strategies for developing and testing reliable and valid indicators across varied cultural contexts. To the extent we incorporate these ideas into our research, we will improve our ability to detect depression in primary care settings and enhance our understanding of the relationship between psychological distress, somatic illness, and help-seeking behavior.

References

Akiskal, H. S. (1979). A biobehavioral approach to depression. In R. A. Depue (ed.), *The psychobiology of the depressive disorders: Implications for the effects of stress* (pp. 409–438). New York: Academic Press.

Akiskal, H. S., & McKinney, W. T. (1975). Overview of recent research in depression: Integration of ten conceptual models into a comprehensive clinical frame. *Archives of General Psychiatry, 32,* 285–305.

American Psychiatric Association (1980). *Diagnostic and statistical manual of mental disorders* (3rd ed.). Washington, D.C.: Author.

Aneshensel, C. S., Clark, V. A., & Frerichs, R. R. (1983). Race, ethnicity and depression: A confirmatory analysis. *Journal of Personality and Social Psychology, 44,* 385–398.

Aneshensel, C. A., & Huba, G. J. (1984). An integrative causal model of the antecedents and consequences of depression over one year. *Research in Community and Mental Health, 4,* 35–72.

Aneshensel, C. A., Estrada, A. L., Hansell, M. H., & Clark, V. A. (1987). Social psychological aspects of reporting behavior: Lifetime depressive episode reports. *Journal of Health and Social Behavior, 28,* 232–246.

Anthony, J. C., Folstein, M., Romanoski, A. J., Von Korff, M. R., Nestadt, G. R., Chahal, R., Muchant, A., Brown, C. H., Shapiro, S., Kramer, M. (1985). Comparison of the lay Diagnostic Interview Schedule and a standardized psychiatric diagnosis. *Archives of General Psychiatry, 42,* 667–675.

Archdeacon, T. J. (1983). *Becoming American: An ethnic history.* New York: Free Press.

Austin, M. A., Criqui, M. H., Barrett-Connor, E., & Holdbrook, M. J. (1981). The effect of response bias on the odds ratio. *American Journal of Epidemiology, 114,* 137–43.

Bartlett, F. C. (1932). *Remembering—A study in experimental and social psychology.* Cambridge: Cambridge University Press.

Beck, A. T., Ward, C. H., Mendelsohn, M., Mock, J. E., & Erbaugh, J. K. (1961). An inventory for measuring depression. *Archives of General Psychiatry, 4,* 561–571.

Beiser, M., & Fleming, J. A. E. (1986). Measuring psychiatric disorder among Southeast Asian refugees. *Psychological Medicine, 16,* 627–639.

Berry, J. W. (1969). On crosscultural comparability. *International Journal of Psychology, 4,* 119–128.

Bower, G. (1981). Mood and memory. *American Psychologist, 36,* 129–148.

Boyd, J. H., & Weissman, M. M. (1981). Epidemiology of affective disorders: A re-examination and future directions. *Archives of General Psychiatry,* 38, 1039–1046.

Boyd, J. H., & Weissman, M. M. (1982). Epidemiology. In E. S. Paykel (ed.), *Handbook of affective disorders* (pp. 109–125). New York: Guilford Press.

Boyer, L. (1964). Folk psychiatry of the Apaches of the Mescalero Indian Reservation. In A. Kiev (ed.), *Magic, faith and healing* (pp. 384–419). New York: Free Press.

Bradburn, N. M., Rips, L. J., & Shevell, S. K. (1987). Answering autobiographical questions: The impact of memory and inference on surveys. *Science, 256,* 157–161.

Bradburn, N. M., Sudman, S., & Associates (1979). Reinterpreting the Marlowe-Crowne Scale. In N. M. Bradburn, S. Sudman, & E. Blair, (eds.), *Improving interview method and questionnaire design* (pp. 85–106). San Francisco: Jossey-Bass Publishers.

Breier, A., Charney, D. S., & Heninger, G. R. (1985). The diagnostic validity of anxiety disorders and their relationships to depressive illness. *American Journal of Psychiatry, 142,* 787–797.

Breslau, N. (1985). Depressive symptoms, major depression, and generalized anxiety: A comparison of self-reports on CES-D and results from diagnostic interviews. *Psychiatry Research, 15,* 219–229.

Breslau, N., & Davis, G. C. (1985). Further evidence on the doubtful validity of generalized anxiety disorder. *Psychiatry Research, 16,* 177–179.

Breslau, N., Davis, G. C., & Prabucki, K. (1987). Searching for evidence on the validity of generalized anxiety disorder: Psychopathology in children of anxious mothers. *Psychiatry Research, 20,* 285–297.

Brislin, R. D. (ed.) (1976). *Translation: Applications and research.* New York: Gardner Press.

Brislin, R. W., Lonner, W. J., & Thorndike, R. M. (1973). *Crosscultural research methods.* New York: John Wiley & Sons.

Bromet, E., Dunn, L., Connell, M., Dew, M., & Schulberg, H. (1986). Long-term reliability of diagnosing lifetime major depression in a community sample. *Archives of General Psychiatry, 43,* 435–440.

Burnam, M. A., Karno, M., Hough, R. L., Escobar, J. I., & Forsythe, A. B. (1983). The Spanish Diagnostic Interview Schedule: Reliability and comparison with clinical diagnoses. *Archives of General Psychiatry, 40,* 1189–1196.

Burnam, M. A., Karno, M., Hough, R. L., Escobar, J. I., & Telles, C. A. (1987). Acculturation and lifetime prevalence of psychiatric disorders among Mexican Americans in Los Angeles. *Journal of Health and Social Behavior, 28,* 89–102.

Canino, G. J., Bird, H. R., Shrout, P. E., Rubio-Stipec, M., & Bravo, M. (1987). The Spanish Diagnostic Interview Schedule: Reliability and concordance with clinical diagnoses in Puerto Rico. *Archives of General Psychiatry, 44,* 720–726.

Carter, J. H. (1974). Recognizing psychiatric symptoms in black Americans. *Geriatrics, 26,* 95–99.

Cassem, N. H., & Hackett, T. P. (1971). Psychiatric consultation in a coronary care unit. *Annals of Internal Medicine, 75,* 9–14.

Chambers, J. J., Puig-Antich, J., Hirsch, M., Paez, P., Ambrosini, P. J., Tabrizi, M. A., & Davies,

M. (1985). The assessment of affective disorders in children and adolescents by semistructured interview: Test-retest reliability of the K-SADS-P. *Archives of General Psychiatry, 42,* 696–702.

Clancy, J., Noyes, R., Hoenk, R. P., & Slymen, D. J. (1978). Secondary depression in anxiety neurosis. *Journal of Nervous and Mental Disorders, 166,* 846–850.

Clark, V. A., Aneshensel, C. S., Frerichs, R. R., & Morgan, T. M. (1981). Analysis of effects of sex and age in response to items on the CES-D scale. *Psychiatry Research, 5,* 171–181.

Codina, E., & Roberts, R. E. (1987). A comparison of well-being in the Mexican origin and general populations using National Survey Data. In R. Rodriquez & M. Coleman (eds.), *Mental Health Issues of the Mexican Origin Population In Texas: Proceedings of the Fifth Robert Lee Sutherland Seminar* (pp. 71–88). Austin: Hogg Foundation for Mental Health.

Collyer, J. (1979). Psychosomatic illness in a solo family practice. *Psychosomatics, 20,* 762–767.

Cooper, B., & Morgan, H. G. (1973). *Epidemiological psychiatry.* Springfield, IL: Charles C. Thomas.

Criqui, M. H. (1979). Response bias and risk ratios in epidemiologic studies. *American Journal of Epidemiology, 109,* 394–399.

Cuellar, I., & Roberts, R. E. (1984). Psychological disorders among Chicanos. In J. L. Martinez, Jr. and R. H. Mendoza (eds.), *Chicano psychology* (2nd ed.) (pp. 133–161). Orlando: Academic Press.

Dawes R. M., & Pearson, R. W. (1986). The effects of theory-based schemas on retrospective data. Unpublished manuscript.

Dealy, R. S., Ishiki, D. M., Avery, D. H., Wilson, L. G., & Dunner, D. L. (1981). Secondary depression in anxiety disorders. *Comprehensive Psychiatry, 22,* 612–618.

Del Castillo, J. C. (1970). The influence of language upon symptomatology in foreign-born patients. *American Journal of Psychiatry, 127,* 242–244.

Dohrenwend, B. P. (1966). Social status and psychological disorder: An issue of substance and an issue of method. *American Sociological Review, 31,* 14–34.

Dohrenwend, B. P., & Dohrenwend, B. S. (1982). Perspectives on the past and future of psychiatric epidemiology. *American Journal of Public Health, 72,* 1271–1279.

Dohrenwend, B. P., Oksenberg, L., Shrout, P. E., Dohrenwend, B. S., & Cook, D. (1981). What brief psychiatric screening scales measure. In S. Sudman (ed.), *Health survey research methods: Third Biennial Conference* (pp. 188–189). Washington, D.C.: National Center for Health Services Research.

Dohrenwend, B. P., Shrout, P. E., Egri, G., & Mendelsohn, F. S. (1980). Nonspecific psychological distress and other dimensions of psychopathology. *Archives of General Psychiatry, 37,* 1229–1236.

Downing, R. W., & Rickels, K. (1974). Mixed anxiety-depression: Fact or myth? *Archives of General Psychiatry, 30,* 312–317.

Dutton, D. B. (1978). Explaining the low use of health services by the poor-costs, attitudes, or delivery systems? *American Sociological Review, 43,* 348–368.

Edelbrock, C., Costello, A. J., Dulcan, M. K., Kalas, R., & Conover, N. C. (1985). Age differences in the reliability of the psychiatric interview of the child. *Child Development, 56,* 265–275.

Fabrega, H., Swartz, J. D., & Wallace, C. A. (1968a). Ethnic differences in psychopathology with emphasis on a Mexican American group. *Journal of Psychiatry Research, 6,* 221–225.

Fabrega, H., Swartz, J. D., & Wallace, C. A. (1968b). Ethnic differences in psychopathology with emphasis on clinical correlates under varying conditions. *Archives of General Psychiatry, 19,* 218–226.

Fienberg, S. E., Loftus, E. F., & Tanur, J. M. (1985). Cognitive aspects of health survey methodology: An overview. *Milbank Memorial Fund Quarterly/Health and Society, 63*(3), 547–563.

Frank, J. D. (1973). *Persuasion and healing.* New York: Schocken Books.

Freidenbergs, I., Gordon, W., Hibbard, M., Levine, L., Wolf, C., & Diller, L. (1981–1982). Psychosocial aspects of living with cancer: A review of the literature. *International Journal of Psychiatry in Medicine, 11,* 303–329.

Friedman, R. J. (1974). The psychology of depression: An overview. In R. J. Friedman & M. M. Katz (eds.), *The psychology of depression: Contemporary theory and research* (pp. 281–298). Washington, D.C.: U.S. Government Printing Office.

Geertz, C. (1973). *The Interpretation of cultures.* New York: Basic Books.

Gersh, F. S., & Fowles, D. L. (1979). Neurotic depression: The concept of anxious depression. In R. A. Depue (ed.), *The psychobiology of the depressive disorders: Implications for the effects of stress* (pp. 81–104). New York: Academic Press.

Goldberg, D. (1979). Detection and assessment of emotional disorders in a primary care setting. *International Journal of Mental Health, 8,* 30–48.

Goldberg, D. P., & Bridges, K. W. (1985). Somatic presentations of DSM-III psychiatric disorders in primary care. *Journal of Psychosomatic Research, 29,* 563–569.

Goldberg, D. P., Bridges, K., Duncan-Jones, P., & Grayson, D. (1987). Dimensions of neuroses seen in primary care settings. *Psychological Medicine, 17,* 461–470.

Goldberg, D. P., & Huxley, P. (1980). *Mental illness in the community.* London: Tavistock.

Gonzales, J. R. (1978). Language factors affecting treatment of bilingual schizophrenics. *Psychiatric Annals, 8,* 68–70.

Good, B., & Kleinman, A. (1985). Epilogue: Culture and depression. In A. Kleinman and B. Good (eds.), *Culture and depression—Studies in the anthropology and cross-cultural psychiatry of affect and disorder,* (pp. 491–505). Berkeley: University of California Press.

Gove, W., & Geerken, M. R. (1977). Response bias in surveys of mental health: An empirical investigation. *American Journal of Sociology, 82,* 1289–1317.

Greenland, S. (1977). Response and follow-up bias in cohort studies. *American Journal of Epidemiology, 106,* 184–187.

Greenland, S., & Criqui, M. H. (1981). Are case-control studies more vulnerable to response bias? *American Journal of Epidemiology, 114,* 175–177.

Guze, S. B., Woodruff, R. A., & Clayton, P. J. (1971). Secondary affective disorders: A study of 95 cases. *Psychological Medicine, 1,* 426–428.

Hankin, J., & Oktay, J. S. (1979). *Mental disorder and primary care* (DHEW Publication No. ADM 78–661). Washington, D.C.: U.S. Government Printing Office.

Hannerz, U. (1969). *Soulside: Inquiries into ghetto culture and community.* New York: Columbia University Press.

Hanson, B., Klerman, G., & Tanner, J. (1973). Clinical depression among black and white women. Unpublished manuscript, Boston State Hospital, Massachusetts.

Harwood, A. (ed.) (1981). *Ethnicity and medical care.* Cambridge: Harvard University Press.

Heiman, E. M., & Kahn, M. W. (1977). Mexican-American and European-American psychopathology and hospital course. *Archives of General Psychiatry, 34,* 167–170.

Helzer J. (1975). Bipolar affective disorder in black and white men. *Archives of General Psychiatry, 32*, 1140–1143.

Helzer , J. E., Robins, L. M., McEvoy, L. T., Spitznagel, E. L., Stoltzman, R. K., Farmer, A., & Brocking, I. F. (1985). A comparison of clinical and Diagnostic Interview Schedule diagnoses. *Archives of General Psychiatry, 42* (7), 657–666.

Hirschfeld, R. M. A., & Cross, L. K. (1982). Epidemiology of affective disorders. *Archives of General Psychiatry, 39*, 35–46.

Hoeper, E., Nycz, G., Cleary, P., Regier, D., & Goldberg, I. D. (1979). Estimated prevalence of RDC mental disorder in primary care. *International Journal of Mental Health, 8*, 6–15.

Huapaya, L., & Onanth, J. (1980). Depression associated with hypertension: A review. *Psychiatric Journal of the University of Ottawa, 5*, 58–62.

Hui, C. H., & Triandis, H. C. (1985). Measurement in crosscultural psychology. *Journal of Crosscultural Psychology, 16*, 131–152.

Jabine, T. B. (1985). Reporting chronic conditions in the National Health Interview Survey: A review of findings from evaluation on studies and methodological tests (DHHS Publication No. 85A04165001D). Unpublished manuscript.

Jabine, T. B., Straf, M. L., Tanur, J. M., & Tourangeau, R. (1984). *Cognitive aspects of survey methodology: Building a bridge between disciplines.* Washington, D.C.: National Academy Press.

Johnson, D., & Johnson, C. (1965). Totally discouraged: A depressive syndrome of the Dakota Sioux. *Transcultural Psychiatric Research Review, 2*, 141–143.

Kaplan, G. A., Roberts, R. E., Camacho-Dickey, T., & Coyne, J. C. (1987). Psychosocial predictors of depression: Prospective evidence from the Human Population Laboratory studies. *American Journal of Epidemiology, 125*, 206–220.

Katon, W., Ries, R., & Kleinman, A. (1984). The prevalence of somatization in primary care. *Comprehensive Psychiatry, 25*, 208–215.

Keesing, R. M. (1974). Theories of culture. *Annual Review of Anthropology, 3*, 73–97.

Kessler, L. G., Cleary, P. D., & Burke, J. D., Jr. (1985). Psychiatric disorders in primary care. *Archives of General Psychiatry, 42*, 583–587.

Kessler, R. C., & Neighbors, H. W. (1986). A new perspective on the relationship among race, social class, and psychological distress. *Journal of Health and Social Behavior, 27*, 107–115.

Kinzie, J. D., & Manson, S. M. (1987). The use of self-rating scales in crosscultural psychiatry. *Hospital and Community Psychiatry, 38*, 190–196.

Klassen, D., Hornstra, R. K., & Anderson, P. B. (1975). Influences of social desirability on symptom and mood reporting in a community survey. *Journal of Consulting and Clinical Psychology, 43*, 448–452.

Klein, D. F. (1974). Endogenomorphic depression: A conceptual and terminological revision. *Archives of General Psychiatry, 34*, 447–454.

Kleinman, A., & Good, B. (1985). Culture and depression: Introduction to the problem. In A. Kleinman & B. Good (eds.), *Culture and depression—Studies in the anthropology and crosscultural psychiatry of affect and disorder* (pp. 1–33). Berkeley: University of California Press.

Kleinman, A., & Kleinman, J. (1985). Somatization: The interconnections in Chinese society among culture, depressive experiences, and the meanings of pain. In A. Kleinman & B. Good (eds.), *Culture and depression-studies in the anthropology and crosscultural psychiatry of affect and disorder* (pp. 429–490). Berkeley: University of California Press.

Kolody, B., Vega, W., Meinhardt, K., & Bensussen, G. (1986). The correspondence of health complaints and depressive symptoms among Anglos and Mexican Americans. *The Journal of Nervous and Mental Disease, 174,* 221–228.

Langner, T. S. (1962). A twenty-two item screening score of psychiatric symptoms indicating impairment. *Journal of Health and Social Behavior, 3,* 269–276.

Lawson, H. H, Kahn, M. W., & Heiman, E. M. (1982). Psychopathology, treatment outcome, and attitude toward mental illness in Mexican-American and European patients. *International Journal of Psychiatry, 28,* 20–26.

Lenski, G. (1966). *Power and privilege: A theory of social stratification.* New York: McGraw-Hill.

Lessler, J. T., & Sirken, M. G. (1985). Laboratory-based research on the cognitive aspects of survey methodology: The goals and methods of the National Center for Health Statistics Study. *Milbank Memorial Fund Quarterly/Health and Society, 63,* 565–581.

Lewinsohn, P. M., & Rosenbaum, M. (1987). Recall of parental behavior by acute depressives, remitted depressives, and nondepressives. *Journal of Personality and Social Psychology, 52,* 611–619.

Linden, W., Paulhus, D. L., & Dobson, K. S. (1986). Effects of response styles on the report of psychological and somatic distress. *Journal of Consulting and Clinical Psychology, 54,* 309–313.

Link, B., & Dohrenwend, B. P. (1980). Formulation of hypotheses about the true prevalence of demoralization in the United States. In B. P. Dohrenwend, B. S. Dohrenwend, M. S. Gould, B. Lind, R. Neugebauer, & R. Wunsch-Hitzig (eds.), *Mental illness in the United States: Epidemiological estimates* (pp. 133–149). New York: Praeger.

Lonner, W. J. (1980). The search for psychological universals. In H. Triandis & W. Lambert (eds.), *Handbook of crosscultural psychology* (vol. 1) (pp. 139–159). Boston: Allyn and Bacon.

Manson, S. M., Shore, J. H., & Bloom, J. D. (1985). The depressive experience in American Indian communities: A challenge of psychiatric theory and diagnosis. In A. Kleinman & B. Good (eds.), *Culture and depression—Studies in the anthropology and cross-cultural psychiatry of affect and disorder* (pp. 331–368). Berkeley: University of California Press.

Marcos, L. R., Urcuyo, L., Kesselman, M., & Alpert, M. (1973). The language barrier in evaluating Spanish-American patients. *Archives of General Psychiatry, 29,* 655–659.

Marden, C. F., & Meyer, G. (1962). *Minorities in American society.* New York: American Book Co.

Marquis, A. V., Marquis, M. S., & Polich, J. M. (1986). Response bias and reliability in sensitive topic surveys. *Journal of American Statistical Association, 81,* 381–389.

Marsella, A. J. (1980). Depressive experience and disorder across cultures. In H. C. Triandis & J. G. Draguns (eds.), *Handbook of crosscultural psychology* (vol. 6) (pp. 237–289). Boston: Allyn and Bacon.

Marsella, A. J., Brennan, J., Kameoka, V., & Shirzuru, L. (1974). Personality correlates of clinical depression: II. Body image. Unpublished manuscript. University of Hawaii, Honolulu.

Marsella, A. J., Kinzie, D., & Gordon, P. (1973). Ethnic variations in the expression of depression. *Journal of Crosscultural Psychology, 4,* 435–458.

Marsella, A. J., Sartorius, N., Jablensky, A., & Fenton, F. R. (1985). Crosscultural studies of depressive disorders: An overview. In A. Kleinman & B. Good (eds.), *Culture and depression—Studies in the anthropology and cross-cultural psychiatry of affect and disorder* (pp. 299–324). Berkeley: University of California Press.

Marsella, A. J., Shirzuru, L., Brennan, J., & Kameoka, V. (1974). Personality correlates of clinical depression in different ethnic groups: I. Self concept. Unpublished manuscript. University of Hawaii, Honolulu.

Marsella, A. J., & Tanaka-Matsumi, J. (1976). Baselines of depressive symptomatology among normal Japanese nationals, Japanese-Americans, and Caucasian-Americans. Unpublished manuscript. University of Hawaii, Honolulu.

Mausner, J. S., & Bahn, A. K. (1974). *Epidemiology: An introductory text.* Philadelphia: W. B. Saunders.

McLaughlin, B., Rickels, K., Abidi, M., & Toro, R. (1969). Meprobamatebenactazine (Deprol) and placebo in two depressed outpatient populations. *Psychosomatics, 10,* 73–81.

Meadow, A., & Stoker, D. (1965). Symptomatic behavior of hospitalized patients. *Archives of General Psychiatry, 12,* 267–277.

Mirowsky, J., & Ross, C. E. (1984). Mexican culture and its emotional contradictions. *Journal of Health and Social Behavior, 25,* 2–13.

Myers, J. K., & Weissman, M. M. (1980). Use of a self-report symptom scale to detect depression in a community sample. *American Journal of Psychiatry, 137,* 1081–1084.

National Institute of Mental Health (1987). *Psychosocial screening of school-age children in pediatric settings: Report of an invitational conference* (NIMH Contract No. 86M020284301D). Rockville, MD: Division of Biometry and Applied Sciences.

Newmann, J. P. (1984). Sex differences in symptoms of depression: Clinical disorder or normal distress? *Journal of Health and Social Behavior, 25,* 136–159.

Novak, M. (1977). *Further reflections on ethnicity.* Middletown, PA: Jednota Press.

Noyes, R., Clancy, J., Hoenk, P. R., & Slymen, D. J. (1980). The prognosis of anxiety neurosis. *Archives of General Psychiatry, 37,* 173–178.

Paffenberger, R. S., & McCabe, L. J. (1966). The effect of obstetric and perinatal events on risk of mental illness in women in childbearing age. *American Journal of Public Health, 56,* 400–407.

Parkes, K. R. (1980). Social desirability, defensiveness and self-report psychiatric inventory scores. *Psychological Medicine, 10,* 735–742.

Patterson, O. (1975). Context and choice in ethnic allegiance: A theoretical framework and Caribbean case study. In N. Glazer & D. P. Moynihan (eds.), *Ethnicity: Theory and experience,* (pp. 305–349). Cambridge: Harvard University Press.

Paulhus, D. L. (1984). Two-component models of socially desirable responding. *Journal of Personality and Social Psychology, 46,* 598–609.

Petty, F., & Nasrallah, H. A. (1981). Secondary depression in alcoholism: Implications for future research. *Comprehensive Psychiatry, 22,* 587–595.

Petty, F., & Noyes, R., Jr. (1981). Depression secondary to cancer. *Biological Psychiatry, 16,* 1203–1220.

Philippus, M. J. (1971). Successful and unsuccessful approaches to mental health services for an urban Hispano-American population. *American Journal of Public Health, 61,* 620–631.

Pitt, B. (1982). Depression and childbirth. In E. S. Paykel (ed.), *Handbook of affective disorders* (pp. 361–378). New York: Guilford Press.

Pokorny, A. D., & Overall, J. E. (1970). Relationship of psychopathology to age, sex, ethnicity, education, and marital status in state hospital patients. *Journal of Psychiatric Research, 7,* 143–152.

Post, F. (1962). *The significance of affective symptoms in old age* (Maudsley Monographs, No. 10). London: Oxford University Press.

Prange, A. (1973). The use of drugs in depression: Its theoretical and practical basis. *Psychiatric Annals, 3,* 55–75.

Price, C. S., & Cuellar, I. (1981). The effects of language and related variables on the expression of psychopathology in Mexican-American psychiatric patients. *Hispanic Journal of Behavioral Science, 3,* 145–160.

Pugh, T. F., Jerath, B. K., Schmidt, W. M., & Reed, R. B. (1963). Rates of mental disease related to childbearing. *New England Journal of Medicine, 268,* 1224–1228.

Pulver, A. E., & Carpenter, W. T., Jr. (1983). Lifetime psychotic symptoms assessed with the DIS. *Schizophrenia Bulletin, 9,* 377–382.

Rabkin, J. G., Charles, E., & Kass, F. (1983). Hypertension and DSM-III depression in psychiatric outpatients. *American Journal of Psychiatry, 140,* 1072–1074.

Radloff, L. S. (1977). The CES-D scale: A self-report depression scale for research in the general population. *Applied Psychological Measurement, 1,* 385–401.

Raskin, A., Crook, T. H., & Herman, K. D. (1975). Psychiatric history and symptom differences in black and white depressed patients. *Journal of Consulting and Clinical Psychology, 43,* 73–80.

Regier, D., Goldberg, I. D., & Taube, C. H. (1978). The de facto U.S. mental health service system. *Archives of General Psychiatry, 35,* 685–693.

Riessman, C. K. (1979). Interviewer effects in psychiatric epidemiology: A study of medical and lay interviewers and their impact on reported symptoms. *American Journal of Public Health, 69,* 485–491.

Roberts, R. E. (1980). Reliability of the CES-D Scale in different ethnic contexts. *Psychiatry Research, 2,* 125–134.

Roberts, R. E. (1981). Prevalence of depressive symptoms among Mexican Americans. *Journal of Nervous and Mental Disease, 169,* 213–219.

Roberts, R. E. (1987a). An epidemiologic perspective on the mental health of people of Mexican origin. In R. Rodriquez and M. Coleman (eds.), *Mental health issues of the Mexican origin population in Texas: Proceedings of the Fifth Robert Lee Sutherland Seminar* (pp. 55–70). Austin: Hogg Foundation for Mental Health.

Roberts, R. E. (1987b). Epidemiological issues in measuring preventive effects. In R. F. Muñoz (ed.), *The prevention of depression: Research directions* (pp. 45–75). Washington, D.C.: Hemisphere Publishing.

Roberts, R. E., & Vernon, S. W. (1981). Usefulness of the PERI Demoralization Scale to screen for psychiatric disorder in a community sample. *Psychiatry Research, 5,* 183–193.

Roberts, R. E., & Vernon, S. W. (1983). The Center for Epidemiologic Studies Depression Scale: Its use in a community sample. *American Journal of Psychiatry, 140,* 41–46.

Roberts, R. E., & Vernon, S. W. (1984). Minority status and psychological distress re-examined: The case of Mexican Americans. In J. R. Greenley (ed.), *Research in community and mental health* (vol. 4) (pp. 131–164). Greenwich, CT: JAI Press.

Roberts, R. E., Vernon, S. W., & Rhoades, H. M. (1988). Effects of language and ethnic status on the DIS. Unpublished manuscript.

Robins, A. H. (1976). Are stroke patients more depressed than other disabled subjects? *Journal of Chronic Disease, 29,* 479–482.

Robins, E., & Guze, S. (1972). Classification of affective disorders: The primary-secondary, the endogeneous-reactive, and the neurotic-psychotic concepts. In T. A. Williams, M. J. Katz, & J. A. Shields (eds.), *Recent advances in the psychobiology of the depressive illnesses* (pp. 283–293). Washington, D.C.: U.S. Government Printing Office.

Robins, L. N. (1985). Epidemiology: Reflections on testing the validity of psychiatric interviews. *Archives of General Psychiatry, 42,* 918–924.

Robins, L. N., Helzer, J. E., Croughan, J., & Ratcliff, K. S. (1981). National Institute of Mental Health Diagnostic Interview Schedule: Its history, characteristics, and validity. *Archives of General Psychiatry, 38,* 381–389.

Ruiz, E. J. (1975). Influence of bilingualism on communication in groups. *International Journal of Group Psychotherapy, 25,* 391–395.

Sackheim, H. A., & Gur, R. C. (1978). Self-deception, self-confrontation and consciousness. In G. E. Schwartz & D. Shapiro (eds.), *Consciousness and self-regulation: Advances in research* (vol. 2) (pp. 139–197). New York: Plenum Press.

Schermerhorn, R. A. (1969). *Comparative ethnic relations: A framework for theory and research.* New York: Random House.

Schulberg, H. C., Saul, M., McClelland, M., Ganguli, M., Christy, W., & Frank, R. (1985). Assessing depression in primary medical and psychiatric practice. *Archives of General Psychiatry, 42,* 1164–1170.

Seiler, L. H. (1973). The 22-item scale used in field studies of mental illness: A question of method, a question of substance and a question of theory. *Journal of Health and Social Behavior, 14,* 252–264.

Shrout, P. E., & Fleiss, J. L. (1981). Reliability and case detection. In J. K. Wing & P. Bebbington (eds.), *What is a case? The problem of definition in psychiatric community surveys* (pp. 117–128). London: Grant & McIntyre.

Simon, R., Fleiss, J., Gurland, B., Stiller, P., & Sharpe, L. (1973). Depression and schizophrenia in hospitalized black and white mental patients. *Archives of General Psychiatry, 28,* 509–512.

Singer, K. (1975). Depressive disorders from a transcultural perspective. *Social Science and Medicine, 9,* 289–301.

Spiro, H. R., Siassi, I., & Crocetti, G. M. (1972). What gets surveyed in a psychiatric survey? *Journal of Nervous and Mental Disease, 154,* 105–114.

Spitzer, R. L., Endicott, T., & Robins, E. (1978). Research diagnostic criteria: Rationale and reliability. *Archives of General Psychiatry, 35,* 773–782.

Spitzer, R. L. & Williams, J. B. W. (1983). *Instruction manual for the Structured Clinical Interview for DSM-III (SCID).* New York: New York State Psychiatric Institute.

Steadman, H. J. (1981). Critically reassessing the accuracy of public perception of the dangerousness of the mentally ill. *Journal of Health and Social Behavior, 22,* 310–316.

Stein, H. F., & Hill, F. R. (1977). *The ethnic imperative: Examining the new White ethnic movement.* University Park: Pennsylvania State University Press.

Stoker, D. H., Zurcher, L. A., & Fox, A. (1968–1969). Women in psychotherapy: A crosscultural comparison. *International Journal of Psychiatry, 15,* 5–22.

Storey, P. B. (1967). Psychiatric sequelae of subarachnoid hemorrhage. *British Medical Journal, 3,* 261–266.

Swidler, A. (1986). Culture in action: Symbols and strategies. *American Sociological Review, 51,* 273–286.

Tanaka-Matsumi, J., & Marsella, A. J. (1977). Ethnocultural variations in the subjective experience of depression: Semantic differential. Unpublished manuscript. University of Hawaii, Honolulu.

Tonks, C., Paykel, E., & Klerman, G. (1970). Clinical depressions among Negroes. *American Journal of Psychiatry, 127,* 329–335.

U.S. Bureau of the Census (1984). *Detailed population characteristics. Part 1, United States Summary PC80-1-D1-A.* Washington, D.C.: U.S. Government Printing Office.

Vernon, S. W. (1980). An investigation of the reliability and validity of the Center for Epidemiologic Studies Depression Scale in three ethnic groups. Unpublished doctoral dissertation, University of Texas School of Public Health, Houston.

Vernon, S. W., & Roberts, R. E. (1981). Further observations on the problem of measuring nonspecific psychological distress and other dimensions of psychopathology. *Archives of General Psychiatry, 38,* 1239–1247.

Vernon, S. W., Roberts, R. E., & Lee, E. S. (1982). Response tendencies, ethnicity, and depression scores. *American Journal of Epidemiology, 116,* 482–495.

Veroff, J., Douvan, E., & Kulka, R. A. (1981). *The inner American.* New York: Basic Books.

Von Korff, M., Shapiro, S., Burke, J. D., Teitlebaum, M., Skinner, E. A., German, P., Turner, R. W., Klein, L., & Burns, B. (1987). Anxiety and depression in a primary care clinic: Comparison of the Diagnostic Interview Schedule, General Health Questionnaire, and practitioner assessments. *Archives of General Psychiatry, 44,* 152–156.

Weiss, C. H. (1975). Interviewing in evaluation research. In E. L. Struening & M. Guttentag (eds.), *Handbook of evaluation research* (vol. 1) (pp. 355–395). Beverly Hills: Sage Publications.

Weissman, M. M. (1987). Advances in psychiatric epidemiology: Rates and risks for major depression. *American Journal of Public Health, 77,* 445–451.

Weissman, M. M., & Klerman, G. L. (1977). Sex differences and the epidemiology of depression. *Archives of General Psychiatry, 34,* 98–111.

Weissman, M. M., & Klerman, G. L. (1978). Epidemiology of mental disorders: Emerging trends in the United States. *Archives of General Psychiatry, 35,* 705–712.

Wheaton, B. (1982). Uses and abuses of the Langner Index: A re-examination of findings on psychological and psychophysiological distress. In D. Mechanic (ed.), *Symptoms, illness behavior, and help-seeking* (pp. 25–54). New York: Prodist.

Whybrow, P., & Palatore, A. (1973). Melancholia, a model in madness: A discussion of recent psychobiologic research into depressive illness. *International Journal of Psychiatry in Medicine, 4,* 351–378.

Widmer, R. B., Cadoret, R. J., & North, C. S. (1980). Depression in family practice: Some effects on spouses and children. *Journal of Family Practice, 10,* 45–81.

Winokur, G. (1972). Family history studies VIII. *Diseases of the Nervous System, 33,* 94–99.

Wing, J. K., Cooper, J. E., & Sartorius, N. (1974). *The measurement and classification of psychiatric symptoms.* London: Cambridge University Press.

Wishnie, H. A., Hackett, T. P., & Cassem, N. H. (1971). Psychological hazards of convalescence following myocardial infarction. *Journal of American Medical Association, 215,* 1291–1296.

Woodruff, R. A., Murphy, G. E., & Herjanic, M. (1967). The natural history of affective disorders— I: Symptoms of 72 patients at the time of index hospital admission. *Journal of Psychiatric Research, 5,* 255–263.

Wynn, A. (1967). Unwarranted emotional distress in men with ischemic heart disease. *The Medical Journal of Australia and New Zealand, 2,* 847–851.

Yancey, W. L., Ericksen, E. P., & Juliani, R. N. (1976). Emergent ethnicity: A review and reformulation. *American Sociological Review, 41,* 391–403.

Zung, W. W. K. (1965). A self-rating depression scale. *Archives of General Psychiatry, 12,* 63–70

14

Depressive Symptomatology in Older American Indians with Chronic Disease: Some Psychometric Considerations

Anna E. Barón, Spero M. Manson, Lynn M. Ackerson and Douglas L. Brenneman

Physical illnesses, both chronic and acute, constitute one of the largest problems facing the American Indian and Alaska Native populations. Among older Indians and Natives, the impact of these illnesses is evidenced by high rates of disability or inability to perform daily activities, and by much higher rates of depression when compared to older non-Indian and non-Native people (U.S. Government Accounting Office, 1978; National Indian Council on Aging, 1981). Both of these factors contribute to decreased longevity in this group compared to the general population (Hill & Spector, 1971; Sievers & Fisher, 1981) and even to other ethnic minorities (U.S. Department of Health and Human Services, 1985).

In the general population of elderly, estimates of the prevalence of depression range from 10% to 65% (Gurland & Cross, 1982) and are much higher for older persons suffering from chronic disease (Ouslander, 1982). Often, it is difficult to distinguish between somatic symptoms of depression that may result from the illness itself and those that do not. In a study of older whites with chronic disease (Berkman et al., 1986), analyses were performed to determine whether endorsement of the somatic items on the Center for Epidemiologic Studies—Depression Scale (CES-D) occurred with greater frequency among individuals with higher levels of disability compared to those with lower levels of disability. Physical disability was associated with almost every item on the CES-D, not just the somatic items, as one might expect. From these results, it was concluded that disability resulting from a chronic disease does not reduce the validity of the CES-D in measuring depressive symptomatology.

While depression has been one of the most studied psychiatric problems, along with suicide and alcoholism, among American Indians and Alaska Natives, little is known about the validity and reliability of screening and diagnostic instruments for assessing depression in this cultural context (Shore & Manson, 1981). Indigenous concepts of depression have been studied in a variety of tribal settings (Devereux, 1961; Devoto, 1953; Johnson & Johnson, 1965; Lewis, 1975; Miller & Schoenfeld, 1971; Parker, 1960). Western psychiatric interpretations have tended to view cultural manifestations of these concepts as simply variations on major psychiatric disorders. In contrast, Manson, Shore, and Bloom (1985) used Kleinman's (1980) explanatory model (EM) framework to elicit indigenous concepts of depression and the major affective disorders to develop the Indian Depression Schedule (IDS), a modified version of the Diagnostic Interview Schedule (DIS) that uses criteria from the DSM-III, Feighner, and Research Diagnostic Criteria (RDC) to obtain a diagnosis. The IDS allows one to examine instrument validity from several points of view: specifically, the local cultural construction, the Western psychiatric perspective, and their intersection.

It is evident from the paucity of available data that more research is needed to develop and validate instruments that are culturally sensitive and meaningful for assessing depression among Indians and Natives. However, investigators need not assume that cultural distinctions automatically invalidate instruments such as the CES-D or the DIS, which were developed in general community settings, especially in the absence of empirical evidence to this effect. Evaluating the generalizability or external validity of these screening and diagnostic instruments across a variety of cultural settings is an important task that should be pursued with similar urgency.

The study described in this chapter provides some insight into this latter issue. The data are used to evaluate various psychometric properties of the CES-D for screening depression among older American Indians with chronic disease. The data also increase our understanding of the epidemiology of depression across culturally different populations.

Methods

This study is part of a more extensive, ongoing research project designed to test a preventive intervention targeted to older American Indians at high risk for depression as a consequence of chronic physical health problems and attendant stressors (Manson, Moseley, & Brenneman, in press). The data reported in this chapter were generated by a health screening that was conducted as a means of identifying participants for a prospective intervention.

Study Sites

The communities participating in this study include four Pacific Northwest reservation populations served by three IHS service units: specifically, the Confederated Tribes of the Warm Springs Indian Reservation, the Yakima Indian Nation, the Lummi Nation, and the Nooksack tribe.

Confederated Tribes of Warm Springs

The Warm Springs reservation is located in the north central part of Oregon, sixty miles southeast of Portland. Its western boundary extends along the summit of the Cascade Range and descends eastward to a wide plateau that is cut deeply by several tributaries to the Deschutes River. The two principal communities are Warm Springs (pop. 1,600) and Simnasho (pop. 200). Madras is the nearest town off reservation, some fifteen miles south of Warm Springs. Tribal enrollment numbers 2,771, with approximately 2,200 members actually residing on reservation. Membership is comprised of three distinct tribes: the Sahaptin, Wasco, and Paiute. Most of the elderly live on reservation close to support services, the health clinic, and tribal facilities. According to a recent tribal census, 623 members are 45 years of age or older.

Yakima Indian Nation

The Yakima reservation covers terrain in south-central Washington that is very similar to its Oregon counterpart. Toppenish, the agency town, has a population of 5,000. Approximately 30,000 individuals live on reservation, 7,480 of whom are Indian. Like Warm Springs, the Yakima represent a confederated nation of fourteen closely related Plateau tribes. The IHS health clinic and Yakima Area Agency on Aging are located in Toppenish; the latter offers a full spectrum of social and home services to the 400 tribal members age 60 and older.

Lummi Nation and Nooksack Tribe

The Lummi live on a reservation just north of Bellingham in northwestern Washington, nestled along the shores of the Puget Sound and inlets of the rivers that empty into it. The Nooksack are located slightly east of the Lummi on scattered homesteads close to traditional village sites, occupying the rich riverine land that stretches briefly between Puget Sound and the Cascade Mountains. Both belong to the coastal Salish language group. Approximately 1,445 Lummi tribal members live on or adjacent to the reservation, 559 of whom are estimated to be 45 years of age and older. The Nooksack number 520 tribal members, 109 of whom are 45 years or more of age. Both tribes share the same IHS health facility, but maintain independent support services for their respective elderly populations.

Sample

With the support and participation of the Portland Area Office of the Indian Health Service (IHS) and its respective service units, a search was conducted of the Ambulatory Patient Care (APC) information system, the IHS's computerized record of health clinic utilization. The search criteria included: (a) individuals 45 years of age or older seen at one of the study sites' three service units during the 1984 calendar year (Lummi and Nooksack share the same facility); (b) a designated first visit during the year in question for one or more of a series of physical illnesses that fell into the diabetes, rheumatoid arthritis, and coronary heart disease diagnostic groupings, and (c) tribal membership. The age criterion was chosen on the basis of the results of a 1979–1980 survey conducted by the National Indian Council on Aging, which demonstrated economic, social, psychological, physical health, and functional equivalences between rural American Indians 45 years of age or older and urban whites 62 years of age or older (National Indian Council on Aging, 1981).

Field staff then reviewed each service unit's medical records to confirm subject eligibility according to these criteria, noted contact information, and mailed letters inviting participation in the health screening. The initial APC search identified 1,112 potential subjects. Subsequent review of service unit medical records revealed that 26 individuals in fact did not meet the eligibility criteria. This discrepancy was the result largely of errors in APC entries with respect to subject age and diagnosis. Another 96 potential subjects were found to have died since their qualifying service visit. Letters of invitation were sent to the 990 subjects who remained eligible for study. Failing a response within ten working days, field staff attempted to contact potential subjects either by telephone or face to face. One hundred and sixty-two individuals had moved or could not be located by staff. Of the remaining pool of 828 subjects, 314 (38%) agreed to participate in the health screening and were interviewed between August and November 1985. A comparison of the characteristics of the refusers and participants indicates that men are significantly overrepresented among those who declined to be interviewed. There are no differences by subject age or diagnosis.

Procedure

Three to four tribal members from each of the participating communities were chosen and trained to conduct the health screening interviews. Those selected as interviewers tended to be older and were experienced in working with older adults from their respective reservations. The interview was scheduled at a time and place convenient to the subject, typically his or her home. It required approximately forty-five minutes to one hour to administer. Subjects were paid ten dollars for consenting to be interviewed. Several questions were asked at the close of the screening as a means of evaluating the interview process. Overall, subjects exhibited good ($n = 84$, 26.8%) to excellent ($n = 212$, 67.5%) degree of cooperation and had trouble with either none ($n = 115$, 36.6%) or a few ($n = 170$, 54.1%) of the questions. Another person was present during about one-third ($n = 109$, 34.7%) of the interviews and either gave no help ($n = 57$, 52%) or assisted only with factual information ($n = 31$, 28%).

Measures

The health screening interview consisted of 103 questions covering: (a) basic sociodemographic items, (b) Marlowe-Crowne Social Desirability Scale, (c) subjective health status, (d) aspects of daily living affected by the health problem, (e) Health Locus of Control Scale and illness attribution, (f) indices of perceived pain, (g) health care utilization and satisfaction, (h) CES-D, (i) Life Satisfaction Index-A, and (j) social support. The results of the health screening using the CES-D are the focus of this chapter.

The CES-D was chosen to assess the presence of dysphoria as well as other cognitive, affective, psychophysiological, and behavioral symptoms of depression. This self-report instrument was constructed from other, widely used depression scales (Radloff, 1977) and was intended specifically for community-based applications. It consists of twenty items that inquire about the frequency with which these symptoms were experienced by subjects during the week prior to administration. Algorithms have been developed to transform CES-D responses into approximate DSM-III and RDC diagnoses (Noh, Wood, & Turner, 1984). However, its 16-point cut-off has been shown to produce a high number of false positives when used for purposes of case identification (Craig & Van Natta, 1976; Myers & Weissman, 1980; Noh et al., 1984; Roberts & Vernon, 1983). Variations in sensitivity and specificity with a varying cut-off value are examined in this chapter.

Radloff reported an internal consistency coefficient of .85 for the CES-D; alpha has been employed in this chapter to determine if the scale is internally consistent for the population at hand. In addition to internal consistency, the CES-D has been factor analyzed to determine which items on the scale are correlated with each other. The factors are estimated for this sample and compared to those obtained by Radloff (1977). Roberts (1980), with a multi-ethnic community, and Berkman et al. (1986), with an older white population, reported factors very similar to those of Radloff. Individual items and total scores on the CES-D also are examined for response patterns by sex, age, subjective health status, perceived pain, and life activities affected by chronic illness. Finally, frequency of endorsement of somatic items on the CES-D is compared to that of nonsomatic items in order to determine if CES-D scores are inflated by symptoms which may be related to chronic health problems.

Results

Table 14.1 presents the characteristics of the study sample, which is predominantly female ($n = 220$). The distribution over the three diagnostic groupings is: rheumatoid arthritis, $n = 127$ (40%), coronary heart disease, $n = 95$ (30.3%), and diabetes, $n = 80$ (25.5%). There are no age or sex differences with respect to physical diagnosis. The median age is 59 years, ranging from 45 to 92 years old. The vast majority of subjects is married ($n = 152$, 48.4%); a large proportion is widowed ($n = 89$, 28.3%). Relatively few are still single ($n = 22$, 7%), separated ($n = 18$, 5.7%), or divorced ($n = 32$, 10.2%). About 16% ($n = 49$) of the sample has six years or less of formal education; nearly 58% ($n = 180$)

Table 14.1. Characteristics of the Study Sample

	Number	Percentage
Sex		
Females	220	70
Males	94	30
Age		
45—64 yrs	205	66
65—74	71	23
75 +	34	11
Chronic condition		
Diabetes	80	26
Coronary heart disease	95	32
Arthritis	127	42
Education		
0—6 yrs	49	16
7—12	184	60
>12	75	24
Employment status		
Full-time	46	15
Part-time	24	8
Unemployed	95	30
Retired	102	32
Other	46	15
Marital status		
Single	22	7
Married	141	45
Living as married	11	4
Divorced/Separated	50	16
Widowed	89	28

completed high school and/or postsecondary training. One-third of the sample is retired (n = 102, 32.5%); nearly another third is unemployed (n = 95, 30.3%); 22% (n = 70) of the subjects is employed either full or part time.

Table 14.2 presents descriptive results on the CES-D for the sample as a whole and by sex, age, and physical diagnosis. Chi-square analyses of the two-way classifications for the CES-D with these characteristics show that individuals exceeding the threshold score of 16 on the CES-D are significantly more likely to be female than male. No differences with respect to age or physical diagnosis in CES-D outcome scores were detected.

The estimated internal consistency for the CES-D in this sample is 0.86. Table 14.3 shows the cross-classifications of the CES-D outcome with the derived DSM-III and RDC diagnoses for depression. The sensitivity of the CES-D is 100% in each case, but the specificity is 73% and 71% relative to the DSM-III and RDC, respectively. Figure 14.1 presents a plot (known as an ROC curve;

Table 14.2. Presence of Depressive Symptoms Using the CES-D

Group	Median CES-D Score		Range	% 16+
All	10		0—51	32

	CES-D Score	
	< 16	16+
	N (%)	N (%)
Sex		
Females	135 (62)	85 (38)*
Males	78 (81)	16 (19)
Diagnosis		
Diabetes	51 (71)	21 (29)
CHD	68 (72)	27 (28)
Arthritis	85 (67)	42 (33)
Age		
45—64	135 (66)	70 (34)
65—74	53 (75)	18 (25)
75+	22 (65)	12 (35)

* $p < .01$

Murphy et al., 1987) of the sensitivity versus one minus the specificity, or false-positive rate, with varying cut-off values for the CES-D relative to the RDC and DSM-III criteria. Points along the curve correspond to an increment (move left along curve) or decrease (move right along curve) of cut-off value relative to the traditional cut-off of 16 (marked by an asterisk). A sensitivity of 100% can be maintained and the specificity increased to about 85% by moving left to the point at which the curve drops to less than 100% sensitivity. This corresponds to a cut-off of 24 on the CES-D using the RDC criteria. The RDC and DSM-III criteria produce very similar ROC curves at very low and very high cut-off values. Minor deviations are observed in the intermediate range of cut-off values, but there is no strong evidence for a preference of one set of criteria over the other.

Table 14.4 presents the factor loadings for four factors estimated from the data using principal factor analysis with varimax rotation (Radloff, 1977). These

Table 14.3. Comparison of the CES-D with Approximated Diagnoses for Depression

		DSM-III		RDC	
		+	−	+	−
CES-D	16+	24	77	15	86
	<16	0	213	0	213

Sensitivity = 100%	Sensitivity = 100%
Specificity = 73%	Specificity = 71%

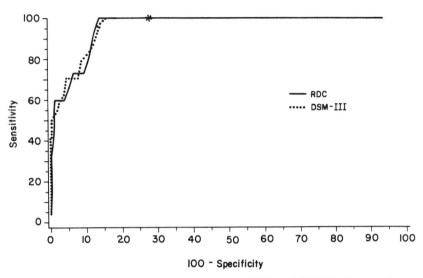

Figure 14.1. ROC Curves for the CES-D versus RDC and DSM-III Criteria. Curve evaluated for discrete values of CES-D.

Table 14.4. Factor Loadings for the CES-D Scale

	Item	Factor 1	Factor 2	Factor 3	Factor 4	Communalities
1.	Bothered	.59	.15	.13	−.10	.39
2.	Appetite	.58	.12	.30	.10	.46
3.	Blues	.65	.32	.22	−.01	.58
4.	Good	.06	.08	.82	−.08	.69
5.	Mind	.62	.06	−.06	.13	.41
6.	Depressed	.75	.27	.10	.05	.65
7.	Effort	.50	−.10	−.02	.36	.39
8.	Hopeful	.10	−.03	.68	.31	.57
9.	Failure	.27	.41	.14	.24	.32
10.	Fearful	.37	.55	−.04	.03	.45
11.	Sleep	.60	.23	.03	.15	.44
12.	Happy	.35	.12	.22	.56	.50
13.	Talk	.42	.16	.10	.10	.22
14.	Lonely	.48	.49	.03	.16	.50
15.	Unfriendly	.06	.65	.20	.16	.49
16.	Enjoy	.00	.25	.03	.75	.62
17.	Cry	.47	.57	.05	−.20	.60
18.	Sad	.63	.45	−.02	−.06	.61
19.	Dislike	.14	.64	−.09	.13	.45
20.	Get going	.58	.04	−.09	.23	.40

factors together explain only 49% of the variation in the data. Inspection of this matrix indicates that factor 1 is a nonspecific factor, including affective and somatic items, and explains 30% of the variance; 12 of the 20 items on the scale have loadings greater than .40. In contrast, the other three factors include only a few items meeting that criterion.

Table 14.5 presents response patterns in the CES-D by age and sex. Females differ from males in this sample in their responses to a number of items, specifically those pertaining to negative affect and interpersonal elements. It is worth noting that no differences in response patterns on the positive affect items are observed between males and females. Nor did age appear to have a relationship with any special response pattern for items on the CES-D in this study.

Table 14.6 presents CES-D outcome by perceived pain, subjective health status, and life activities affected by chronic illness. CES-D outcome is significantly related to responses to questions about pain associated with the illness; those with a higher level of perceived pain were more likely to have exceeded a score of 16 on the CES-D than those with a lower level of pain reported. Similarly, for health status, those who perceive their health to be fair or poor, or worse than

Table 14.5 Relative Frequency of Positive* Response on Individual CES-D Items by Sex and Age

		Sex		Age		
		Females	Males	45—64	65—74	75+
1.	Bothered	.28**	.13	.27	.23	.09
2.	Appetite	.23*	.11	.20	.14	.27
3.	Blues	.22**	.07	.20	.14	.12
4.	Good	.85	.89	.87	.82	.91
5.	Mind	.27**	.10	.20	.23	.30
6.	Depressed	.28*	.10	.25	.17	.21
7.	Effort	.33	.31	.32	.27	.47
8.	Hopeful	.82	.88	.84	.85	.81
9.	Failure	.10	.05	.09	.07	.06
10.	Fearful	.16*	.07	.13	.10	.21
11.	Sleep	.38*	.23	.37	.23	.35
12.	Happy	.82	.88	.81	.86	.94
13.	Talk	.29	.23	.26	.28	.39
14.	Lonely	.25*	.13	.21	.21	.21
15.	Unfriendly	.08	.02	.06	.04	.09
16.	Enjoy	.90	.91	.92	.87	.85
17.	Cry	.15**	.04	.12	.13	.12
18.	Sad	.26**	.11	.20	.20	.29
19.	Dislike	.08*	.01	.05	.06	.12
20.	Get going	.27	.21	.27	.20	.27

* Positive response is defined as an answer of "occasionally" *or* "most or all of the time."

* p < .05

** p < .01

Table 14.6. Association of CES-D Outcome with Perceived Pain, Subjective Health Status, and Activities of Daily Living Affected by Chronic Condition

	CES-D Total Score	
	< 16	≥ 16
Variable	N (%)	N (%)
Perceived Pain		
General pain experienced in association with illness		
None or not much	91 (44)	30 (30)
A fair amount or a lot	118 (57)	70 (70)*
Pain experienced during the last week		
None or not much	130 (62)	41 (41)
A fair amount or a lot	90 (38)	59 (59)**
Subjective Health Status		
Expectation of illness 6 months from now		
Much or somewhat better	79 (38)	40 (42)
About the same	108 (53)	42 (44)
Somewhat or much worse	18 (9)	14 (14)
Health compared to people one's own age		
Much or somewhat better	113 (56)	48 (50)
About the same	71 (35)	31 (32)
Somewhat or much worse	18 (9)	18 (18)*
Overall health rating		
Excellent	23 (11)	3 (3)
Good	86 (41)	29 (30)
Fair	81 (39)	48 (49)
Poor	18 (9)	18 (18)*
Activities of Living Affected by chronic Condition *		
Caring for self	79 (36)	56 (56)**
Caring for others	80 (38)	53 (53)*
Eating habits	83 (40)	52 (52)*
Sleeping habits	81 (39)	59 (59)**
Household chores	82 (39)	56 (56)**
Going shopping	74 (35)	49 (49)*
Visiting friends	59 (28)	41 (41)*
Enjoying hobbies	65 (31)	44 (44)*
Working	93 (45)	50 (50)
Maintaining friendships	50 (24)	40 (40)*

  * Percentages are of responses that illness has affected activity "a fair amount," "a great deal," or "no longer able to do this activity."

  * $p < .05$

  ** $p < .01$

that of their peers are more likely to score above 16 on the CES-D. Expectation about health status six months from now is not associated with outcome on the CES-D. Finally, CES-D outcome is positively associated with levels of impairment on all but one of the activities of daily living affected by the respondents' chronic conditions, namely, working.

Table 14.7 presents the partial correlations of two sets of items within the CES-D—the subtotal of the seven somatic items and the subtotal of the thirteen nonsomatic items—with perceived pain, subjective health status, and life activities. The somatic items are: bothered, appetite, mind, effort, sleep, talk, and get going. The correlations for the somatic items subtotal are adjusted for the nonsomatic items subtotal and vice versa. It is readily observed that the partial correlations between the somatic items subtotal and the illness-related variables are much higher than the partials of the nonsomatic items subtotal. All but one of the correlations for the somatic items are significant, whereas only one of the correlations is significant for the nonsomatic items.

Table 14.7. Partial Correlations of the Somatic Items Subtotal and Nonsomatic Items Subtotal with Perceived Pain, Subjective Health Status, and Activities of Daily Living

| | Partial Correlations* | |
| | Somatic Items Subtotal | Nonsomatic Items Subtotal |
Variable		
Perceived Pain		
General pain experienced in association with illness	.20**	−.04
Pain experienced during the last week	.20**	.02
Subjective Health Status		
Expectation of illness 6 months from now	.10*	−.11
Health compared to people one's own age	.04	.06
Overall health rating	.13*	.11*
Activities of Living Affected by Chronic Condition		
Caring for self	.11*	.04
Caring for others	.15**	−.01
Eating habits	.14**	−.004
Sleeping habits	.16**	.09
Household chores	.14**	.05
Going shopping	.18**	−.01
Visiting friends	.16**	.06
Enjoying hobbies	.18**	−.01
Working	.14**	−.01
Maintaining friendships	.16**	.06

* Correlation between the somatic items subtotal and the nonsomatic item subtotal is .67.

* p < .05

** p < .01

Discussion

No data have been reported previous to this study on the internal consistency of the CES-D as completed by American Indians. The alpha coefficient of .86 obtained herein is consistent with estimates obtained by the developers of the CES-D in community settings and indicates that the CES-D is an internally consistent measure of depressive symptomatology in this group of older American Indians with chronic disease. The prevalence estimates for depression generated in this study are higher than those obtained in a previous study of older whites with chronic illnesses, where estimates ranged from 9% to 31% (Berkman et al., 1986).

The higher prevalence reported in this study for females compared to males is consistent with well-documented sex differences in reporting of depressive symptoms that have appeared in the literature. Specifically, the response patterns examined on individual items within the CES-D in this sample reflect tendencies towards higher reporting by females of negative affect and interpersonal difficulties, rather than underreporting of positive affect.

The CES-D cut-off of 16 or above is demonstrated to be 100% sensitive but not highly specific for depression in this sample. The low specificity is consistent with reports in the literature. Perfect sensitivity of the CES-D was reported previously by Noh, et al. (1984) in an older population, but other authors have reported much lower sensitivities (Myers & Weissman, 1980; Roberts & Vernon, 1983).

While other psychometric properties of the CES-D were replicated, the estimated factor structure was substantially different. In particular, no "somatic" factor, as such, is identified here; and the "positive" factor identified by Radloff separates into two factors, factor 3 (includes feeling as good as others and feeling hopeful about the future) and factor 4 (includes feeling happy and enjoying life). Factor 2 is similar to the "interpersonal" factor estimated by Radloff, but includes many items that are in the affective domain of depression: crying and feeling fearful, lonely, and sad.

The positive relationships between depressive symptomatology and pain, health status, and activities affected are consistent with results of Berkman et al. (1986). The latter examined CES-D scores and levels of impairment in older whites with chronic disease and found higher scores among those with greater functional disabilities. A concern in looking at depression in older age groups is that somatic complaints related to age and physical condition may dominate the reports of depressive symptoms. Age was seen to have no association with responses to items on the CES-D. However, it appears that the somatic items on the CES-D explain much of the variability in the variables used here as measures of impairment, even after adjusting for the nonsomatic items. The opposite is not true. After adjusting for the somatic item subtotal, the nonsomatic items subtotal explains a trivial amount of the variability in the impairment variables. This is not consistent with the findings of Berkman et al. (1986), who examined the relationship between functional ability and response to individual items on the CES-D. The positive association was not restricted to the somatic items, but included the negative and positive affect and interpersonal items as well. The same was observed in this study (not shown). But the partial correlation analysis indicates that the positive association between nonsomatic depressive complaints and functional disability disappears after taking into account the positive association of the latter with somatic depressive complaints.

Conclusion

The CES-D was developed as a screening instrument and not as a diagnostic tool. The use of the CES-D for diagnostic purposes may thus be considered suspect. Furthermore, the application of the transformational algorithms creates a circular, rather than external, relationship between the derived DSM-III and RDC outcomes and the CES-D score. Nevertheless, important information is obtained by the respective cross-classifications.

The lack of false negatives provides support for use of the CES-D as a screening tool for a preventive intervention, as it was used in this study. The high percentage of false positives, however, could be costly in such a context, suggesting the use of additional criteria for establishing eligibility for intervention, such as a second screening with a diagnostic protocol as recommended by Shrout and Fleiss (1981). An alternative suggested by the results of this study is the use of a higher cut-off score, 24 rather than 16, which maintains high sensitivity and reduces the false-positive rate.

Differences between the factor analytic results obtained in this study relative to other studies call into question an aspect of the external validity of the previous results. The differences may be attributed to the composition of this sample, particularly its cultural disparity relative to those in other studies. Further investigation of this finding is indicated.

Perceived pain and limitations placed on daily activities are related to the reporting of depressive symptoms. In this study, these appear to be related through the expression of somatic complaints. This provides some evidence that the internal validity of the CES-D is compromised in this chronically ill population of older American Indians. More research is needed with aging populations and other American Indian groups in order to assess fully the strengths and limitations of the CES-D in measuring depressive symptomatology and its use as a screening instrument.

References

Berkman, L. F., Berkman, C. S., Kasl, S, Freeman, D. H., Leo, L., Ostfeld, A. M., Cornoni-Huntley, J., & Brody, J. A. (1986). Depressive symptoms in relation to physical health and functioning in the elderly. *American Journal of Epidemiology, 124,* 372–388.

Craig, T. J., & Van Natta, P. (1976). Presence and persistence of depressive symptoms in patient and community populations. *American Journal of Psychiatry, 133,* 1426–1429.

Devereux, G. (1961). *Mohave ethnopsychiatry.* Washington, D.C.: Smithsonian Institution Press.

DeVoto, B. (Ed.) (1953). *The Journals of Lewis and Clark.* Boston: Houghton Mifflin.

Gurland, B., & Cross, P. S. (1982). Epidemiology of psychopathology in old age. *Psychiatric Clinics of North America, 5* (1), 11–26.

Hill, C. A., & Spector, M. I. (1971). Natality and mortality of American Indians compared with U.S. whites and nonwhites. *HSHA Reports, 86,* 29–246.

Johnson, D. L., & Johnson, C. A. (1965). Totally discouraged: A depressive syndrome of the Dakota Sioux. *Transcultural Psychiatric Research, 1,* 141–143.

Kleinman, A. (1980). *Patients and healers in the context of culture.* Berkeley: University of California Press.

Lewis, T. H. (1975). A syndrome of depression and mutism in the Oglala Sioux. *American Journal of Psychiatry, 132,* 753–755.

Manson, S. M., Moseley, R., & Brenneman, D. (in press). Physical illness, depression, and older American Indians: A preventive intervention trial. In T. Owan & M. Silverman (eds.), *Special populations: Preventive intervention concerns—A new beginning.* Washington, D.C.: U.S. Government Printing Office.

Manson, S. M., Shore, J. H., & Bloom, J. D. (1985). The depressive experience in American Indian communities: A challenge for psychiatric theory and diagnosis. In A. Kleinman & B. Good (eds.), *Culture and depression* (pp. 331–368). Berkeley: University of California Press.

Miller, S. J., & Schoenfeld, L. (May 1971). Grief in the Navajo: Psychodynamics and culture. Paper presented at the annual meeting of the American Psychiatric Association, Washington, D.C..

Murphy, J. M., Berwick, D. M., Weinstein, M. C., Borus, J. F., Budman, S. H., & Klerman, G. L. (1987). Performance of screening and diagnostic tests—Application of Receiver Operating Characteristic analysis. *Archives of General Psychiatry, 44,* 550–555.

Myers, J. K., & Weissman, M. M. (1980). Use of a self-report symptom scale to detect depression in a community sample. *American Journal of Psychiatry, 137,* 1081–1084.

National Indian Council on Aging. (1981). *American Indian elderly: A national profile.* Albuquerque: National Indian Council on Aging.

Noh, S., Wood, D. W., & Turner, R. J. (1984). Depression among the physically disabled: Somatic and psychological contributions. Unpublished manuscript.

Ouslander, J. G. (1982). Physical illness and depression in the elderly. *Journal of the American Geriatrics Society, 30* (9), 593–599.

Parker, S. (1960). The Windigo psychosis in the context of Ojibwa personality and culture. *American Anthropologist, 62,* 603–623.

Radloff, L. S. (1977). The CES-D scale: A self-report depression scale for research in the general population. *Journal of Applied Psychological Measurement, 1,* 385–401.

Roberts, R. E. (1980). Reliability of the CES-D Scale in different ethnic contexts. *Psychiatry Research, 2,* 125–134.

Roberts, R. E., & Vernon, S. W. (1983). The Center for Epidemiologic Studies Depression Scale: Its use in a community sample. *American Journal of Psychiatry, 140,* 41–46.

Shore, J. H., & Manson, S. M. (1981). Cross-cultural studies of depression among American Indians and Alaska Natives. *White Cloud Journal, 2,* 5–12.

Shrout, P. E., & Fleiss, J. L. (1981). Reliability and case detection. In J. K. Wing & P. Bebbington (eds.), *What is a case? The problem of definition in psychiatric community survey* (pp. 117–128). London: Grant & McIntyre.

Sievers, M. L., & Fisher, J. R. (1981). Diseases of North American Indians. In H. Rothschild (ed.), *Biocultural aspects of disease* (pp. 191–252). New York: Academic Press.

U.S. Department of Health and Human Services (1985). *Report of the Secretary's Task Force on Black and Minority Health*. Washington, D.C.: U.S. Government Printing Office.

U. S. Government Accounting Office (1979). Special report.

15

Depression Prevention Research: The Need for Screening Scales that Truly Predict

Jeanne Miranda, Ricardo F. Muñoz, and Martha Shumway

The major task of primary care physicians is health maintenance and prevention of disease. Although guidelines for the prevention of physical disease in primary care have been written, little has been written about prevention of psychiatric disorders in this population. Yet, the coexistence of depression and physical disorders has been recognized for several decades. A current challenge is to decrease the high incidence of depressive disorders in primary care. This chapter will examine a necessary step in meeting that challenge, the development of screening scales that truly predict to depression. First, we will discuss guidelines that should be met if screening for depression is to become a routine practice in primary care. Next, we will consider the need for prevention of depression in primary care and discuss our research in this area. Finally, we will discuss screening scales that truly predict depression.

Criteria for Screening of Depression

Depression has generally been treated only during symptomatic stages. Persons who are at risk for depression remain undetected and untreated. Although generally accepted screening criteria exist for a variety of physical disorders, they have not been applied to depressive disorders. However, they may serve as models upon which to build intervention guidelines for depressive disorders.

The following are generally accepted criteria to justify the implementation of screening protocols for physical disorders:

1. The incidence of the condition must be sufficient to justify the cost of screening.

2. The condition must have a significant effect on the quality or quantity of life.

3. Acceptable methods of treatment must be available.

4. Tests that are acceptable to patients must be available at reasonable cost to detect the condition in the asymptomatic period.

5. The condition must have an asymptomatic period during which detection and treatment significantly reduce morbidity or mortality.

6. Treatment in the asymptomatic phase must yield a therapeutic result superior to that obtained by delaying treatment until symptoms appear.

These same criteria may be applied to determine whether or not to screen routinely for depression in primary care.

Depression clearly meets the first criterion of sufficient incidence. Studies of depression in primary care using standardized psychiatric diagnostic instruments have revealed prevalence rates near 6% for major depressive disorder (Hoeper, Nycz, Cleary, Regier, & Goldberg, 1979; Schulberg et al., 1985). Furthermore, the presence of significant depressive symptomatology (as indexed by depression screening scores) in primary care is exceptionally high. The frequency of significant depressive symptomatology has been estimated to range as high as 32% (Kathol & Petty, 1981) and reached 55% in our sample of low-income and minority patients from public medical clinics (Muñoz, Ying, Armas, Chan, & Gurza, 1987). This presence of significant depressive symptomatology may indicate high risk for development of a depressive episode. Thus, depressive disorders and depressive symptomatology are frequent enough in primary care populations to justify screening.

Depressive disorders also meet the second criterion of exerting a significant negative effect on quantity and quality of life to justify screening. In fact, clinical depression may be one of the most painful of human experiences. According to a recent study, depressed psychiatric inpatients with a history of life-threatening physical illnesses considered the pain of depression to be worse than that of physical disorders (Osmond, Mullaly, & Bisbee, 1984). Furthermore, depression has significant negative sequelae, including: (a) increased frequency of medical visits (Hankin et al., 1982; Hoeper et al., 1980; Mumford, Schlesinger, & Glass, 1981; Weissman, Myers, & Thompson, 1981); (b) psychological impairment (Sternberg & Jarvik, 1976); (c) impaired life-functioning (Nicholi, 1967; Whitney, Cadoret, & McClure, 1971); (d) increased general morbidity (Murphy, Monson, Olivier, Sobol, & Leighton, 1987); and (e) increased risk of suicide (Guze & Robins, 1970). The long-term risk for suicide in persons who are depressed is between 10 and 15% (Teuting, Koslow, & Hirschfeld, 1981). In sum, depression is significantly detrimental and screening in order to prevent and treat the disorder is thus justified.

Currently, there are no acceptable tests to detect depression in an asymptomatic phase. Although a fair amount of work has been done on high-risk factors for depression (Akiskal, 1987; Boyd & Weissman, 1982; Hirschfeld & Cross, 1981; Roberts, 1987), these high-risk factors are generally derived from lifetime prevalence studies rather than from incidence studies. This means that they are helpful in predicting which groups of people are more likely to become clinically depressed sometime during their lives. They are not as helpful in identifying imminent onset of depression. Scales that would identify those who are currently depressed and those who are currently at high-risk for depression are needed. These scales could be used to identify three groups of patients: (a) those who currently meet criteria for major depression, (b) those who are at high-risk for depression, and (c) those who are at low-risk for depression. Ideally, those who are depressed would be referred for assessment and treatment. Those who are at risk for depression would be referred to a preventive intervention. Finally, those who are at low-risk for developing depression would need no intervention. Table 15.1 provides an overview of treatment that could be offered at different stages of depressive symptomatology.

The next three criteria necessary to include screening for depression as an integral part of primary care refer to treatment outcome. First, acceptable methods of treatment for depression are available. Recent evidence suggests that both psychological and pharmacological treatments for depression are effective (see narrative review by Weissman, 1979; and meta-analysis by Steinbrueck, Maxwell, & Howard, 1983). The final two criteria for treatment state that treatment in an asymptomatic phase must reduce morbidity or mortality and that such preventive treatment must produce results superior to those achieved in the symptomatic phase. These criteria point to the need for randomized, controlled prevention trials to determine the outcome and efficacy of preventing onset of major depression. Although the results of such trials are not currently available, preliminary results of our work on prevention of depression will be reviewed.

The San Francisco Mood Survey Project

Our initial work on prevention of depression involved a community-wide intervention. One of the desiderata of prevention programs is their ability to reach large portions of the community. Our first attempt at such an intervention investigated the effectiveness of a televised miniseries educating the public on preventing depression (Muñoz, Glish, Soo-Hoo, & Robertson, 1982). A series of ten four-minute segments depicting cognitive-behavioral methods to control depression was shown during the noon, six o'clock, and eleven o'clock news hour over the course of two weeks. The week before the segments were aired, a random sample of adults from the white pages of the San Francisco telephone book were contacted and administered the Center for Epidemiological Studies-Depression Scale (CES-D; Radloff, 1977), a twenty-item self-report scale frequently used in epidemiological studies. The same people were recontacted after the segments were shown, and the CES-D was again administered. Among those who were initially symptomatic (i.e., CES-D of 16 or above), there was a significant decrease in depression following the televised intervention. Those who had not watched the segments had an average score of 22 at pretest and 17 at posttest, whereas, those who had watched had a mean score of 24 at pretest and 11 after.

This study suggests that cognitive-behavioral methods that teach ways to increase control over thoughts and activities can have beneficial effects in reducing depressive symptomatology. Furthermore, as depressive symptomatology is reduced, one would expect that fewer persons would subsequently reach the threshold of clinical depression. Thus, these methods offer promise for preventing incidence of major depressive disorder.

The Depression Prevention Research Project

Before describing our own work, we should note other research efforts to prevent depression. At least two other studies presently in progress were designed to look at preventive effects on the incidence of depression across randomly assigned study groups. Vega and his colleagues (Vega, Valle, Kolody, & Hough, 1987) are conducting a randomized depression prevention trial in San Diego focused on Spanish-speaking women. The most impressive aspect of this study is the epidemiological basis for sample selection. The persons meeting study inclusion criteria in the community in which the study is being conducted were enumerated, so that the sample is a representative sample of that community. Spero Manson (ch. 14) is also conducting a randomized trial with an Indian population; his work is described further in this volume.

Methodology

Our own study, the Depression Prevention Research Project, is a randomized, controlled prevention trial (Muñoz et al., 1987). The high-risk population being studied includes low-income and minority medical outpatients at public primary care clinics associated with the University of California, San Francisco. The study is being conducted in English, Spanish, Cantonese, and Mandarin. Preliminary results from English- and Spanish-language groups will be presented at this time. Subjects who participated were between 18 and 69 years of age and had been registered clinic patients for at least six months prior to the initial interview. Those who agreed to participate were screened to determine that they were literate, not receiving mental health treatment, not terminally ill, and able to attend classes at predetermined times. During an initial screening in the clinics, demographic information was obtained, and the CES-D was administered.

The second screening interview was scheduled approximately one week after primary care visits and consisted of the Beck Depression Inventory (BDI) (Beck, Ward, Mendelsohn, Mock, & Erbaugh, 1961) and the NIMH Diagnostic Interview Schedule (DIS) (Robins, Helzer, Croughan, & Ratcliff, 1981). The latter produced DSM-III diagnoses, including major depression and dysthymia. Participants were paid ten dollars for this interview.

Participants were also paid ten dollars for a third screening interview during which they completed measures assessing cognitive behavior variables considered

Table 15.1. Intervention Guidelines for Affective Disorders.

Severity	No symptoms	Few symptoms	Significant symptoms	Clinical Levels (DSM-III-R Dx)	Maintainance
Public Health Level of Intervention	[------Primary prevention------] Interventions to prevent significant symptoms or later disorder.		[------Secondary prevention------] [Early identification and intervention to prevent diagnosable disorder.	[------Tertiary prevention------] [Treatment to shorten duration, reduce disability, and prevent reoccurrence.	]
Description of Individual	Energetic, optimistic	Transient dysphoria	Bothersome dysphoria	Daily functioning impaired Minor----------incapacitated	Generally back to normal mood & activity level.
Areas to Examine:					
1. Aloneness	Self-sufficient, comfortable	Lonely, needy	Low self-efficacy, suffers alone		Baseline
2. Relationships	Balanced, assertive	Resentful, misunderstood	Burdened by others, unloved		Baseline
3. Work	Productive	Reduced productivity, "burned out"	Takes great effort to keep up, immobilized		Baseline
Helpful Measures: (recommended cutoff scores)	[------Center for Epidemiologic Studies-Depression Scale (CES-D) (Radloff, 1977)------]				
	{------CES-D < 16------}		{--CES-D > 15------}		
	[------Beck Depression Inventory (BDI) (Beck et al., 1961)------]				
	{--BDI<11------} {--10<BDI<17------}		}{--BDI>16------}		

236

Table 15.1. Intervention Guidelines for Affective Disorders (*continued*).

Severity Type of Intervention:	No symptoms	Few symptoms	Significant symptoms	Clinical Levels (DSM-III-R Dx)	Maintainance
	[--Educational ————————————————————————————]				
		[--Supportive interventions —————————————————]			
				[Treatment of DSM-III-R disorder] [--Maintenance--] (Outpatient----Hospitalization) (For recurrent or bipolar)]	
		[--Social system or environmental strategies —————————————]			
Modality: Psychological	[--Educational-supportive preventive interventions ————]		[--Verbal and/or behavioral therapy ——————————————————— (At severe levels, combine with medications)]		
	(Self-control approaches, skill-learning, self-efficacy, competency-building interventions, "growth therapies," economic, social, community empowerment approaches)		(Cognitive, behavioral, psychodynamic interventions)		(Self-control-oriented interventions)
Medical	[--None indicated (yet) ————————————]		[--Antidepressants —————————————— [Other meds, e.g., MAO inhibitors) [--ECT————] [--For bipolar, manic, or recurrent unipolar: lithium, or if non-responsive, other medications, e.g. carbamazepine] (--If manic, or with psychotic features, antipsychotics may be indicated at first]		

important intervening variables to depressive disorder. At this interview, participants once again completed the CES-D.

Persons who met criteria for a current (within the last six months) diagnosis of depression (major depression or dysthymia), mania, schizophrenia, drug or alcohol abuse or dependence, organic brain syndrome, or were judged to be in need of immediate treatment were not accepted into the study. This ensured that the randomized trial was a preventive trial and not a therapy outcome study. Those who were symptomatic at the time were referred to community mental health clinics for treatment.

Representativeness of the Random Sample

Prior to determining the efficacy of the preventive intervention, we examined the representativeness of our sample and the utility of our measures within ethnic subgroups of our sample. San Francisco, like most major urban centers, is a socially, racially, and linguistically diverse city. Care was taken to establish liaisons with clinics that reflected the demographic characteristics of the city, and pilot studies were conducted early in the process to prepare to do the study in Spanish and Chinese.

Our sample was ethnically diverse, as Table 15.2 indicates. These data were obtained during the first interviews done in the clinics. Next to this, the percentage of each ethnic group represented in the randomized sample is presented. We were concerned that the rigorous interview procedures that were part of screening for this study might bias our randomized sample. As can be seen, our randomized sample remained ethnically representative of the sample contacted during the initial screening.

Ethnic and Language Differences in
Screening for Depression

Next, we examined the utility of our measures within the ethnic and language subgroups of our sample. During the past two decades, several methods for

Table 15.2. Ethnic Representativeness of Sample

	Prior to Screening		Randomized Sample	
Ethnicity	n	%	n	%
Asian	105	14.0	40	23.0
Black	145	19.4	34	19.0
Latino	178	23.8	38	22.0
White	268	35.8	63	36.0
Other	53	7.0		

making reliable diagnoses of depression with majority populations have been developed (e.g., Schedule for Affective Disorders and Schizophrenia [SADS], DIS, DSM-III; for review see Leber, Beckham, & Danker-Brown, 1985). However, diagnosis of depression in ethnic minority individuals is less well defined. Members of ethnic minorities report more symptoms of depression than do whites (for blacks see Comstock & Helsing, 1976; Eaton & Kessler, 1981; Neff & Husaini, 1980; Roberts, Stevenson, & Breslow, 1981; Warheit, Holzer, & Avery, 1975; for Hispanics see Dohrenwend & Dohrenwend, 1969; Fredrichs, Aneshensel, & Clark, 1981; Vernon & Roberts, 1982; and for Chinese see Kleinman & Lin, 1981; Kuo, 1984); however, the prevalence of clinical depression as measured by standardized interviews does not appear to vary as a function of ethnicity (Blazer et al., 1985; Robins et al., 1984; Weissman & Myers, 1978). This discrepancy may occur because of several factors: (a) Members of ethnic minority groups may respond differently to standardized instruments than do whites; (b) depression may vary in its symptomatology crossculturally; or (c) the differences may reflect sampling biases in the groups studied.

In order to determine the sensitivity and specificity of our screening measures for predicting diagnoses of major depression, we used receiver operating characteristic analyses (ROC; Murphy et al., 1987). The sensitivity and specificity values of a test for a single threshold score do not represent the complete performance of the test over the entire range of potential scores. ROC analysis, however, plots the sensitivity and specificity of the test across all potential scores. All possible pairs of sensitivity and specificity values are joined into one curve by plotting the true-positive rates (sensitivity) on the vertical axis and the false-positive rates (one minus specificity) on the horizontal axis. Finally, we estimated the area under the curve (AUC) produced by our screening measures, which may be interpreted as an estimate of the probability that a randomly chosen person with DIS-diagnosed major depression will, at each threshold, have a higher test score than a randomly chosen person. An AUC of .50 would suggest that the screening scale has no information value, and an AUC of 1.0 suggests that the screen perfectly predicts to the diagnosis of major depression.

Preliminary ROC analyses were calculated to determine which of the screening scales best predicted to DIS-diagnosed major depression: (a) the CES-D given during the initial screening session, (b) the BDI given at the second screening session, or (c) the repeat CES-D given at the third screening session. Figures 15.1a, 15.1b, and 15.1c represent the ROC curves comparing these three measures with the diagnosis of depression. The AUC for the first CES-D is .76 (se = .036); the AUC for the BDI is .86 (se = .021); and the AUC for the repeat CES-D is .86 (se = .028). The AUC for the BDI and the repeat CES-D is significantly better than for the first CES-D ($p = .002$ for both). However, there is no difference between the BDI and the second CES-D ($p = .69$) in predicting the DIS diagnoses of major depressive episode. Thus, the initial CES-D given at

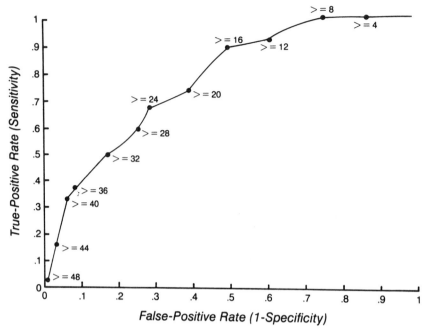

Figure 15.1a. Receiver Operating Characteristic (ROC) Curve: Initial CES-D for All DPRP Subjects

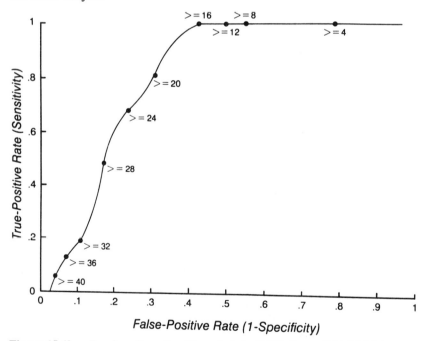

Figure 15.1b. Receiver Operating Characteristic (ROC) Curve: Initial BDI for All DPRP Subjects

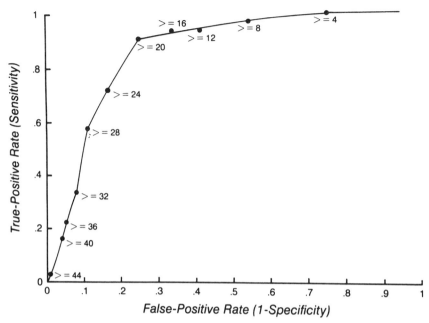

Figure 15.1c. Receiver Operating Characteristic (ROC) Curve: Second CES-D for All DPRP Subjects

primary care clinic visits was less useful in screening for major depression than are subsequently administered screening scales. We use the scores for the repeat administration of the CES-D for all remaining analyses.

Next, we compared the language comparability of the repeat CES-D in predicting to DIS diagnosis of major depressive episode. Great attention was paid to the development of both linguistically and culturally appropriate translation of all research and intervention materials. Research and diagnostic instruments currently available were developed for and normalized on mainstream populations. Translations do not assure conceptual or psychometric equivalence.

The AUC analyses for the CES-D in English and Spanish are presented in Figures 15.2a and 15.2b. The AUC for the English CES-D is .87 (*se* = .025), and the AUC for the Spanish CES-D is .83 (*se* = .07). There is no difference between the Spanish and English AUC (*p* = .67) in predicting to DIS diagnosis of major depressive episode. Thus, translation of the measures into Spanish did not attenuate the prediction of major depression by the screening scales.

To determine ethnic differences in the efficacy of the CES-D administered at the third interview for predicting DIS diagnosis of major depressive episode, the AUC was computed separately for blacks, Latinos, and whites. Figures 15.3a, 15.3b, and 15.3c depict these analyses. The AUC for blacks is .94 (*se* = .032); the AUC for Latinos is .84 (*se* = .067); and the AUC for whites is .81 (*se* = .044). The AUC does not differ between blacks and Latinos (*p* = .19) or between

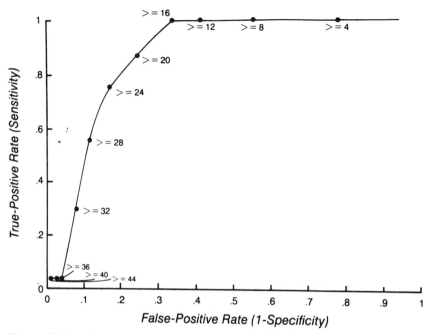

Figure 15.2a. Receiver Operating Characteristic (ROC) Curve: Second CES-D for English-Speaking DPRP Subjects

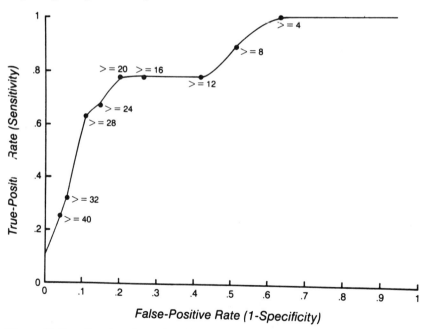

Figure 15.2b. Reveiver Operating Characteristic (ROC) Curve: Second CES-D for Spanish-Speaking DPRP Subjects

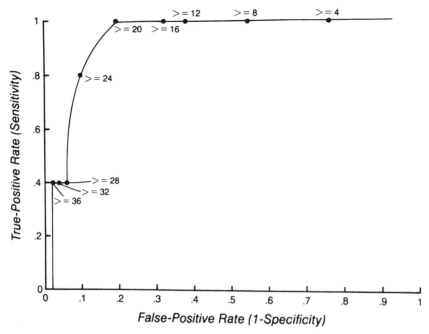

Figure 15.3a. Receiver Operating Characteristic (ROC) Curve: Second CES-D for Black DPRP Subjects

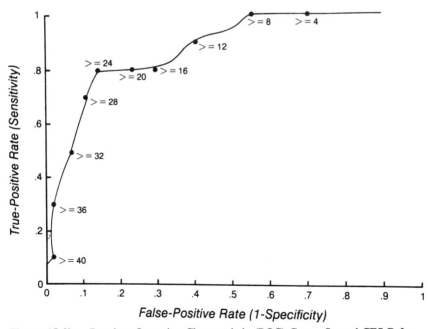

Figure 15.3b. Receiver Operating Characteristic (ROC) Curve: Second CES-D for Latino DPRP Subjects

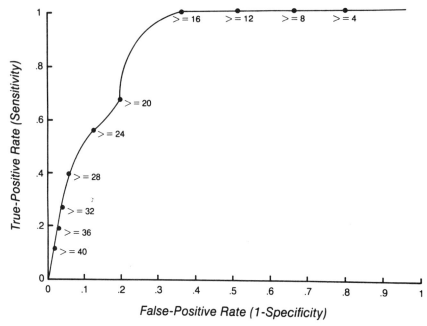

Figure 15.3c. Receiver Operating Characteristic (ROC) Curve: Second CES-D for White DPRP Subjects

Latinos and whites ($p = .69$). The AUC does differ significantly between blacks and whites; the CES-D predicts diagnosis of depression better for black than for white participants in our sample.

In sum, the Depression Prevention Research Project was successful in recruiting and maintaining ethnic representation in the randomized sample of the project. Furthermore, translation of materials into Spanish did not appear to attenuate the relationship between the CES-D screen for depression and DIS diagnosis of major depressive episode. Finally, there were ethnic differences in the relationship of the CES-D screen and the diagnosis of depression. However, the difference was not in the expected direction. That is, the screen predicted better in one ethnic minority group, the black sample, than it did in the white sample. There were no other ethnic differences in performance of the screen in predicting major depressive episode.

The Depression Prevention Course

Following screening, persons eligible for the study were randomly assigned to one of two conditions: half to the class condition and half to the control conditions. For English-speaking participants, the control condition was divided into two equal groups: one received a forty-minute videotape presentation that briefly covered the methods and ideas presented in the class and thus served as an "information only" control, and the other was a "no intervention" control group. The Spanish and Chinese samples had only the "no intervention" control conditions.

The Depression Prevention Course is an eight-week, two-hour-per-week intervention, in which groups of eight to ten persons are taught a number of social learning, self-control techniques of the type used in behavioral and cognitive therapies for depression. The course is based on *Control Your Depression* (Lewinsohn, Muñoz, Youngren, & Zeiss, 1986).

All randomized participants were administered the outcome measures at posttesting. Follow-ups occurred six months after screening and included the outcome measures. Twelve months after screening, these measures plus the DIS were re-administered.

Results of the Prevention Trial

The intervention was intended to change thoughts and behavior, which were then expected to affect future levels of depression as well as the occurrence of clinical episodes of depression. To determine the effects of the intervention, repeated measures analyses of covariance, with the prescores as covariates, and the posttesting, six-month, and one-year scores as the dependent variables were conducted.

Of the six instruments assessing cognitive-behavioral variables, the Pleasant Activities Schedule showed significant results in the predicted direction $(F [1,118] = 6.57, p = .012)$. The BDI showed a significantly greater decrease than did the CES-D in the level of depressive symptoms in those persons randomized for the cognitive-behavioral intervention $(F [1,115] = 5.8, p = 0.12)$.

The above repeated measures analyses reduced our sample size because only participants with data at all assessment periods were used. Since treatment assignment did not interact with time, we averaged the available postintervention data points (post, six months, and twelve months) into a single postintervention score. We then conducted analyses of covariance with these mean scores as the dependent variables. These more powerful analyses yielded significant differences between class and control for both the CES-D $(F [1,117] = 3.82, p = .02)$ and the BDI $(F = [1,120] 4.91, p < .01)$, as well as for the Pleasant Activities score $(F [1,116] = 5.62, p < .01)$.

To examine whether changes in the mediating variables related to changes in depression level, a correlation between the residualized postscores for Pleasant Activities and for the BDI was computed. As hypothesized, the correlation was significant $(r = .34; p = .0001)$, suggesting that changes in numbers of pleasant activities engaged in mediated the lowering of depression following the intervention.

The aim of this intervention was to lower the incidence, that is, the occurrence, of new episodes of clinical depression in the one year following recruitment into the study. None of the 42 individuals who completed the intervention met criteria for major depression during that year, as compared to 6 out of 97 who were either assigned to the control condition (4 new cases out of 72 controls) or who did not attend the intervention (2 new cases out of 25 dropouts). This finding, although encouraging, is not statistically significant. The incidence was not as high as we had expected, and thus we are presently following up the sample after three years, to see if the trend continues and reaches significance as more new cases develop.

The development of a screening instrument that identifies a subgroup of primary care patients who are at even higher risk for depression than their peers would facilitate the implementation of primary prevention research. Specifically, higher risk identification would increase the expected incidence of depression within a sample during a specified period of time, thus reducing the sample size needed to obtain adequate statistical power in a randomized primary prevention trial.

Conclusions

To return to our original task, that of determining whether or not depression meets the generally accepted guidelines for screening for disorders in primary care, we will review all findings. Again, depression is both pervasive and serious enough to justify screening. Evidence from preventive intervention trials suggests that we may be able to intervene early and prevent onset of depressive episodes. However, at the current time, research efforts must clearly delineate two additional factors: (a) In order to adequately determine the effectiveness of screens for depression in primary care, we must first determine the course of depressive disorders in primary care populations; and (b) screening scales that truly predict to depression must be developed. These two issues will be considered below.

Depression in any population is etiologically complex, involving genetic factors, environmental factors, life events, and secondary response to substance abuse (Akiskal & McKinney, 1975). Depression in those who utilize medical settings is particularly complex. Depression may be the cause of physical symptoms that mimic illness, a reaction to illness, secondary to pathological changes of disease, or a side effect of medical treatment (Goldberg, Comstock, & Hornstra, 1979; Hollister, 1980; Kolivakis & Ananth, 1980; Weissman et al., 1983). Assessment of depression in medical patients must take into account the fact that many physical disorders cause symptoms similar to those of depression (Kathol, 1985) and that many symptoms of depression are similar to those of physical disorders. Research is needed to identify the course of disorder in primary care patients who (a) meet criteria for major depression and (b) are highly symptomatic but do not meet criteria for depression. Currently, we are conducting a follow-up study of persons who met criteria for major depressive episode or dysthymia according to the DIS interviews in our initial interviews. These patients were not involved in the preventive intervention and are currently being examined to determine the course and consequences of depression over a three- to four-year period. Symptomatic patients who did not meet criteria for depressive disorder and served as control subjects for the preventive intervention trial are also being evaluated. These data will help determine whether our screening and assessment procedures evaluate serious psychopathological depressive disorders in primary care populations or whether they reflect transient disorders that might be secondary to medical illnesses.

Finally, screening scales that truly predict depression should be developed. Ideally, these scales would be used routinely in primary care settings. Patients would then be categorized into one of three groups: (a) currently depressed, (b) at high risk for depression, and (c) at low risk for depression. Those who are depressed would be referred for further clinical assessment and treatment and would offer a clear instance of secondary prevention. Those who are at risk for depression would be offered a referral to a preventive intervention. Those who are at low risk for depression would not be contacted further and would be spared unnecessary intervention.

We believe that depression meets generally accepted standards for routine screening in primary care settings. The disorder is both severe and prevalent enough to warrant such efforts. Current evidence suggests that early intervention efforts will be worthwhile, but final results are still pending. In order for progress to be made, there is a need to develop high-risk screening scales that truly predict depression. Identifying people who are at imminent risk for depression as well as identifying individuals who are currently depressed will allow for a combined primary and secondary prevention project.

References

Akiskal, H. S. (1987). Overview of biobehavioral factors in the prevention of mood disorders. In R. F. Muñoz (ed.), *Depression prevention: Research directions* (pp. 263–280). Washington, D.C.: Hemisphere.

Akiskal, H., & McKinney, W. (1975). Overview of depression: Integration of ten conceptual models into a comprehensive clinical frame. *Archives of General Psychiatry, 32,* 285–305.

Beck, A. T., Ward, C. H., Mendelsohn, M., Mock, J. E., & Erbaugh, J. K. (1961). An inventory for measuring depression. *Archives of General Psychiatry, 4,* 561–571.

Blazer, D., George, L., Landerman, R., Pennybacker, M., Melville, M., Woodbury, M., Manton, K., Jordan, K., & Locke, B. (1985). Psychiatric disorders: A rural/urban comparison. *Archives of General Psychiatry, 42,* 651–656.

Boyd, J. H., & Weissman, M. M. (1982). Epidemiology. In E. S. Paykel (ed.), *Handbook of affective disorders* (pp. 109–125). New York: Guilford.

Comstock, G., & Helsing, K. (1976). Symptoms of depression in two communities. *Psychological Medicine, 6,* 551–563.

Dohrenwend, B., & Dohrenwend, B. (1969). *Social status and psychological disorder.* New York: John Wiley and Sons.

Eaton, W., & Kessler, L., (1981) Rates of symptoms of depression in a national sample. *American Journal of Epidemiology, 114,* 528–538.

Fredrichs, R., Aneshensel, C., & Clark, V. (1981). Prevalence of depression in Los Angeles County. *American Journal of Epidemiology, 113,* 691–699.

Goldberg, E., Comstock, G., & Hornstra, R. (1979). Depressed mood and subsequent physical illness. *American Journal of Psychiatry, 136,* 530–534.

Guze, S. B., & Robins, E. (1970). Suicide and primary affective disorders. *British Journal of Psychiatry, 117,* 437–438.

Hankin, J., Steinwachs, D., Regier, D., Burns, B., Goldberg, I., & Hoeper, E. (1982). Use of general medical care services by persons with mental disorders. *Archives of General Psychiatry, 39,* 225–231.

Hirschfeld, R. M. A., & Cross, C. K. (1981). Psychosocial risk factors for depression. In D. A. Regier & G. Allen (eds.), *Risk factor research in the major mental disorders* (pp. 55—66) (DHHS Publication No. ADM 81–1068). Washington, D.C.: U.S. Government Printing Office.

Hoeper, E. W., Nycz, G. R., Cleary, P., Regier, D., & Goldberg, I., (1979). Estimated prevalence of RDC mental disorder in primary care. *International Journal of Mental Health, 8,* 6–15.

Hoeper, E. W., Nycz, G. R., Regier, D., Goldberg, I., Jacobson, A., & Hankin, J. (1980). Diagnosis of mental disorder in adults and increased use of health services in four outpatient settings. *American Journal of Psychiatry, 137,* 207–210.

Hollister, L. E. (1980). Depressed medical patients: Diagnostic and treatment challenges. In F. Ayd (ed.), *Clinical depressions: Diagnostic and therapeutic challenges* (pp. 92–102). Baltimore: Ayd Medical Communications.

Kathol, R. G. (1985). Depression associated with physical disease. In E. E. Beckham & W. R. Leber (eds.), *Handbook of depression: Treatment assessment and research* (pp. 745–762). Homewood: Dorsey Press.

Kathol, R., & Petty, F. (1981). Relationship of depression to medical illness: A critical review. *Journal of Affective Disorders, 3,* 111–121.

Kleinman, A., & Lin, K. (eds.) (1981). *Normal and abnormal behavior in Chinese culture.* Dordrecht, Holland: Reidel.

Kolivakis, T., & Ananth, J. (1980). Think depression: The signs and symptoms of primary and secondary depression. In F. Ayd (ed.), *Clinical depression: Diagnostic and therapeutic challenges* (pp. 22–32). Baltimore: Ayd Medical Communications.

Kuo, W. (1984). Prevalence of depression among Asian Americans. *Journal of Nervous and Mental Disease, 172,* 449–457.

Leber, W., Beckham, E., & Danker-Brown, P. (1985). Diagnostic criteria for depression. In E. Beckham & W. Leber (eds.), *Handbook of depression* (pp. 343–371). Homewood, IL: Dorsey Press.

Lewinsohn, P. M., Muñoz, R. F., Youngren, M. A., & Zeiss, A. M. (1986). *Control your depression* (rev. ed.). New York: Prentice-Hall.

Mumford, E., Schlesinger, H., & Glass, G. (1981). Reducing medical costs through mental health treatment. In A. Broskowski, E. Marks, & S. H. Budman (eds.), *Linking health & mental health (2)* (pp. 257–273). Beverly Hills: Sage Publications.

Muñoz, R. F., Glish, M., Soo-Hoo, T., & Robertson, J. (1982). The San Francisco Mood Survey Project: Preliminary work toward the prevention of depression. *American Journal of Community Psychology, 10,* 317–329.

Muñoz, R. F., Ying, Y., Armas, R., Chan, F., & Gurza, R. (1987). The San Francisco Depression Prevention Research Project: A randomized trial with medical outpatients. In R. F. Muñoz, (ed.), *Depression prevention: Research directions* (pp. 199–215). Washington, D.C.: Hemisphere.

Murphy, J. M., Berwick, D. M., Weinstein, M. C., Borus, J. F., Budman, S. H., & Klerman, G. L. (1987). Performance of screening and diagnostic tests: Receiver Operating Characteristic analysis. *Archives of General Psychiatry, 44,* 550–555.

Murphy, J. M., Monson, R. R., Olivier, D. C., Sobol, A. M., & Leighton, A. H., (1987). Affective disorder and mortality. *Archives of General Psychiatry, 44*(5), 473–480.

Neff, J., & Husaini, B. (1980). Race, socioeconomic status, and psychiatric impairment: A research note. *Journal of Community Psychology, 8,* 16–19.

Nicholi, A. (1967). Harvard dropouts: Some psychiatric findings. *American Journal of Psychiatry, 124,* 651–658.

Osmond, H., Mullaly, R., & Bisbee, C. (1984). The pain of depression compared with physical pain. *Practitioner, 228,* 849–853.

Radloff, L. S. (1977). The CES-D scale: A self-report depression scale for research in the general population. *Applied Psychological Measurement, 1,* 385–401.

Roberts, R. E. (1987). Epidemiological issues in measuring preventive effects. In R. F. Muñoz (ed.), *Depression prevention: Research directions* (pp. 45–75). Washington, D.C.: Hemisphere.

Roberts, R. E., Stevenson, J., & Breslow, L. (1981). Symptoms of depression among blacks and whites in an urban community. *Journal of Nervous and Mental Disorders, 169,* 212–219.

Robins, L. N., Helzer, J. E., Croughan, J., & Ratcliff, K. S. (1981). National Institute of Mental Health Diagnostic Interview Schedule: Its history, characteristics, and validity. *Archives of General Psychiatry, 38,* 381–389.

Robins, L., Helzer, J., Weissman, M., Orvaschel, H., Gruenberg, E., Burke, J., & Regier, D., (1984). Lifetime prevalence of specific psychiatric disorders in three sites. *Archives of General Psychiatry, 41,* 949–958.

Schulberg, H., Saul, M., McClelland, M. Ganguli, M., Christy, W., & Frank, R. (1985). Assessing depression in primary medical and psychiatric practices. *Archives of General Psychiatry, 42,* 1164–1170.

Steinbrueck, S., Maxwell, S., & Howard, G. (1983). A meta-analysis of psychotherapy and drug therapy in treatment of unipolar depression with adults. *Journal of Consulting and Clinical Psychology, 51,* 856–863.

Sternberg, D., & Jarvik, M. (1976). Memory functions in depression. *Archives of General Psychiatry, 33,* 219–224.

Teuting, P., Koslow, S. H., & Hirschfeld, R. M. A. (1981). *Special report on depression research* (DHHS Publication No. ADM 81–1085). Washington, D.C.: U.S. Government Printing Office.

Vega, W. A., Valle, R., Kolody, B., & Hough, R. (1987). The Hispanic Social Network Prevention Intervention Study: A community-based randomized trial. In R. F. Muñoz (ed.), *Depression prevention: Research directions* (pp. 217–231). Washington, D.C.: Hemisphere.

Vernon, S., & Roberts, R. (1982). Prevalence of treated and untreated psychiatric disorders in three ethnic groups. *Social Science and Medicine, 16,* 1575–1582.

Warheit, G., Holzer, C., & Avery, S. (1975). Race and mental illness: An epidemiologic update. *Journal of Health and Social Behavior, 16,* 243–256.

Weissman, M. (1979). The psychological treatment of depression. *Archives of General Psychiatry, 36,* 1261–1269.

Weissman, M., & Myers, J. (1978). Rates and risks of depressive symptoms in a United States urban community. *Acta Psychiatrica Scandanavia, 57,* 219–231.

Weissman, M., Myers, J., & Thompson, W. (1981). Depression and its treatment in a United States urban community, 1975–1976. *Archives of General Psychiatry, 38,* 417–421.

Weissman, M., Myers, J., Tischler, G., Orvaschel, H., Holzer, C., & Leaf, P. (1983). Depression and physical illness in an urban community. In L. Temoshok, C. Van Dyke, & L. Zegans (eds.), *Emotions in health and illness: Theoretical and research foundations* (pp. 51–60). New York: Grune & Stratton.

Whitney, W. Cadoret, R., & McClure, J. (1971). Depressive symptoms and academic performance in college students. *American Journal of Psychiatry, 128,* 766–770.

16

Screening for Depression in Primary Care: A Clinician's Perspective

John Matthew

Many studies suggest that more than 20% of patients attending a primary care practice have a depressive disorder (Barrett, Barrett, Oxman, & Gerber, 1988; Daniels, Linn, Ward, & Leake, 1986; Diamond, Eping, & Gage, 1987; Gray, 1988; Hankin & Locke, 1983; Nielsen & Williams, 1980; Rosenthal, Goldfarb, Lepiolis-Carlson, Sagi, & Balaban, 1987), that the overwhelming majority of depression presents in primary care practice settings (Sacramella, 1977), and that depression is underrecognized (Gray, l988; Schulberg et al., 1985) as well as undertreated (Ketai, 1976). The primary care clinician is faced with the challenge of identifying depression in outpatients within the context of ongoing care. In day-to-day practice the physician will see a spectrum of patients, both established and new, ranging from the newborn to the frail elderly and presenting with a variety of problems encompassing the panorama of medical possibilities. Which are depressed and which are not? Most of those who are depressed are unaware of the nature of their difficulties, and few, indeed, come in with a primary complaint of depression. Many have somatic or vegetative symptoms rather than dysphoric and cognitive symptoms (Gray, 1988), causing the depression to be masked from the clinician's detection. Most research on depression takes place in university settings and often in specialty practices. Consequently, there is a dearth of information concerning the presentation of depression in nonacademic primary care practices. The physician will not find this information collated or well presented in one particular reference or text. There are substantial gaps in most documents or volumes that purport to teach the recognition of depression. For some clinical situations there is little if any published data—and most practices have not collected and analyzed their own data. What follows, then, is a distillation of practical experience rather than of data-gathering. While experiential learning lacks the quantification and exactness of more formal research, there is practical information to be gained from such an analysis. The purpose of this chapter is to describe the diagnostic approach to depression of one practitioner.

The clinical assessment method does not primarily involve a paper and pencil screening device. While there is little doubt that such devices may serve an alerting function and aid in uncovering depression otherwise missed by physicians

(Rosenthal et al., 1987), the integration of such screening questionnaires in the real world of everyday practice is difficult.

Most studies of the use of screening questionnaires involve relatively short-term interventions at single visits of relatively homogenous outpatient populations who are, one gathers, literate. The published studies involve concentration on a single, albeit common and important, area of distress, with a psychological emphasis, and are set up with extra support staff or at least extra staff training for the study interval. Often the studies are conducted in academically based practices operating at a relatively slow pace. The clinicians, or at least the study staff, have special interests and skills in dealing with depression.

In contrast, real world practice involves long-term relationships with patients in ongoing care with multiple visits over time and includes patients seen in nursing homes, private homes, and hospitals, as well as those seen in office practice. Not all of these patients are literate, some may be put off by questionnaires, and most focus on somatic matters during their visit. Most primary care practices have little extra support-staff time. The office staff is busy with everything from lacerations to fielding phone calls and operates at a relatively fast pace. The clinicians involved have no study staff to promote an emphasis on clinical depression and may or may not have special skills or interests in dealing with depression.

This having been said, it is clear that primary care physicians miss depressive conditions, whether "depression" is conceived of as major depression (Nielsen & Williams, 1980), the more common various minor depressions, or depression mixed with anxiety. While paper and pencil screening devices for depression are, in my view, inappropriate for some practices and large proportions of the patient population seen in primary care, screening for depression is, nonetheless, an important function for all primary care practitioners. This chapter advocates an unstructured method of screening that does not involve a questionnaire and that is applied, insofar as possible, at every encounter with the patient.

The pitfalls of unstructured screening methods are several. Lack of application in the pell-mell of daily practice, failure to get below a veneer of defensiveness or compensation, and being so familiar with a patient that new formulations are crowded out by familiar ongoing concerns are among the more obvious.

So, while the unstructured method of screening this chapter espouses works well in terms of "yield" and fitting into office encounters, there is no doubt that it is not in itself entirely sufficient or optimal, since it is a common experience to uncover, recognize, or stumble over depression after a number of visits with the patient (Widmer & Cadoret, 1978) at which the diagnosis was often assuredly—in retrospect—missed. It may be that a screening questionnaire intended to serve as a "flag" or "thermometer" by alerting the clinician to the possibility of depression ought to be incorporated into a well-care schedule for periodic completion much as occult blood tests or pap smears are employed. This would provide a second line of defense against missing this important diagnosis, but cannot, in my estimation, substitute for the attention to depression at *every* encounter as outlined in this chapter.

Depression, as used in this discussion, is not synonymous with major depression described in psychiatric literature. The primary care physician deals with a much broader spectrum of depressive distress, which includes not only major depression, but also many permutations of depression and combinations of depression intertwined with other medical disorders (Lubin, 1988). Symptoms of and clues to depression—some of which are not emphasized in the psychiatric literature (Wilson, Widmer, Cadoret, & Judiesch, 1983)—are detected, more or less easily, depending on circumstances. Symptoms will vary in number, severity, chronicity, and impact on the individual and may stem from a variety of causes. After finding "depression," the primary care clinician must sort out etiology (or etiologies) insofar as possible, then decide on a course of treatment.

Depressions which do not meet DSM-III-R criteria for major depressive episode may still significantly impact on the quality of patients' lives (Fahy, 1974; Johnson & Mellor, 1977; Sireling, Freeling, Paykel, & Rao, 1985; Sireling, Freeling, Payne, & Rao, 1985). These depressions will include many less severe but perhaps more chronic or intermittently symptomatic cases that appear very similar to major depression in character and response to treatment. There will also be depressions coupled with anxiety or panic disorders (Katon et al., 1986) and depressive symptoms associated with or due to a number of illnesses such as hypothyroidism or cerebrovascular accidents. In many of these instances the depressive symptoms respond to pharmacologic therapy with antidepressants, whether or not the depression is intertwined with medical problems or is of sufficient intensity and impact to satisfy psychiatric diagnostic criteria.

The key to a physician's adequate recognition of depression in an accurate, efficient, and effective manner is a method of screening that can be modulated and tuned to fit the individual circumstance of each encounter, which is often limited by necessity to fifteen or twenty minutes.

The method involves considering the possibility that every patient seen might have depression, just as one must consider that every heart listened to might have a murmur. If clues are apparent on initial probing, then questioning, which follows normally in the clinical setting from a concerned physician, becomes more specific and/or directive. The physician may have a checklist in mind, but often has no time to present a paper and pencil screening questionnaire.

While caring for patients' acute problems, the clinician must maintain a high index of suspicion for affective disorder. He or she must also maintain both an efficient clinical method for scouting for depression and a posture that enables him or her to intervene effectively if depression is found. The physician must be vigilant, suspecting and probing for clues to the diagnosis, while maintaining the flow of patients in the office schedule.

As the clinician approaches the various individuals who attend the practice on any one day, he or she will need to alter approach, vocabulary, and manner of speech to be most effective with a logger at one moment and with a lawyer the next. A new patient with whom the physician has little rapport or an established patient with whom he or she has an extensive friendly working relationship might be depressed. One patient may be prepared to accept whatever the physician says, while another must be convinced that the diagnosis is correct. One depressed person may be relieved to learn that what is suspected is indeed true, while another may be highly resistant to the acceptance of this diagnosis. How one goes about detecting depression to a large extent may determine not only whether the individual, particularly the resistant or unconvinced person, can be brought into a working therapeutic alliance.

Depression is often found by the company it keeps. I find it useful to be particularly aware of the possibility of a patient's having depression in the various clinical situations in which the likelihood of depression is increased, to look for depression in persons with certain associated conditions, and to expect depression in association with certain life circumstances.

Having been alert for the situations, conditions, and circumstances often associated with depression, I find that a few questions often suffice to screen persons who are not obviously probable depressives from their presentation.

I utilize questions that scout for the somatic, rather that psychological, manifestations of depression first, then go on to the "psych" questions if my index of suspicion is raised by the response to these first inquiries. This approach seems best because it does not offend patients sensitive or oblivious to psychological distress and draws them into cooperating with further questioning if the physician has detected (or appeared insightful in recognizing) these safer and more easily discussed problems. Few patients are put off by questions concerning sleep, energy, aches and pains, or unusual irritability. If I come across a warm trail, I often present the later, more sensitive questions concerning mood, interests, pleasure, and so on as matters of possible association with the unrefreshing sleep, lack of energy, symptoms of fibromyalgia, or unusual irritability detected by initial questioning. I allow the patient to consider the more psychological aspects of depression as symptoms some people may have, if they have some of the four somatic symptoms, almost as if these are options to choose from. The more sensitive questions can thus be indirectly asked, thereby avoiding a frontal assault on sadness, lack of libido, crying, and the like.

Thus, the method I advocate for screening for depression involves first the recognition that depression in its various forms is extremely common and that anyone who walks into a primary care office might be depressed. It is, in fact, much more likely that he or she will have depression than it is that hypertension, diabetes, or a number of other common medical conditions will be found.

The method also involves asking a few questions about somatic matters—unrefreshing sleep and fatigue being the least intrusive—which seem to be almost invariable concomitants of depressions that are not recognized as such by the patient or manifestly obvious to the clinician. Third, it involves concentrating on the patients who present with certain clinical situations or findings, conditions, and/or circumstances that appear to be most frequently associated with the masked depression.

A number of clinical situations are often associated with depression. These include clinical complaints of chronic or multiple pain, fatigue, sleep disorders, appetite problems, and abdominal symptoms. Similarly, certain clinical findings are associated with depression. These include fibromyalgia, irritability, carbohydrate or chocolate craving, anxiety or panic, and the use of certain medications.

Pain. A good rule of thumb is that anyone who reports a pain of duration of a year or longer is depressed until proven otherwise. Whether a primary cause of pain, such as an accidental injury, eventuates in depression, or, as I am disposed to believe, depression is at the root of continuing pain, persons with chronic pain constitute a group with a very high likelihood of being depressed (Patterson, 1987). Pain reported at multiple sites should also raise one's index of suspicion for depression (Dworkin, Von Korff, & LeResche, 1987).

Fatigue. For every anemia or undiagnosed infection such as mononucleosis or hepatitis found to explain fatigue, there will be several cases of depression found presenting as lack of energy, tiredness, "weakness," or the like. This presentation, perhaps because it is more socially acceptable than other complaints or is apparent even to those with little insight into their emotions, is one of the most common ways the depressed come to the attention of primary care physicians (Cadoret, Widmer, & North, 1980).

Sleep Disorders. Many depressed persons present with complaints of sleep disorders of various sorts or complain of not being refreshed after a night's sleep. This is a useful "handle" for diagnosing depression in persons, most often men, who may have difficulty recognizing or admitting to having depression. Sleep disorders may also lead to secondary depression (Gilleminault, 1984). There are a number of causes of disordered sleep, but two stand out due to their frequency of occurrence and ease of treatment. One of these is sleep apnea syndrome. While the literature describes obese middle-aged men with marked sleep apnea, often obstructive in nature and resulting in cardiac dysrhythmia, there is no question but that there is a spectrum of sleep apnea severity, including quite a few persons with mild to moderate disease, which may result in or be associated with some combination of fatigue, depression, hypertension, and headache (Waldhorn, 1985). The other frequent cause of poor deep sleep is the rest cramp or restless legs syndrome, which can interfere substantially with sleep and lead to depression.

Appetite Problems. Anorexia nervosa, bulimia, or the unexpected loss of weight in persons of any age (including the elderly) may point to depression (Johnson, Stuckey, & Mitchell, 1983). More commonly overlooked is the high incidence of depression in the overweight population (Wurtman & Wurtman, 1989). Sensitive questioning of these individuals frequently results in findings of depression, often of the "atypical" type with hypersomnia, but also often of a pattern mixing increased appetite and/or carbohydrate craving with the more "typical" depression sleep disorders.

Abdominal Symptoms. Chronic abdominal symptoms are often due to depression (Young, Alpers, Norland, & Woodruff, 1976). While one certainly does not want to overlook the diagnosis of a pancreatic carcinoma or bowel tumor, a good number of the people presenting with abdominal symptoms ranging from dyspepsia to constipation will prove to have depression with no organic gastrointestinal disease. There will certainly be times when it is warranted to try treating the patient's depression, once it is obvious to the physician, before undertaking a prolonged GI investigation, with the contingency of doing the GI work-up if treatment of the depression fails to eliminate the gastrointestinal complaints. Rather than depression being the last diagnosis on the list with many rule-outs above it, it may be better medicine to put what appears most likely at the top of the list, with a "pursue if persists" approach to the GI symptoms found to exist in association with depression.

Fibromyalgia. The central cause of this disorder, which presents with diffuse or focal aching discomfort, is lack of adequate deep sleep (Goldenberg, 1987). While this lack of delta-wave sleep may result from causes other than depression, such as the rest cramps or restless legs syndrome, often the presentation of diffuse aching, tender neck and shoulder muscle spasm, temporomandibular joint (TMJ) syndrome, or chronic back pain is the first clue on a trail that leads to the diagnosis of depression. The demonstration by sleep researchers that a primary sleep disorder may cause a mild to profound secondary depression indistinguishable from primary depression causes some chicken and egg questions to arise, however.

Irritability. While sadness and crying typify depression in the lay mind, irritability, hostility, and/or easy anger are also frequent markers for depression. Individuals with these symptoms are often overlooked as potentially depressed. Before getting one's hackles up at the complaining, irritable, never-pleased patient, or the parent who is irritable with children in the office, or the man who blows up because the front desk needs a new registration completed—look for depression. These individuals are more likely to admit to nonrestorative sleep or fatigue or poor concentration, particularly if they are men, than they are to admit to sadness or poor libido. But they often have most if not all of the DSM-III-R criteria under their prickly surfaces.

Carbohydrate Craving. In the nonoverweight as well as in the overweight, craving for carbohydrate appears to correlate with depression in many instances (Wurtman & Wurtman, 1989). Carbohydrate cravers may present in disguise, thinking that they have "hypoglycemia" because intervals of irritability, fatigue, anxiety, or poor concentration seem to improve with eating carbohydrates. These symptoms usually do not, however, develop in a characteristic time frame after eating high carbohydrate meals, exercising, or drinking alcohol, as do the symptoms in the far less common (but overdiagnosed) reactive hypoglycemia, insulinomia, or inhibition of gluconeogenesis by alcohol. The demonstration that carbo-hydrate ingestion stimulates or augments central serotonin release (Lieberman, Corken, Spring, Gowdun, & Wurtman, 1984) at least provides an explanation for the hypoglycemia folklore, which is encountered so frequently that there has to be some physiology behind the myth.

Chocolate. Similarly, chocolate craving correlates with depression (Cassem, 1985; Liebowitz & Klein, 1979) in some patients. These individuals, in response to direct questioning, often reveal that chocolate makes them feel better. Other than the carbohydrate content, the phenylethelamine in chocolate seems to serve as a mild surrogate neurotransmitter or catecholamine releaser, having a mild, but real and substantial, effect on the mood of some persons. Chocolate's long-term popularity, like that of caffeine and, in some settings, chewing of cocoa leaves, perhaps derives from its mood-altering effects, not its flavor alone. I certainly do not run across many people who crave artificially flavored chocolate pudding. Everyone who craves chocolate is not depressed, but many are.

Anxiety. The large population of persons with anxiety, panic, and agoraphobia includes many persons with depression. They may suffer either depression per se, primarily manifested as anxiety or in an overlap syndrome of panic disorder and a degree of depression (Klein, 1986; Wilson et al., 1983). Of the four main varieties of depression (retarded, hostile, anxious, and agitated), physicians seem to recognize the retarded type best. Like the hostile depression referred to above, the anxious and agitated subtypes of depression often get overlooked.

Medications. Persons under treatment with any of the numerous medications that may cause or aggravate depression (Gelenberg & Donaldson, 1986; Schraw-Solie, 1986) should be actively questioned concerning the symptoms of depres-sion, even when they present no complaint that leads to suspicion. In fact, often persons who have slowly developed depression over months while on an offending medication not only do not recognize the connection, but also may not recognize their depression, even when questioned about it directly. Particularly insidious are lipid soluble beta blockers such as Propanalol, Timolol eye drops, and other medications used chronically, such as antihypertensives and medication for Parkinson's Disease. Because the list of potentially offending medications is long and difficult to remember, it may be useful to make up a prepared list of medica-tions with depressant effects as a reminder.

There are also a number of conditions with which depression is often associated. These include headaches, alcoholism, irritable bowel syndrome, premenstrual syndrome, dementia, cerebrovascular accidents, hypothyroidism, and cigarette smoking.

Headache. Migraine headache is thought to have a central "cause" related to deficient activity of serotonin in certain central nervous system (CNS) areas (Scheif & Hills, 1980). Depression involves deficient catecholamine or serotonin activity in other loci within the brain. Upon careful questioning a great number of persons with what are superficially "nonmigraine" headaches prove to have histories compatible with vascular headache, and a good number of such migraine patients and a smaller but substantial percentage of individuals with nonvascular headache prove on questioning to have depression also.

Alcoholism. The vast numbers of persons who are alcohol abusers include a good number of primary depressives (Frazier, 1986). While alcohol is obviously a CNS depressant and destroys deep sleep, leading to depression by an alternative and complimentary route, the prealcohol (and postalcohol, dry) profile of the alcoholic often reveals clear-cut affective disorder. While arguments and moral posturing rage over whether 14% or 35% or 50% of alcoholics have co-existent "endogenous" depression, the primary care physician, faced with the grave risk to health and happiness that alcohol poses and our meager success at helping alcoholics stop drinking alcohol and not return to it, would do well to look for depression in every alcoholic. When underlying depression is found and treated, my experience is that the alcoholic is much less prone to return to alcohol. Of course, there will also be persons with bipolar disease and anxiety/panic disorders in the heterogenous alcoholic group. Identifying and addressing the underlying medical problem when there is one are essential to ending alcohol abuse.

Irritable Bowel Syndrome. This most common gastrointestinal diagnosis in primary care—and probably in the practice of gastroenterology as well—often is tied to intermittent or chronic anxiety as a component of primary depression (Clouse & Alpers, 1986).

Premenstrual Syndrome. Premenstrual Syndrome is a very useful clue to depression. Some women appear to have primary depression that is aggravated premenstrually. Others appear to have depression only at the premenstrual portion of their menstrual cycle. A number of these women prove on thyrotropin-releasing factor (TRF) stimulation testing to have hypothyroidism (Brayshaw & Brayshaw, 1986).

Dementia. Certain patients who appear demented may have only pseudodementia of depression, entirely "fixable" with proper medication. A very large percentage of persons who are demented are also depressed. No one should be written off as having organic brain disorder (OBS) without consideration of depression as an etiologic factor or complicating component in his or her presentation. Use of stimulant "diagnostic probes" with methylphenidate or low dose amphetamine may be of great help in sorting out what is depression and what is dementia (Cassem, 1985).

After CVAs. The incidence of depression after cerebral vascular accidents (CVAs) is quite high. This is a biological phenomenon that correlates with CVA location, but is quite common after cortical strokes in any distribution (Sinyor et al., 1986). For anterior dominant side infarction the incidence may be as high as 65%.

Hypothyroidism. Hypothyroidism is very common and often causes or aggravates depression. Because it develops gradually, even the more obvious of its manifestations may go undetected. It may be the accompanying physical signs and symptoms that finally attract the attention of the patient or physician, although presentation with typical features of depression is common. These signs and symptoms may include cystic and tender breasts; menstrual flow changes, particularly heavy flow; "puffy" peri-orbital edema; reduction of sexual hair; greater sensitivity to cold than others; leg cramps; premenstrual syndrome; loss of scalp hair; elevated cholesterol; bradycardia; or changes in voice. If the physical complaints are most obvious, these may attract the physician's attention and enable finding of the depression as well. The importance of finding hypothyroidism cannot be over emphasized, since it is an easily treated cause not only of substantial depression, but also of widespread somatic disorders some of which, such as elevated cholesterol, have cumulative long term deleterious effects. TRF stimulation testing, because of the prevalence of hypothyroidism with a normal baseline thyroid-stimulating hormone (TSH) (Valenota & Elias, 1983) but causing considerable depression, is an extremely useful diagnostic tool in our office practice.

Smokers. By no means are all smokers depressives, but it certainly seems that affective and anxiety disorders are more commonly found in smokers than in the general population.

Finally, certain life circumstances or stages are associated with depression with sufficient frequency such that one's index of suspicion should be quite high when approaching persons in these circumstances. These include those with family history of depression, youths, women who have had postpartum depression, persons with marital troubles, women who are menopausal, persons suffering grief, those who are elderly, and those who are unemployed, socially marginalized, or in the social underclass.

Family History. One major advantage in family practice may be having knowledge of the medical history of members of a family. Depression involves a great genetic component, to be sure. I make it a practice to tell persons with affective disorders to talk with members of their family: parents, siblings, children, etc. This is effective in locating some cases in families, but over time the physician's knowledge of families having depression is a great boon. If grandfather, aunt, and mom have been plagued by depression, it is none too soon to begin watching the children, particularly after puberty, for signs of depression (Puig-Antich, 1984).

Postpartum Depression. Women who have a history of postpartum depression constitute a small group of individuals at higher than usual risk for subsequent depression. The postpartum depression itself is "biologic" in origin, but this event also marks these women as being at increased risk for future depression, which may not occur, at least in its most manifest form, until some years later.

Youth. The six-month prevalence of affective disorders, anxiety disorders, and substance abuse in persons age 18 to 21 was 21% in the NIMH Epidemiologic Catchment Area (ECA) Studies (Weissman, 1986), but depression in teenagers is approximately as common (Kashani et al., 1987; Ryan & Puig-Antich, 1986).

This group of sufferers is often overlooked, the manifestations of mood disorders being dismissed as part of growing up or rebellion or the like. While mood disorders certainly occur in children (Carlson & Kashani, 1988), these problems, often with an apparent pubertal velocity boost, flare up in adolescence (Puig-Antich, 1984). Mood disorders in this age group often present in a different manner from those in other age groups. Youth who are affected may have problems in school, such as failing grades or behavioral problems, or present problems at home, such as temper outbursts or withdrawal, or manifest problems in the community, such as encounters with the police, vandalism, reckless driving, or drug abuse (Biederman & Hoge, 1985). A keen eye must be kept on these young people, since they are quite unlikely to recognize and even less to articulate dysphoric moods if these are experienced. This group presents more of a challenge than the "macho" male or hostile female depressive in terms of recognition by the clinician.

Marital Disorder. Well over one-third of women reporting problems getting along with a spouse are depressed (46% in the recent ECA studies) (Weissman, 1986). Often the history reveals that at least some of the marital discord appears to result from her fatigue in the face of the substantial demands married life places on a woman. Or her irritability, anhedonia, and/or diminished libido may be playing a part in a deteriorating relationship. I think men are similarly affected in marital relationships by their mood disorders, but men are substantially less adept at recognizing their "feelings," less prone to talk with a physician about their marriage, and far less apt to admit to or recognize depression in themselves when it does exists. So this circumstantial red flag is of less value in the case of men.

Menopause. Women who are experiencing hot flashes and night sweats may have sleep disturbances and depression (Lobo, 1987), often with anxiety dominating their clinical presentation. The literature contains no clear indication that postmenopausal women without vasomotor symptoms have an increased incidence of depression, but it is my impression that at least some of these women, when they are depressed, have an appreciable response in terms of becoming less anxious, manifesting less depression, and improving their "sense of well being" when begun on estrogen replacement therapy. There have been hypotheses offered making this connection via anabolic affect of estrogen "enabling" the enzymatic synthesis of central catecholamines or of estrogen reducing monoamine oxidase activity (Meeks, 1986). Whatever the mechanism, some women seem to respond. A similar response appears to occur in the case of the much less common hypogonad male who starts testosterone replacement. In both sexes the response seems to be sustained, not short-lived.

Persons Suffering Grief. Persons suffering a loss such as death of a loved one may not be at increased risk of becoming depressed, but because they appear to have a good reason for being depressed, the illness may go untreated in such persons—or be unrecognized by the patient, the family, friends, and the physician. One must take care to note when the reaction to loss persists for more than three to six months or involves symptoms such as pain, psychomotor retardation, morbid sense of diminished worth, guilt, pervasive fatigue, or suicidal thoughts. These individuals may well have major depression that is all too easy to explain away by focusing on a loss, however remote.

The Elderly. The prevalence of depressive symptoms in the elderly population is multiple that in the general population, though major depression is not (Blazer, 1987). My opinion is that the genesis of these symptoms is biological, not social, for the most part. The increasing activity of monoamine oxidase with aging, combined with the tendency of cyclic primary depression to occur with increasing frequency over time and the increasing incidence of thyroid failure with aging—perhaps taken together with the effect of estrogen deficiency—results in a large percentage of the elderly population having depressive symptoms, often not meeting criteria for major depression, but often with a gratifying response to antidepressants. Any problem with a point incidence of 10 to 20%, which depressive symptoms exhibit in this population, will be seen with even greater frequency in office practice.

The Unfortunate. Other patients to scrutinize carefully for depression are those who are unemployed, and those who are unsuccessful in life educationally, economically, or socially. It certainly appears to me that not only are the unemployed operating under enormous stress, but that often antecedent/recurrent depression has affected their ability to function and maintain employment. Whatever the survival value of the genes for primary depression that have allowed this inherited disorder to become so prevalent in humankind, energetic, resilient, and enthusiastic people do better in today's job market. Only a limited number of jobs are best filled by the fatigued, the brittle, the irritable, and the withdrawn. Similarly, I believe that the biology of certain families, taken with the enormous impact of family values, traditions, and support on subsequent success, is a major determinant of social class, with cycles of poverty, lack of education, and marginal economic life determined, in an almost Calvinistic sense, by the mood disorders that affect generation after generation of certain families as they cycle on the margins of society (Davis, Nathan, & Cash, 1986).

Having recognized depression—more often than not because of this approach of "screening" for its manifestations—the physician is then faced with the substantial task of sorting out the causes of depression. While the preponderant etiology may be "endogenous," a broad range of possible causes and imitators of depression must be considered (Talley, 1983). These include, in addition to the matters discussed above, such problems as iron deficiency (Freedman, 1986), hypercalcemia, B–12 deficiency (Evans, Edelsohn, & Golden, 1983), and a host of other psychological and social as well as biologic possibilities (Gelenberg & Donaldson, 1986).

Astute recognition of depression, whether by unstructured techniques or a paper and pencil questionnaire, is but the first step in attentive care of this extremely common clinical disorder.

References

Barrett, J. E., Barrett, J. A., Oxman, T. E., & Gerber, P. D. (1988). The prevalence of psychiatric disorders in a primary care practice. *Archives of General Psychiatry, 45,* 1100–1106.

Biederman, J., & Hoge, S. K. (1985). New approaches to childhood depression. *P.A. Update,* 42–52.

Blazer, D. (1987). Depression in later life, myths and realities. *Clinical Report on Aging, 1* (2), 1–10.

Brayshaw, N. D., & Brayshaw, D. D. (1986). Thyroid hypofunction in Premenstrual Syndrome. *New England Journal of Medicine, 315,* 1486–1487.

Cadoret, R. J., Widmer, R. B., & North, C. (1980). Depression in family practice: Long-term prognosis and somatic complaints. *Journal of Family Practice, 10,* 625–629.

Carlson, G. A., & Kashani, J. H. (1988). Phenomenology of major depression from childhood through adulthood: Analysis of three studies. *American Journal of Psychiatry, 145* (10), 1222–1225.

Cassem, E. H. (1985). Meet the professor session, psychopharmacology, American College of Physicians Annual Session, Washington, D.C..

Clouse, R. E., & Alpers, D. H. (1986). Irritable bowel syndrome, five steps for effective management. *Consultant, January,* 123–135.

Daniels, M. L., Linn, L. S., Ward, N., & Leake, B. (1986). A study of physician preference in the management of depression in the general medical setting. *General Hospital, 8,* 229–235.

Davis, T. C., Nathan, R. G., & Cash, M. N. (1986). Diagnosing depression in primary care: A practical interdisciplinary review and call for change. *Southern Medical Journal, 79,* 1273–1279.

Diamond, E. L., Eping, R., & Gage, L. (1987). Estimating the prevalence of depression in family practice using variant methods. *Journal of Family Practice, 24,* 267–273.

Dworkin, S. T., Von Korff, M., & LeResche, L. (June 1980). Pain co-morbidity, depression and somatization. Paper presented at Mental Disorders in General Health Care Settings: A Research Conference, Seattle.

Evans, D., Edelsohn, G., & Golden, R. (1983). Organic psychosis without anemia or spinal cord symptoms in patients with vitamin B–12 deficiency. *American Journal of Psychiatry, 140,* 218–221

Fahy, T. J. (1974). Depression in hospital and general practice: A direct clinical comparison. *British Journal of Psychiatry, 124,* 231–242.

Frazier, S. (April, 1986). Meet the professor session at the American College of Physicians Annual Session, San Francisco.

Freedman, M. L. (1986). Iron deficiency in the elderly. *Hospital Practice, 21,* 115–137.

Gelenberg, A. J., & Donaldson, S. R. (1986). Treating depression, a primer for the nonspecialist. *Medical Times, 114,* 33–43.

Gilleminault, C. (April, 1984). Panel on sleep disorders. Presented at the American College of Physicians Annual Session, Atlanta.

Goldenberg, D. L. (1987). Fibromyalgia syndrome an emerging but controversial condition. *Journal of the American Medical Association, 257*(20), 2782–2787.

Gray, F. D. (ed.) (1988). *American College of Physicians Medical Knowledge Self-Assessment Program VIII* (Syllabus Part A, Book 1, p. 13).

Hankin, J., & Locke, B. (1983). Extent of depressive symptomatology among patients seeking care in a prepaid group practice. *Psychological Medicine, 13,* 121–129.

Johnson, C., Stuckey, M., & Mitchell, J. (1983). Psychopharmacological treatment of anorexia nervosa and bulimia: Review and synthesis. *Journal of Nervous and Mental Diseases, 171,* 524–534.

Johnson, D. A., & Mellor, V. (1977). The severity of depression in patients treated in general practice. *Journal of the Royal College of General Practitioners, 27,* 419–422.

Kashani, J. H., Carlson, G. A., Beck, N. C., Hoeper, E. W., Corcoran, C. M., McAllister, J. A., Fallahi, C., Rosenberg, T. K., & Reid, J. C. (1987). Depression, depressive symptom, and depressive mood among a community sample of adolescents. *American Journal of Psychiatry, 144,* 931–934.

Katon, W., Vialiano, P. P., Russo, J., Cormier, L., Anderson, K., & Jones, M. (1986). Panic disorder: Epidemiology in primary care. *Journal of Family Practice, 23,* 233–239.

Ketai, R. (1976). Family practitioners' knowledge about treating depressive illness. *Journal of the American Medical Association, 235* (24), 2600–2603.

Klein, D. L. (1986). *Family Practice News,* May 15–31, p. 62.

Lieberman, H., Corkin, S., Spring, G., Gowdun, J. H., & Wurtman, R. J. (1984). Mood, performance, and sensitivity: Changes induced by food constituents. *Journal of Psychiatric Research, 17,* 135–145.

Liebowitz, M. R., & Klein, D. F. (1979). Hysteroid dysphoria. *Psychiatric Clinics of North America, 2,* 555–575.

Lobo, R. A. (1987). *Family Practice News, 17* (13), 35.

Lubin, M. F. (1988). Depression in internal medicine. *Medical Rounds, 1,* 12–20.

Meeks, G. R. (April 1986). Interview with G. R. Meeks. *Medical Aspects of Human Sexuality,* 88–107.

Nielsen, A. C., & Williams, T. A. (1980). Depression in ambulatory medical patients prevalence by self-report questionnaire and recognition by non-psychiatric physicians. *Archives of General Psychiatry, 37,* 999–1004.

Patterson, W. M. (1987). Paper presented at the annual meeting of the Ohio Academy of Family Practice, Dayton.

Puig-Antich, J. (1984). Clinical and treatment aspects of depression in childhood and adolescence. *Pediatric Annals, 13* (1), 37–45.

Rosenthal, M. P., Goldfarb, N. I., Lepiolis-Carlson, B., Sagi, P. C., & Balaban, D. T. (1987). Assessment of depression in the family practice center. *Journal of Family Practice, 25* (2), 143–149.

Ryan, N. D., & Puig-Antich J. (1986). Affective illness in adolescence. *Annual Review of the American Psychiatric Association, 5,* 420–450.

Sacramella, T. J. (1977). Management of depression and anxiety in primary care practice. *Primary Care, 4,* 67–77.

Scheif, R. T., & Hills, J. R. (1980). Migraine headache: Signs and symptoms, biochemistry and current therapy. *American Journal of Hospital Pharmacy, 37,* 365–374.

Schulberg, H. C., Saul, M., McClelland, M., Ganguli, M., Christy, W., & Frank, R. (1985). Assessing depression in primary medical and psychiatric practices. *Archives of General Psychiatry, 42,* 1164–1170.

Schraw-Solie, J. A. (1986). Diagnosing depression in primary care. *P.A. Outlook, Winter,* 4–12.

Sinyor, D. Jacques, P., Kaloupek, D. G., Becker, R., Goldenberg, M., & Coopersmith, H. (1986). Poststroke depression and lesion location. *Brain, 109,* 537–546.

Sireling, L. I., Freeling, P., Paykel, E. S., & Rao, B. M. (1985). Depression in general practice: Clinical features and comparison with outpatients. *British Journal of Psychiatry, 147,* 119–126.

Sireling, L. I., Freeling, P., Payne, E. S., & Rao, B. M. (1985). Depression in general practice: Case thresholds and diagnosis. *British Journal of Psychiatry, 145,* 113–119.

Talley, J. A. (1983). Depression: Differentiate the endogenous variety from the look alikes. *Consultant, February,* 105–116.

Valenota, L. J., & Elias, A. N. (1983). How to detect hypothyroidism when screening tests are normal—Use of the TRF stimulation test. *Post Graduate Medicine, 74* (2), 267–274.

Waldhorn, R. E. (1985). Sleep apnea syndrome. *American Family Physician, 32*(3), 149–166.

Weissman, M. M. (1986). The NIMH epidemiologic catchment area study. Paper presented at the American Association for the Advancement of Science Symposium, Philadelphia.

Widmer, R. B., & Cadoret, R. J. (1978). Depression in primary care, changes in patterns of patient visits and complaints during a developing depression. *Journal of Family Practice, 7* (2), 293–302.

Wilson, D. R., Widmer, R. B., Cadoret, R. J., & Judiesch, K. (1983). Somatic symptoms, a major feature of depression in a family practice. *Journal of Affective Disorders, 5,* 199–207.

Wurtman, R. J., & Wurtman, J. J. (1989). Carbohydrates and depression. *Scientific American, 260,* 68–75.

Young, S. J., Alpers, D. H., Norland, L. L., & Woodruff, R. A., Jr. (1976). Psychiatric illness and the irritable bowel syndrome: Practical implications for the primary physician. *Gastroenterology, 70,* 162–166.

Part IV
Conclusions, Guidelines, and Recommendations for Clinical Applications and Future Research

In the concluding chapter, Herbert C. Schulberg overviews the volume and distills principles and directions for future research and clinical practice. Schulberg draws conclusions about current knowledge and specifies areas in depression screening needing further research and synthesis. Depression in primary care practice is presented as a major arena for clinical services research that focuses on development of measures and screening instruments, studies of treatment efficacy, and evaluation of innovative clinical diagnostic and treatment alternatives. Such studies will potentially broaden the scope of practice in primary care settings and promote physician sensitivity to the mental health needs of their patients.

17

Screening for Depression in Primary Care: Guidelines for Future Practice and Research

Herbert C. Schulberg

The scientific validity and practical feasibility of screening primary care patients for depression are appropriate concerns in the late 1980s. The disorder's point prevalence of 6 to 8% in an ambulatory medical population, the potentially severe consequences of failing to diagnose and treat depression properly, and the major effort by the National Institute of Mental Health to educate physicians in the disorder's recognition (Regier et al., 1988) highlight the need to scrutinize available screening procedures. Given screening's utility in other facets of daily medical practice, the authors of preceding chapters critiqued this assessment strategy from multiple perspectives. Collectively, they portrayed the state of the art relative to: (a) depression as it is manifested in primary care practice and the relevance of currently available classificatory schema, (b) the diverse purposes of screening and their applicability to depression, and (c) the psychometric properties of existing depression screening instruments. After reviewing the prior analyses of screening's value for depression, what conclusions emerge for clinical practice and what future research priorities are indicated? The following commentary integrates themes implicitly and explicitly addressed in the preceding contributions. Where consensus exists, it is highlighted; where differences persist, they are acknowledged and explored.

Depression and Its Classification

Screening for depression in primary care patients may be pursued for epidemiologic, nosologic, and/or diagnostic purposes. This book focuses primarily upon the ability of screening instruments to inform the clinical management of affective disorders in this population. Given this emphasis, the first issue to be addressed is whether valid classificatory systems and criterion measures exist for assessing an instrument's efficacy in identifying cases and predicting outcomes.

Classificatory systems may have multiple or delimited purposes. Those like International Classification of Diseases–9 (ICD–9) seek to categorize every form of physical and psychiatric morbidity; its groupings are comprehensive, albeit heterogenous. Systems like the Research Diagnostic Criteria (RDC) were constructed for psychiatric research purposes and therefore contain a more limited but highly reliable set of categories. Still other systems like DSM-III-R have essentially clinical purposes; their categories may be limited to those for which knowledge about treatment and/or outcome has been established. Barrett (ch. 4) notes that theoretically all of these purposes may be served by a single nomenclature system, but that is not yet the case.

In American psychiatric practice, the dominant classificatory system is DSM-III-R, which presents distinct and reliable criteria for diagnosing depression. This nomenclature represents a marked advance over the nonspecific indices included within the earlier conceptual frameworks and diagnostic systems reviewed by Akiskal and McKinney (1979). Nevertheless, as Barrett (ch. 4) emphasizes, DSM-III-R categories and measures for mood disorders remain heterogenous in content and state of refinement. For example, the subcategory of major depression has clear-cut indices of duration and symptom type as well as treatment implications. Severe depressions are now recognized as being of fairly long duration and often superimposed upon less severe but chronic forms of the disorder. On the other hand, subcategories of depression like dysthymia, which is highly prevalent among patients with chronic medical conditions, are based upon indices meeting research and planning purposes, but they have vaguer treatment implications. Still other subcategories like adjustment disorder with depressed mood may be viewed as descriptive at best since their criteria and clinical implications remain uncertain (Fabrega, Mezzich, & Mezzich, 1987).

Equally crucial with respect to judging DSM-III-R's relevance as the framework for assessing depression screening instruments in primary care practice is the scope of its mood disorder subtypes. Since DSM-III-R is founded upon disorders exhibited by psychiatric patients, Barrett is concerned about the omission of morbidity patterns predominantly displayed by ambulatory medical patients. Indeed, he has found that while 10% of this population meet criteria for an established type of DSM-III-R mood disorder, another 10% present with a non–DSM-III-R "masked" depression or a mixed anxiety-depression syndrome. Zung (ch. 11) and Roberts (ch. 13) note that the latter syndrome is particularly common in ambulatory medical patients, although its precise and clinical outcome remains indeterminate. For example, it remains unclear whether anxiety and depression truly are distinct disorders as formulated by DSM-III-R, or whether anxiety is a concomitant or subtype of depression whose intensity is influenced by the patient's physical health. Given these dilemmas and complexities, it would appear that when restricted to DSM-III-R's typology of mood disorders, physicians might be unable to diagnose half of their affectively disturbed patients. If this critique is accurate, the DSM-III-R framework is significantly deficient when utilized as the criterion measure for a screening instrument's diagnostic efficacy in primary care practice.

With regard to DSM-III-R's predictive validity, Katon (ch. 5) notes the dearth of outcome studies specific to depressed primary care patients. The assumption that treatment protocols standardized with depressed psychiatric patients are generalizable to ambulatory medical patients thus must be deemed tenuous until empirically validated. Katon stresses that affective disorders in these two cohorts often manifest differing phenomenology and natural histories. Primary care patients focus upon and even amplify somatic components of depression because of various internal and external factors. The former includes the physiologic changes secondary to an organic illness; the latter includes the patient's awareness that physicians typically are more concerned about organic than psychiatric morbidity.

If DSM-III-R classifications of depression are imperfect criterion measures, what alternatives are available? Barrett (ch. 4) suggests consideration of the "triaxial" system, which includes physical, psychological, and social dimensions; the "problem-oriented" approach, which includes similar foci; and the "reason for encounter" system, which encompasses transitions within an episode of care. While conceptually appealing and potentially useful for tracing the course of illness, these additional classificatory frameworks require much field testing before they can serve as valid criterion measures for assessing screening instruments.

In addition to these uncertainties about classification, Roberts (ch. 13) raises the even more complex issue of whether depression is a universal disorder for which a single screening instrument is valid, or whether its characteristics are so culture-specific that unique instruments must be constructed for each cultural setting. Roberts suggests that affective disorder manifests itself differently in Western and non-Western societies. Cognitive and mood disturbances predominate in the former; somatic symptoms prevail in the latter, which lack a Western conception of depression. However, studies controlling for cultural setting have yet to be conducted with primary care patients so as to distinguish depression from somatization and true organic disease. Given these ambiguities, the psychometric properties of screening instruments might well differ depending upon the compatibility between a test's items and a socio-ethnic population's idiom for depression. To avoid such confounding, the Indian Depression Scale was developed to elicit concepts of depression indigenous to this population (Barón et al., ch. 14).

Another concern raised by Roberts regarding the intrinsic nature of depression is the relationship between this disorder and demoralization in the various strata of American society. When controlling for such depression risk factors as social class and social support, what is the prevalence of demoralization in primary care patients prior, during, and after an affective episode? Roberts suggests a 2 × 2 research design utilizing samples with both, one, or none of these conditions, but he stresses that reliable and valid indicators of depression and demoralization among ethnic and minority populations are needed to study this question.

This review by the preceding authors of depression and its classification leads to the conclusion that DSM-III-R categories of affective disorder often are meaningful and reliable criterion measures for assessing the efficacy of a screening instrument. However, these categories lack precision and comprehensiveness when applied to primary care patients and refinements thus are indicated. Such questions as the following warrant future investigation:

1. Which DSM-III-R depressive disorder subtypes are clinically uniform across patient types, and which should be recombined for primary care populations using outcome as the criterion measure in this effort?

2. Should such categories as "masked depression" be included in DSM-III-R so that this subtype of the disorder will be properly assessed and treated in the primary care sector?

3. What is the natural course of untreated depression among ambulatory medical patients, and how does this outcome compare with that for treated episodes, with that for psychiatric patients, etc.?

4. What is the utility of such frameworks as the problem-oriented approach and the triaxial system in classifying depression?

The Value of Screening For Depression

Assuming that depression can be classified within a system that validly encompasses the disorder's varied features as it presents in primary care practice, does detection through screening have clinical value? If the answer is negative, administration of even the most psychometrically sophisticated depression screening instrument is pointless. Given this fundamental concern, the value of screening as judged from diverse and often conflicting perspectives is discussed in several chapters.

The six criteria proposed by Frame (ch. 2) for determining screening's utility comprise a generally acceptable model for this analysis. Thus, most clinicians agree that: (a) Depression significantly affects the quality of life; (b) acceptable treatment methods are available; and (c) the disorder's incidence is sufficient to justify the cost of screening. However, there are markedly diverging views— best explicated by Frame and by Miranda, Muñoz, and Shumway (ch. 15)—as to whether: (d) Depression may be conceived as having an asymptomatic phase during which detection and treatment significantly reduce morbidity and mortality; (e) treatment in the asymptomatic phase produces an outcome superior to that obtained when treatment is delayed until the symptomatic phase; and (f) screening tests are available to detect asymptomatic depression.

Frame does not consider a depressive disorder to meet the latter three criteria. Unlike other illnesses presenting in primary care, the diagnosis of depression is wholly symptom-based. The disorder has few suggestive signs and no confirmatory laboratory tests as yet. Moreover, there is no evidence that treatment of subtle unrecognized symptoms improves outcome over that delayed to the illness' clinical phase. Given these diagnostic and treatment concerns, Frame strongly opposes screening during asymptomatic periods. Instead, he considers screening for depression as a selective and longitudinal process whereby the primary care physician refines the patient's comprehensive data base so that emerging symptoms may be assessed within a proper temporal and clinical context.

While acknowledging the continuing dual lack of biological markers for asymptomatic depression and instruments suited to screening during this phase, Miranda et al. (ch. 15) urge the use of known risk factors for lifetime depression to identify this morbidity in its nonclinical phase. Drawing upon their prior research, Miranda and colleagues contend that persons at high risk for depression who are taught behavioral and cognitive techniques will experience fewer clinical episodes than persons at similar risk who are not provided this preventive intervention. Miranda and colleagues therefore urge the development of a screening instrument that can identify asymptomatic but high-risk cohorts so as to maximize the beneficial impact of preventive interventions.

Miranda, Muñoz, and Shumway's views are conceptually attractive and deserving of further attention. Nevertheless, most clinicians undoubtedly would conclude that screening presently is best used for case identification purposes—i.e., sensitizing physicians to an existing illness that might otherwise be missed in routine practice (Coulehan, Schulberg, & Block, in press). With knowledge of a patient's screening score, the physician can diagnostically redefine presenting symptoms as part of an affective disorder and initiate treatment within the parameters permitted by the patient's attitude toward psychiatric morbidity, his or her insurance coverage, etc., and the physician's expertise in this area. Roberts (ch. 13) also stresses the need for screening to alert physicians to the related state of demoralization. While it rarely has life-threatening implications, demoralization is highly prevalent and the cause of much patient suffering. Thus, early recognition and treatment of depression and demoralization should reduce medical care utilization, particularly unneeded and risky diagnostic procedures.

The use of screening as an alerting/sensitizing procedure implies that knowledge of screening scores will lead physicians to identify and treat depressed patients. Indeed, Barrett (ch. 4) deems the appropriate validity criterion for a screening instrument to be the increased number of instances whereby physicians identify and treat depression with this information compared to clinical practice in its absence. Are there data to support this premise about screening's utility?

The complexity of this premise and the multiple perspectives from which it must be analyzed are evident in several pertinent studies. Rucker, Frye, and Cygan (1986) determined that residents in a general medical clinic judged patient scores on the Beck Depression Inventory useful. For 20% of their patients, this information altered the clinical formulation and treatment plan. Zung and Magruder-Habib (ch. 11) caution, however, that screening scores per se are not capable of improving diagnostic accuracy. As Matthew (ch. 16) notes from his perspective as a primary care physician, the process of clinical decision-making also entails the nature, quality, and timing of pertinent information. Indeed, Yager and Linn (ch. 9) found that chart notations of depression and the nature of treatment initiated after the focal visit are influenced by the timing of screening feedback (prior or subsequent to the visit), the scope of data provided (about one or two disorders), the patient's depressive distress level (mild, moderate, or severe), and the physician's clinical experience level (resident or faculty status).

The complex relationship between a physician's diagnostic and treatment decisions is also highlighted by the findings from research by Zung and his colleagues. They found no significant differences after twelve months in the proportion of patients treated for depression regardless of whether or not physicians knew their Zung Self-Rating Depression Scale (SDS) score. Equally striking was the lack of difference after one year in the SDS score of treated and untreated patients. This pattern is consistent with that reported by Schulberg, McClelland, and Gooding (1987) and raises questions about the efficacy of screening as well as the nature of appropriate treatment for depressed primary care patients as opposed to depressed psychiatric patients (Blacker & Clare, 1988).

What conclusions may be drawn, then, about the value of screening for depression in primary care settings? Most clinicians would restrict administration of suitable instruments to case-finding purposes. While the identification of asymptomatic as well as symptomatic cases is conceptually attractive, there is yet little evidence to support the clinical utility and fiscal costs of such clinical practice. Indeed, it remains equivocal whether there are benefits in sensitizing physicians, via screening scores, to patients whose presenting symptoms may be conceived as part of an affective disorder. At the least, further research is needed to explicate the subtleties of clinical decision making as it pertains to affective disorders among ambulatory medical patients (Schulberg, McClelland, Coulehan, Block, & Werner, 1986).

Screening Instruments and Their Psychometric Properties

Having described selected purposes for which depression screening is judged appropriate, are suitable instruments available for use in these circumstances? Do existing questionnaires meet validity criteria, and are they sufficiently efficient to warrant administration in clinical practice? The following section analyzes these questions at the general level as well as in relation to particular instruments.

As was stated by Barrett and others, the most common criterion of a screening instrument's validity is its ability to identify a true case of morbidity. With regard to depression, which still lacks biological markers, the present gold standard is the diagnostic formulation produced by a structured interview. While this criterion measure is considered superior to clinician judgments, it, too, remains imperfect. Murphy (ch. 6) notes that since the Diagnostic Interview Schedule (DIS), the Schedule for Affective Disorders and Schizophrenia (SADS), and the Present State Exam (PSE) utilize unique conceptions of a diagnosable depressive disorder, each yields differing validities for the same screening instrument. The need to align the content of screening questionnaires with the conceptual framework upon which the criterion measure interview schedule is based has led to the development of such screening scales as the Inventory to Diagnose Depression (IDD) (Zimmerman & Coryell, 1987). Since its items reflect DSM-III-R's criteria for an affective disorder, the IDD's framework is congruent with that employed by the DIS. It is also necessary to insure that the screening instrument and criterion measure assess morbidity for similar time frames—e.g., current or lifetime episodes, past week or past two weeks, etc.

Additional factors affect the structured interview's ability to serve as the criterion measure against which to assess screening instruments. Cleary (ch. 12) emphasizes that the validity of a diagnostic schedule is constrained by its reliability coefficient. For example, data cited by Cleary from the Epidemiologic Catchment Area (ECA) Program and those generated by Bromet, Dunn, Connell, Dew, and Schulberg (1986) from their Three Mile Island community sample demonstrate that respondent reports of a lifetime episode of depression are highly unreliable. Poor interrater reliability is another form of error measurement inherent in a standardized assessment. Roberts (ch. 13) notes that when the DIS serves as the gold standard, diagnostic variations may be associated with mode of administering the schedule since lay interviewers and psychiatric clinicians have been found to derive differing formulations. Still further influences on the gold standard's reliability are the differing conceptions of illness and the need for treatment expressed by patients, providers, and epidemiologists. When comparing each group's unique perspective, ECA researchers found little congruence regarding such indices as subjective appraisal of mental health and level of functional disability due to mental illness.

Thus, a criterion measure's validity and reliability may be confounded in various ways. The more extensive these constraints, the more poorly it serves as the gold standard in determining a screening instrument's psychometric properties. Accepting these caveats about standardized assessment schedules, most researchers nevertheless consider structured interviews like the DIS, the SADS, and the PSE appropriate gold standards at this time.

Turning, then, to screening instruments, what psychometric properties should they exhibit? Relevant indices are reviewed by Shrout (ch. 7), Hough (ch. 10), and Cleary (ch. 12), who highlight the balances that must be struck between sensitivity and specificity so that the test may detect the disorder of concern with maximal efficiency. Optimally, a depression screen should identify patients whose disorder is treatable but who otherwise would have remained undiagnosed and untreated. Furthermore, the screen should have a low misclassification rate so that the costs of a second stage evaluation for false positives do not exceed the benefits produced for true positives. Shrout notes, however, that the quantitative index of screening's benefit—i.e., its utility function—will vary in keeping with the screening program's purpose.

Scoring procedures for achieving the goals of efficient case identification typically are of the "count and cut" method. Murphy (ch. 6) laments that once cut scores are established, they function as a fixed attribute of the scale rather than as a threshold specific to a particular subpopulation with a given prevalence of depression. She and Cleary, therefore, urge the use of receiver operating characteristic (ROC) curves in selecting optimal cutpoints for a given population and/or its subcohorts. Such use of ROC curves would clarify, for example, whether optimal cutpoints established for community samples and psychiatric patients are equally efficient when screening primary care patients. Presently available microcomputer software facilitates calculation of these curves, which also permit comparison of the relative validity of several screening scales. While ROC analyses are useful in selecting a scale's optimal sensitivity and specificity values, they do not clarify which symptoms are integral to rather than associated with the DSM-III-R depressive syndrome. Murphy, therefore, advocates the construction of diagnostic algorithms that have a clear factorial structure and which distinguish the critical dimensions of a mood disorder from its associated concomitants. Such algorithms might also address Yager and Linn's (ch. 9) call for screening instruments that distinguish high scorers whose depressive symptomatology will or will not remit spontaneously.

In addition to a screening instrument's sensitivity and specificity, predictive validity is also essential if the scale is to be used in clinical practice. While the former indices are independent of depression's prevalence in a given population, the latter index is very much affected by this rate. The higher the prevalence, the stronger the screen's potential predictive validity. Given depression's varying prevalence among subpopulations of medical care users (Kessler et al., 1987), screening instruments can most efficiently identify true cases among nonmarried females for whom the prevalence of depression approximates 9%. They will be least efficient for married males whose depression prevalence rate is only about 3%.

A further psychometric feature of screening instruments is their effectiveness. Cleary suggests that while an instrument may adequately discriminate cases from noncases (efficiency), its ultimate impact on the former group's clinical outcome may be minimal (effectiveness). When this occurs, it becomes necessary to assess whether the intervention program was available to referred patients, whether it was implemented properly, whether it was acceptable to patients and physicians, and so on.

Turning from this overview of a screening instrument's needed psychometric properties to the numerous scales available for the assessment of depression (Beckham & Leber, 1985; Marsella, Hirschfeld, & Katz, 1987), what is their conceptual orientation and how can they be utilized in clinical practice? Murphy's (ch. 6) analysis of depression screening instruments distinguishes those founded upon a holistic, unitary, and hierarchical approach to mental illness from those conceiving depression as a categorical and dimensional disorder. The former conception is operationalized in scales such as the General Health Questionnaire wherein depression coexists with other disorders in a hierarchical structure. The latter approach is implemented through instruments like the Beck Depression Inventory, which assesses affective disorder alone. While the trend clearly is towards construction and use of questionnaires specific to depression, Murphy emphasizes the continuing value of scales which assess comorbidity. For example, in primary care patients there may be a close relationship between depression and anxiety, either as epiphenomena or as distinct but closely linked disorders with a common neural biological substrate (Paul, 1988).

Given the available uni- and multi-dimensional symptom scales for screening depression in primary care practice, what is their relative efficiency? Using DIS formulations as the gold standard, Hough (ch. 10) found no differences in the sensitivity and specificity values generated by the Center for Epidemiologic Studies-Depression Scale (CES-D), the GHQ–28, and the 25-item Hopkins Symptom Checklist (HSCL–25). All three instruments were far more sensitive to major depression than dysthymia. However, screening for the more severe diagnosis consistently yielded the highest false-positive rates, particularly when cutpoints were set low enough to achieve the minimal 90% sensitivity standard recommended by Murphy (ch. 6). Conversely, raising cutpoints to better balance sensitivity and specificity produces an excessive false-negative rate on all of the scales. This is an unsatisfactory situation from either the clinical or cost-benefit perspectives.

In light of these patterns, Hough concluded that none of the three tested questionnaires warrants use for routine primary care screening purposes. However, they are efficient in screening selected subgroups such as females, the young, and persons with lower class socioeconomic characteristics—i.e., cohorts among whom depression's prevalence exceeds that for the population at large. This strategy of assessing specified high-risk populations is consistent with Shapiro et al.'s (1987) finding that patient characteristics influence screening's effectiveness in primary care practice. In general, however, Hough calls for a new generation of instruments that more perfectly reflect DSM-III-R criteria for affective disorder. Since the existing instruments are more efficient and have greater utility with severe rather than minor depressions, Hough recommends that psychometric initiatives focus primarily on the former conditions.

The previously described IDD developed by Zimmerman and Coryell (1987) represents such a new generation, DSM-III-R—based screening instrument. Most investigators, however, are refining existing scales to incorporate this nomenclature's diagnostic criteria. This latter approach may be seen in RAND's modification of the CES-D. Burnam and Wells (ch. 8) reported that this scale's twenty items could be reduced to six when an alternative scoring approach is utilized and two DIS items assessing the persistence of dysphoric mood are included. When thus modified, the CES-D achieved a sensitivity of 85% and a positive predictive value of at least 33%. The latter measure of efficiency surpasses that reported for the full scale by Schulberg et al. (1985). Not surprisingly, Burnam and Wells found the modified CES-D to identify major depressive disorders and dysthymia more efficiently than other psychiatric conditions. They concluded that the RAND-modified CES-D efficiently detects affective morbidity even in populations where its prevalence is low.

The RAND procedures illustrate scoring modifications for improving the efficiency of screening instruments. However, additional psychometric concerns must be addressed in determining the validity and utility of the CES-D and other scales. These include the effects of medical patient response style on total score, whether the diagnosis and prevalence of depression are affected by the sequence in which the screening instrument and criterion measure are administered, and the clinical significance of test-retest score changes on scales that appear ordinal but may not truly be so.

As further research clarifies such still unstudied concerns, investigators should also study the factorial structure underlying screening instruments. This knowledge is critical for interpreting scores of persons from varying socio-cultural backgrounds. For example, Barón et al. (ch. 14) analyzed CES-D responses of American Indians and found their factor structure to differ substantially from that of other populations. No specific "somatic" factor could be identified in the Native American responses, but the "nonspecific" factor accounting for 30% of the variance did include somatic as well as affective items. Barón et al., therefore, caution that the internal validity of the CES-D is compromised when depression is expressed through somatic complaints—e.g., by such subgroups as the elderly and persons with chronic physical illness. Similar concern about the CES-D's factor structure was expressed by Roberts (ch. 13). Finding that gender is associated with variations on the factor loadings and differences in patterns of interitem, interscale correlations, Roberts conjectures whether the CES-D measures unique phenomena in men and women.

Summary

Kamerow (ch. 3) questioned whether screening for mental health problems has utility in family practice. He concluded with a "less than resounding probably." This blend of affirmation and caution equally well depicts the thinking of other chapter authors about the benefits of screening for depression in primary care. They are impressed with screening's potential for identifying depression in its early phases and intervening with state of the art treatments of demonstrated efficacy. However, they remain equally cognizant of unresolved problems in pursuing this clinical strategy. The conclusion to be drawn, therefore, is that depression questionnaires should not be routinely administered to ambulatory medical patients. There is merit, however, to such assessment practice in selected circumstances and with well-defined populations.

A major concern in the detection of depressed primary care patients is whether present diagnostic systems permit physicians to classify the clinical phenomena encountered in their daily practice appropriately. If not, screening instruments would be irrelevant. There is agreement that DSM-III-R categories for affective illness are valid and reliable with regard to major depressive disorders but far less so for minor depressions, adjustment disorders with depressed mood, intermittent depression, and masked depression so prevalent in ambulatory medical settings. Since no alternative classificatory system is presently available, the DSM-III-R framework continues to be used in daily primary care practice. However, affective disorders should be reorganized in DSM-IV to include the forms of this illness commonly manifested by primary care patients (a task the American Psychiatric Association will be shortly undertaking).

As was noted previously, screening's major value is thought to be clinical case identification rather than the detection of asymptomatic forms of depression. This conclusion is based on inadequate evidence demonstrating that vulnerable persons experience fewer subsequent episodes when provided interventions during asymptomatic periods. Equally ambiguous, however, is the evidence regarding a physician's willingness to use screening information even for case identification and treatment purposes. Thus, when the possible purposes of screening for depression are examined within the framework typically applied to the screening of other illnesses, further research still must delineate those circumstances when depression screening has the greatest utility.

Turning finally to the issue of whether psychometrically valid scales are available for the screening of depression, it is clear that any questionnaire's validity coefficient depends upon the choice of criterion measure. Structured diagnostic interviews are the current gold standard, but each such instrument's conception and definition of affective disorder differ somewhat. In addition to variations in validity produced by the criterion measure, the depression screening scale's validity may also be influenced by its structural type—i.e., holistic or unidimensional. Designers of unidimensional scales increasingly are incorporating items keyed to DSM-III-R criteria for depression so as to improve the screen's positive predictive value. Efficiency is also being enhanced through the calculation of ROC curves that specify the most efficient cutpoints for given populations. Given these developments, future research should be able to clarify which depression screening instruments have the greatest utility for which purposes in primary care practice.

References

Akiskal, H., & McKinney, W. (1979). Depressive disorders: Toward a unified hypothesis. *Science, 182,* 20–29.

Beckham, E., & Leber, W. (eds.) (1985). *Handbook of depression: Treatment, assessment and research.* Homewood, IL: Dorsey Press.

Blacker, C., & Clare, A. (1987). Depressive disorder in primary care. *British Journal of Psychiatry, 150,* 737–751.

Bromet, E., Dunn, L., Connell, M., Dew, M., & Schulberg, H. (1986). Long-term reliability of lifetime major depression in a community sample. *Archives of General Psychiatry, 43,* 435–440.

Coulehan, J., Schulberg, H., & Block, M. (in press). The efficiency of depression questionnaires for case finding in primary medical care. *Journal of General Internal Medicine.*

Fabrega, H., Mezzich, J., & Mezzich, A. (1987). Adjustment disorder as a marginal or transitional illness category in DSM-III. *Archives of General Psychiatry, 44,* 567–572.

Kessler, L., Burns, B., Shapiro, S., Tischler, G., George, L., Hough, L., Bodision, D. S., & Miller, R. (1987). Psychiatric diagnoses of medical service users: Evidence from the Epidemiology Catchment Area Program. *American Journal of Public Health, 77,* 18–24.

Marsella, A., Hirschfeld, R., & Katz, M. (eds.) (1987). The measurement of depression. New York: Guilford Press.

Paul, S. (1988). Anxiety and depression: A common neuralbiological substrate. *Journal of Clinical Psychiatry, 49* (Oct. Suppl. 10), 13–16.

Regier, D., Hirschfeld, R., Goodwin, F., Burke, J., Lazar, J., & Judd, L. (1988). The NIMH Depression Awareness, Recognition, and Treatment Program. Structures, aims, and scientific basis. *American Journal of Psychiatry, 145,* 1351–1357.

Rucker, L., Frye, E., & Cygan, R. (1986). Feasibility and usefulness of depression screening in medical outpatients. *Archives of Internal Medicine, 146,* 729—731.

Schulberg, H., Saul, M., McClelland, M., Ganguli, M., Christy, W., & Frank, R. (1985). Assessing depression in primary medical and psychiatric practice. *Archives of General Psychiatry, 42,* 1164–1170.

Schulberg, H., McClelland, M., Coulehan, J., Block, M., & Werner, G. (1986). Psychiatric decision-making in family practice: Future research directions. *General Hospital Psychiatry, 8,* 1–6.

Schulberg, H., McClelland, M., & Gooding, W. (1987). Six-month outcomes for medical patients with major depressive disorders. *Journal General Internal Medicine, 2,* 312–317.

Shapiro, S., German, P., Skinner, E., Von Koff, M., Turner, R., Klein, L., Teitelbaub, M., Kramer, M., Burke, J., & Burns, B. (1987). An experiment to change detection and management of mental morbidity in primary care. *Medical Care, 25,* 327–339.

Zimmerman, M., & Coryell, W. (1987). The Inventory to Diagnose Depression (IDD): A self-report scale to diagnose major depressive disorder. *Journal of Consulting and Clinical Psychology, 55,* 55–59.

Index

Abdominal symptoms, 256, dyspepsia, constipation, 256
see Somatic complaints
Absenteeism, (job) 43
Adjustment disorder with depression, 32, 36, 268, 277
Adolescence, 260
Affect, 3; descriptor, 185; disorder, 87, 100, 112, 149, 253, 258–259, 269, 271–277; illness, 44–45, 50, 58, 277; positive, 228
African ethnic groups, 205, *see* Black Americans
Aging, 261, aging populations, 229, *see* elderly
Agitation, 186–188
Agoraphobia, 257
Alaska native, 217
Alcohol, 18; abuse, 45, 57, 132–133, 146–147, 177; dependence, 30, 146–147
Alcoholism, 18, 50, 188, 198, 217, 257–258
American Indian, 181, 186, 217–218, 228–229, 276
Amphetamine, (low dose), 258
Anger, 47, (easy) 256
Anhedonia, 185, 260
Anorexia nervosa, 132, 177, 255, *see* bulimia
Anti-depressants, 21, 23–24, 30, 35–38, 40, 54–55, 135, 159, 166, 261; Amitriptyline, 56, *see* medications, *see* tricyclic anti-depressant
Antihypertensives, 257

Anxiety, 68, 71–72, 75, 78, 80, 117–118, 128–132, 140, 149, 160–161, 166, 187–189, 191, 193–194, 196–198, 252–253, 255–260, 268, 275
Appetite, 3, 5, 52, 78, 100, 123, 185, 189, 227, 255–256
Area under the curve (AUC), 74–79, 239, (analysis) 241, 244
Arthritis, 6, 222
Asian refugee groups, 197, (Chinese) 186–187, 239, 245, (Laotians) 186, (Southeast Asian) 186, (Vietnamese) 186
Asymptomatic, 16, 272; forms of depression, 277; period, 13, 232–233; persons, 21; phase, 21, (stage) 22, 233–234, 270; population, 17
Ataque de nervios, 187
AUC, *see* area under the curve
Autonomic arousal, (increased) 46

B-12 deficiency, 261
Back pain, 48, (problems) 6, 47, 51
Balanced Inventory of Desirability Responding (BIDR), 202
BDI, *see* Beck Depression Inventory
Beck Depression Inventory (BDI), 18, 23–24, 46, 66–68, 70, 105, 190, 202, 235–236, 239–240, 245, 271, 275
Behavioral therapy, 237, 245, *see* psychotherapy
Bereavement, 132, 185, 259–260, *see* grief
Bias, 203, (source of) 183
BIDR, *see* Balanced Inventory of Desirability Responding

Contributors

C. Clifford Attkisson, Ph.D.
Professor of Medical Psychology
Department of Psychiatry
University of California, San Francisco

Jane M. Zich, Ph.D.
Assistant Clinical Professor & Assistant Research Psychologist
University of California, San Francisco

Paul Frame, M.D.
Clinical Assistant Professor of Family Medicine
University of Rochester School of Medicine and Medical Director
Tri-County Family Medicine Program

Douglas B. Kamerow, M.D., M.P.H.
Director, Clinical Preventive Services Staff
Office of Disease Prevention and Health Promotion
U.S. Department of Health and Human Services

James Barrett, M.D.
Research Professor of Community & Family Medicine & Psychiatry
Dartmouth Medical School

Wayne Katon, M.D.
Associate Professor of Psychiatry
University of Washington, Seattle

Michael Von Korff, Sc.D.
Group Health Cooperative
Center for Health Studies
Seattle, WA

Jane M. Murphy, Ph.D.
Chief, Psychiatric Epidemiology Unit
Massachusetts General Hospital &
Associate Professor
Department of Psychiatry
Harvard Medical School

Patrick E. Shrout, Ph.D.
College of Physicians & Surgeons
Columbia University

M. Audrey Burnam, Ph.D.
Associate Research Psychologist
The Rand Corporation

Kenneth B. Wells, M.D.
Associate Professor of Psychiatry
UCLA and
Senior Researcher
The Rand Corporation

Joel Yager, M.D.
Professor in Residence
Department of Psychiatric and Biobehavioral Sciences
University of California, Los Angeles

Lawrence S. Linn, Ph.D.
Adjunct Professor & Research Sociologist
Department of Medicine
University of California, Los Angeles

Richard L. Hough, Ph.D.
Professor of Sociology
San Diego State University

John A. Lansverk, Ph.D.
Professor of Sociology
San Diego State University and
Director of Research
Center for Child Protection
Children's Hospital

Gerald F. Jacobson, M.D. (deceased)
Director
Didi Hirsch Community Mental Health Center
Los Angeles, CA

William W. K. Zung, M.D.
Professor of Psychiatry
Department of Community and Family Medicine
Duke University Medical Center

Kathryn Magruder-Habib, M.P.H., Ph.D.
Assistant Professor
Department of Community and Family Medicine
Duke University Medical Center

John R. Feussner, Ph.D.
Director
Health Services Research and Development
Durham, NC

Paul Cleary, Ph.D.
Associate Professor of Social Medicine and Health Policy
Harvard Medical School

Robert E. Roberts, Ph.D.
Professor
School of Public Health
University of Texas Health Sciences Center
Houston, TX

Anna E. Barón, Ph.D.
Assistant Professor and Biostatistician
National Center for American Indian and Alaska Native Mental Health Research
University of Colorado, Denver

Spero Manson, Ph.D.
Associate Professor and Director
National Center for American Indian and Alaska Native Mental Health Research
University of Colorado, Denver

Lynn M. Ackerson, Ph.D.
Professional Research Associate and Data Manager
National Center for American Indian and Alaska Native Mental Health Research
University of Colorado, Denver

Douglas L. Brenneman, B.S.
Professional Research Assistant and Project Manager
National Center for American Indian and Alaska Mental Health Research
University of Colorado, Denver

Jeanne Miranda, Ph.D.
Assistant Clinical Professor
Department of Psychiatry
University of California, San Francisco

Ricardo Muñoz, Ph.D.
Professor of Medical Psychology
Department of Psychiatry
University of California, San Francisco

Martha Shumway, B.A.
Staff Research Associate
San Francisco General Hospital
San Francisco

John Matthew, M.D.
ASPEN Health Center
Plainfield, VT

Herbert C. Schulberg, Ph.D.
Professor of Psychiatry & Psychology
University of Pittsburgh